T0226843

Spinal Cord Diseases

Editors

ALIREZA MINAGAR
ALEJANDRO A. RABINSTEIN

NEUROLOGIC CLINICS

www.neurologic.theclinics.com

Consulting Editor
RANDOLPH W. EVANS

February 2013 • Volume 31 • Number 1

ELSEVIER

1600 John F. Kennedy Boulevard • Suite 1800 • Philadelphia, Pennsylvania 19103-2899

http://www.theclinics.com

NEUROLOGIC CLINICS Volume 31, Number 1
February 2013 ISSN 0733-8619, ISBN-13: 978-1-4557-7121-9

Editor: Donald Mumford

Neurologic Clinics (ISSN 0733-8619) is published quarterly by Elsevier Inc., 360 Park Avenue South, New York, NY 10010–1710. Months of issue are February, May, August, and November. Periodicals postage paid at New York, NY, and additional mailing offices. Subscription prices are $285.00 per year for US individuals, $470.00 per year for US institutions, $140.00 per year for US students, $359.00 per year for Canadian individuals, $564.00 per year for Canadian institutions, $397.00 per year for international individuals, $564.00 per year for international institutions, and $199.00 for Canadian and foreign students/residents. To receive student/resident rate, orders must be accompanied by name of affiliated institution, date of term, and the *signature* of program/residency coordinator on institution letterhead. Orders will be billed at individual rate until proof of status is received. Foreign air speed delivery is included in all *Clinics* subscription prices. All prices are subject to change without notice. **POSTMASTER:** Send address changes to *Neurologic Clinics*, Elsevier Health Sciences Division, Subscription Customer Service, 3251 Riverport Lane, Maryland Heights, MO 63043. **Customer Service: Telephone: 1-800-654-2452 (U.S. and Canada); 314-447-8871 (outside U.S. and Canada). Fax: 314-447-8029. E-mail: journalscustomerservice-usa@elsevier.com (for print support); journalsonlinesupport-usa@elsevier.com (for online support).**

Reprints. For copies of 100 or more of articles in this publication, please contact the Commercial Reprints Department, Elsevier Inc., 360 Park Avenue South, New York, New York, 10010-1710; Tel.: (+1) 212-633-3812; Fax: (+1) 212-462-1935, and E-mail: reprints@elsevier.com.

Neurologic Clinics is also published in Spanish by Nueva Editorial Interamericana S.A., Mexico City, Mexico.

Neurologic Clinics is covered in *Current Contents/Clinical Medicine, MEDLINE/PubMed (Index Medicus), EMBASE/Excerpta Medica, and PsycINFO, and ISI/BIOMED.*

Printed and bound by CPI Group (UK) Ltd, Croydon, CR0 4YY

Transferred to digital print 2012

Contributors

CONSULTING EDITOR

RANDOLPH W. EVANS, MD
Clinical Professor, Department of Neurology, Baylor College of Medicine, Houston, Texas

GUEST EDITORS

ALIREZA MINAGAR, MD, FAAN
Professor, Department of Neurology, LSU Health Sciences Center, Shreveport, Louisiana

ALEJANDRO A. RABINSTEIN, MD, FAAN
Professor of Neurology, Divisions of Critical Care Neurology and Cerebrovascular Neurology, Department of Neurology, Mayo Clinic, Rochester, Minnesota

AUTHORS

J.D. BARTLESON, MD
Associate Professor of Neurology, Department of Neurology, Mayo Clinic College of Medicine, Rochester, Minnesota

SHIN C. BEH, MD
Department of Neurology and Neurotherapeutics, University of Texas Southwestern Medical Center, Dallas, Texas

ORHAN BICAN, MD
Department of Neurology, Louisiana State University Health Sciences Center, Shreveport, Louisiana

MAIKE BLAYA, MD
Assistant Professor of Neurology, Department of Neurology, Tulane University School of Medicine, New Orleans, Louisiana

GIUSEPPE CICCOTTO, MD, MPH
Resident in Neurology, Department of Neurology, Tulane University School of Medicine, New Orleans, Louisiana

EOIN P. FLANAGAN, MBBCh
Assistant Professor of Neurology, Department of Neurology, Mayo Clinic, Minnesota

ELLIOT M. FROHMAN, MD, PhD
Department of Neurology and Neurotherapeutics; Department of Ophthalmology, University of Texas Southwestern Medical Center, Dallas, Texas

TERESA FROHMAN, PA-C
Department of Neurology and Neurotherapeutics, University of Texas Southwestern Medical Center, Dallas, Texas

BENJAMIN M. GREENBERG, MHS, MD
Department of Neurology and Neurotherapeutics, University of Texas Southwestern
Medical Center, Dallas, Texas

BHARAT GUTHIKONDA, MD
Assistant Professor, Director of Skull Base Research, Department of Neurosurgery, LSU
HSC Shreveport, Shreveport, Louisiana

JUSTIN HAYDEL, MD
Department of Neurosurgery, LSU HSC Shreveport, Shreveport, Louisiana

KENDRICK JOHNSON, BS
Department of Neurosurgery, LSU HSC Shreveport, Shreveport, Louisiana

B. MARK KEEGAN, MD, FRCP(C)
Associate Professor of Neurology, Department of Neurology, Mayo Clinic, Rochester,
Minnesota

ROGER E. KELLEY, MD
Professor and Chairman of Neurology, Department of Neurology, Tulane University
School of Medicine, New Orleans, Louisiana

LASZLO L. MECHTLER, MD
Medical Director, Dent Imaging and Neuro-Oncology Center, Dent Neurologic Institute;
Chief of Neuro-Oncology, Roswell Park Cancer Institute, Buffalo, New York; President,
American Society of Neuro-Imaging, Minneapolis, Minnesota

ALIREZA MINAGAR, MD, FAAN
Department of Neurology, Louisiana State University Health Sciences Center, Shreveport,
Louisiana

KAVEER NANDIGAM, MD
Neuro-Imaging Fellow, Dent Neurologic Institute, Buffalo, New York

AMY A. PRUITT, MD
Associate Professor of Neurology, Department of Neurology, University of Pennsylvania,
Philadelphia, Pennsylvania

ALEJANDRO A. RABINSTEIN, MD
Professor of Neurology, Divisions of Critical Care Neurology and Cerebrovascular
Neurology, Department of Neurology, Mayo Clinic, Rochester, Minnesota

ERNST-WILHELM RADUE, MD
Medical Image Analysis Center, University Hospital, Basel, Switzerland

KOUROSH REZANIA, MD
Assistant Professor, Department of Neurology, University of Chicago Medical Center,
Chicago, Illinois

MEGAN B. RICHIE, MD
University of Pennsylvania, Philadelphia, Pennsylvania

RAYMOND P. ROOS, MD
Marjorie and Robert C. Straus Professor in Neurologic Science, Department of Neurology,
University of Chicago Medical Center, Chicago, Illinois

MARK N. RUBIN, MD
Instructor of Neurology, Department of Neurology, Mayo Clinic, Rochester, Minnesota

MOHAMMAD ALI SAHRAIAN, MD
Sina MS Research Center, Iranian Center for Neurological Research, Sina Hospital, Tehran, Iran

ROBERT N. SCHWENDIMANN, MD
Professor of Clinical Neurology, Department of Neurology, LSU Health-Shreveport, Shreveport, Louisiana

WILLIAM SHEREMATA, MD, FRCP(C), FACP, FAAN
Professor Emeritus of Clinical Neurology, Department of Neurology, Multiple Sclerosis Center of Excellence, University of Miami Miller School of Medicine, Miami, Florida

JEFFREY A. STROMMEN, MD
Department of Physical Medicine and Rehabilitation, Mayo Clinic, Rochester, Minnesota

MICHEL TOLEDANO, MD
Department of Neurology, Mayo Clinic College of Medicine, Rochester, Minnesota

JAMIE TOMS, BS
Department of Neurosurgery, LSU HSC Shreveport, Shreveport, Louisiana

LETICIA TORNES, MD
Instructor of Clinical Neurology, Fellow in Multiple Sclerosis, Department of Neurology, Multiple Sclerosis Center of Excellence, University of Miami Miller School of Medicine, Miami, Florida

RISHI WADHWA, MD
Department of Neurosurgery, LSU HSC Shreveport, Shreveport, Louisiana

SHIHAO ZHANG, MD
Department of Neurosurgery, LSU HSC Shreveport, Shreveport, Louisiana

Contents

resulting in paresis, a sensory level, and autonomic (bladder, bowel, and sexual) impairment below the level of the lesion. Etiologies for TM can be broadly classified as parainfectious, paraneoplastic, drug/toxin-induced, systemic autoimmune disorders, and acquired demyelinating diseases. We discuss the clinical evaluation, workup, and acute and long-term management of patients with TM. Additionally, we briefly discuss various disease entities that may cause TM and their salient distinguishing features, as well as disorders that may mimic TM.

Neuromyelitis optica (NMO) is a severe inflammatory demyelinating disease of the central nervous system with distinguishing features from multiple sclerosis. Understanding of clinical presentation, immunopathology, and imaging features has changed during the last decade. The identification of NMO immunoglobulin G and aquaporin 4 as the target antigen in this disease helped to define the NMO spectrum of disorders and showed that NMO is an autoimmune channelopathy of the central nervous system. Several types of brain involvement have been described in patients with NMO. This article discusses the epidemiology, clinical manifestations, and immunopathogenesis of the disease with an emphasis on neuroimaging.

Vascular disease affecting the spinal can cause substantial neurologic morbidity. Several vascular spinal cord ailments present as neurologic emergencies, and should thus be recognizable to the practicing neurologist. We review the epidemiology, presentation, management strategies, and prognosis of various pathologies, including infarction, dural arteriovenous fistula, arteriovenous malformation, cavernous malformation, compressive epidural hematoma, vasculitis, and genetic abnormalities.

Spine trauma is a devastating clinical condition that affects many people annually on a worldwide basis. Management of spinal trauma has become much more surgically oriented with advances in stabilization techniques over the past two decades. The degree of injury to the spinal cord dictates the prognosis of the patient in cervical and thoracolumbar trauma. Traumatic spinal cord injury is a major area of socioeconomic burden and, as such, is a burgeoning area of ongoing research interest.

This review article identifies and describes the clinical manifestations of various metabolic, nutritional, and toxic conditions that result in symptoms of myelopathy and, in some cases, myeloneuropathy. It includes discussions of the clinical pictures that occur secondary to these causes. Familiarity with the clinical symptoms may lead to accurate diagnosis through laboratory and imaging studies and to treatment with successful identification of the underlying causes.

NEUROLOGIC CLINICS

RELATED INTEREST

Orthopedic Clinics, October 2012
Management of Compressive Neuropathies of the Upper Extremity
Asif M. Ilyas, MD, *Guest Editor*

DOWNLOAD
Free App!

Review Articles
THE CLINICS

NOW AVAILABLE FOR YOUR iPhone and iPad

Preface

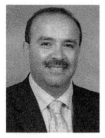 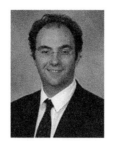

Alireza Minagar, MD, FAAN   Alejandro A. Rabinstein, MD, FAAN
Guest Editors

The human spinal cord is a magnificent wonder of nature, which for centuries has fascinated neuroanatomists, neurophysiologists, and clinical neurologists. This cylindrical structure mainly consists of a complex array of neurons and ascending and descending neuroanatomic pathways. During recent decades, the fundamental structure and function of the spinal cord and the diseases that affect it have been subjects of intense research by neurologists, neurosurgeons, and neuroscientists. Our knowledge of spinal cord pathophysiology is constantly growing and this knowledge is unraveling the causes, mechanisms, and effects of spinal cord diseases. Therefore, we felt that this is an excellent opportunity to review, summarize, and present the current knowledge about the spinal cord.

This issue of *Neurologic Clinics* begins with a brief review of spinal cord neuroanatomy and offers readers discussions on a wide spectrum of spinal cord diseases. Each article expounds on the latest findings about each particular topic, thus providing an updated clinical summary. The contributors to this issue are among the finest neurologists, neurosurgeons, and neuroscientists in the world and have spent their time and effort rendering comprehensive and informative articles. We immensely appreciate their generous contributions. Without their expertise and hard work, this issue would have never materialized. We also received invaluable assistance from Mr Donald Mumford, editor at Elsevier. He has been instrumental in the successful completion of this volume. We hope that it will stimulate more research about the spinal cord and its diseases by our avid and enthusiastic readers.

Neurol Clin 31 (2013) xiii–xiv
http://dx.doi.org/10.1016/j.ncl.2012.09.015
0733-8619/13/$ – see front matter © 2013 Elsevier Inc. All rights reserved.

Alireza Minagar, MD, FAAN
Department of Neurology
LSU Health Sciences Center
1501 Kings Highway
Shreveport, LA 71130, USA

Alejandro A. Rabinstein, MD, FAAN
Department of Neurology
Mayo Clinic
200 First Street–Mayo W8B
Rochester, MN 55905, USA

E-mail addresses:
aminag@lsuhsc.edu (A. Minagar)
rabinstein.alejandro@mayo.edu (A.A. Rabinstein)

Erratum

For *Neurologic Clinics*, May 2012, Volume 30, Issue 2.

In the article "Nerve Conduction Studies: Basic Concepts and Patterns of Abnormalities" by Lyell K. Jones.

The conduction velocity formula provided on page 411 should have been

$$\text{Conduction velocity} = \frac{\text{Distance}}{\text{proximal latency} - \text{distal latency}}$$

instead of

$$\text{Conduction velocity} = \frac{\text{proximal latency} - \text{distal latency}}{\text{distance}}$$

Neurol Clin 31 (2013) xv
http://dx.doi.org/10.1016/j.ncl.2012.11.001
0733-8619/13/$ – see front matter © 2013 Elsevier Inc. All rights reserved.

neurologic.theclinics.com

The Spinal Cord
A Review of Functional Neuroanatomy

Orhan Bican, MD[a], Alireza Minagar, MD[a], Amy A. Pruitt, MD[b],*

KEYWORDS

- Spinal cord anatomy • Dorsal columns • Corticospinal tract
- Lateral spinothalamic tract • Central cord syndrome • Brown-Sequard
- Compressive myelopathy

KEY POINTS

- The spinal cord is located within the spinal canal but does not extend the entire length of the vertebral canal.
- The spinal cord is incompletely divided into 2 halves by a deep anterior median fissure and a shallow posterior median sulcus.
- The anatomic organization of ascending and descending pathways in the spinal cord often allows precise longitudinal and transverse localization of the pathologic process.
- Disproportion between the length of the spinal cord and the length of the bony spinal vertebral column gives rise to longitudinal localization discrepancies.

The spinal cord controls the voluntary muscles of the trunk and upper and lower extremities and receives sensory input from these areas of the body. It is anchored to the dura by the denticulate ligaments and extends from the medulla oblongata to the lower border of the first lumbar vertebra. A basic knowledge of spinal cord anatomy is essential for the interpretation of and understanding of pathologic findings. The blood supply of the spinal cord is discussed elsewhere in this issue. In this article, anatomic structures are correlated with relevant clinical signs and symptoms.

GROSS ANATOMY OF SPINAL CORD

The spinal cord is located within the spinal canal but does not extend the entire length of the vertebral canal. The spinal cord length is about 45 cm in men and 43 cm in women and its width ranges from 1.27 cm in cervical and lumbar regions to 64 mm in the thoracic region. There are 20 or 21 pairs of denticulate ligaments that constitute a surgical landmark for the anterolateral segment of the spinal cord. Caudally, the

[a] Department of Neurology, Louisiana State University Health Sciences Center, Shreveport, LA 71130, USA; [b] Department of Neurology, University of Pennsylvania, 3400 Spruce Street, Philadelphia, PA 19104, USA
* Corresponding author.
E-mail address: pruitt@mail.med.upenn.edu

Neurol Clin 31 (2013) 1–18
http://dx.doi.org/10.1016/j.ncl.2012.09.009   **neurologic.theclinics.com**
0733-8619/13/$ – see front matter © 2013 Elsevier Inc. All rights reserved.

spinal cord is anchored by filum terminale, which is a nonneural membrane arising from the conus medullaris and descending to attach to the coccyx (**Fig. 1**).

The spinal cord has 31 segments (8 cervical, 12 thoracic or dorsal, 5 lumbar, 5 sacral, and 1 coccygeal), each of which (except the first cervical segment, which has only a ventral root) has a pair of dorsal and ventral roots and a pair of spinal nerves. There are no sharp boundaries between the segments within the cord, but the cervical and lumbar enlargements, giving rise to nerve roots for arms and legs, respectively, are clearly apparent. Each dorsal and ventral root joins in the intervertebral foramina to form a spinal nerve. Outside the spinal cord and just proximal to its junction with the ventral root, the dorsal root has an oval enlargement, the dorsal root ganglion, which contains sensory neurons (**Fig. 2A**). The neurons of the sensory ganglia are pseudounipolar nerve cells (ie, the cell body is in the ganglion where a solitary nerve process divides into a long process coming from the periphery as the receptor and

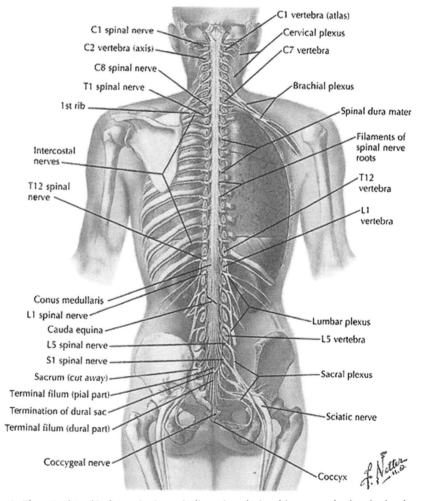

Fig. 1. The spinal cord is shown in situ to indicate its relationship to vertebral and other bony structures. Drawing by Frank Netter, MD. (Netter illustration from www.netterimages.com. © Elsevier, Inc. All rights reserved.)

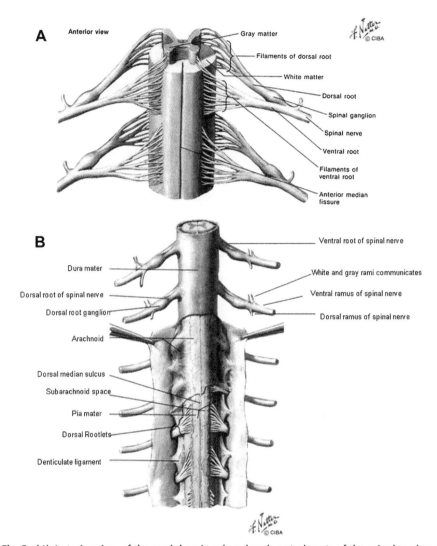

A — Anterior view
- Gray matter
- Filaments of dorsal root
- White matter
- Dorsal root
- Spinal ganglion
- Spinal nerve
- Ventral root
- Filaments of ventral root
- Anterior median fissure

B
- Dura mater
- Dorsal root of spinal nerve
- Dorsal root ganglion
- Arachnoid
- Dorsal median sulcus
- Subarachnoid space
- Pia mater
- Dorsal Rootlets
- Denticulate ligament
- Ventral root of spinal nerve
- White and gray rami communicates
- Ventral ramus of spinal nerve
- Dorsal ramus of spinal nerve

Fig. 2. (*A*) Anterior view of the cord showing dorsal and ventral roots of the spinal cord and formation of the spinal nerves and their dorsal and ventral rami as well as the rami communicantes. Drawing by Frank Netter, MD. (*B*) Posterior view of the cord indicating the meningeal layers, denticulate ligaments, and dorsal root ganglia. Drawing by Frank Netter, MD. (Netter illustration from www.netterimages.com. © Elsevier, Inc. All rights reserved.)

a much shorter process entering the spinal cord). There are no synapses in the dorsal root ganglia. Spinal nerves leave the vertebral canal through the intervertebral foramina. The first cervical nerve emerges from the vertebral canal between the occipital bone and the atlas; the eighth cervical nerve emerges between the seventh cervical (C7) and the first thoracic (T1) vertebrae. All spinal nerves caudal to C7-T1 exit beneath the corresponding vertebrae.

Spinal cord and vertebral column levels do not correspond because of their differences in rates of growth during embryonic development. In the upper cervical region the cord segment corresponds to the like-numbered vertebral body. From C5 to C8 the spinal cord level is 1 level higher than the corresponding vertebral body. Thus, the fifth cervical vertebral body corresponds to the level of the sixth spinal cord segment. In the upper thoracic region, the vertebral spinal process is 2 segments above the corresponding cord segment. In the lower thoracic and upper lumbar regions, the difference between the vertebral and cord level is 2 or 3 segments so that a spinal cord sensory level at T9 would correspond to a pathologic abnormality at the sixth or seventh thoracic vertebral body. Sacral cord levels correspond to vertebral T12-L1 levels. These longitudinal discrepancies should be taken into account when a sensory level is found during clinical examination (see later discussion and **Fig. 3**). As the nerve roots descend to their corresponding vertebral level, they become more oblique from rostral to caudal so that the lumbar and sacral nerves descend almost vertically to reach their points of exit (see **Fig. 1**). The lumbosacral roots below

Spinal Segmental Sensory Innervation

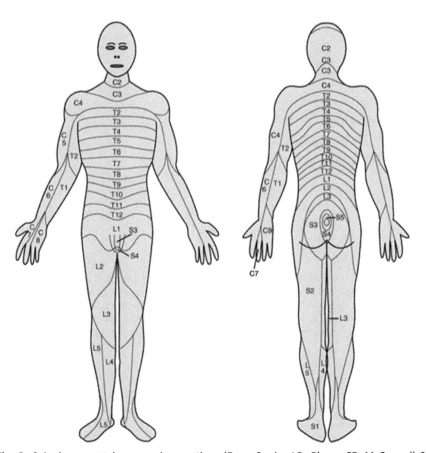

Fig. 3. Spinal segmental sensory innervation. (*From* Squire LR, Bloom FE, McConnell SK, et al. Fundamental neuroscience. 2nd edition. New York: Academic Press; 2003. p. 678; with permission. Copyright © 2002, Elsevier Science (USA), All rights reserved.)

the termination of the spinal cord form the cauda equina. These spinal roots surround the filum terminale and are organized such that caudal-most segments are most centrally located, but this somatotopic organization is not usually of much value in clinical localization.

MENINGES

Dura mater, arachnoid, and pia mater are the membranes covering the spinal cord from the most superficial layer to that closest to the spinal cord, respectively (see **Fig. 2B**). The outer of the 2 cranial dural layers serves as the cranial periosteum and at the foramen magnum the inner layer separates to descend as the dural sleeve of the spinal cord. The epidural space separates dura from the vertebral canal and contains a layer of fat that can be useful as a magnetic resonance imaging landmark. A network of epidural veins called Batson's plexus is also in the epidural space and is believed to be relevant to the spread of infection or metastatic cancer. The subdural space is a potential space between the dura mater and the arachnoid space. The subarachnoid space is a clinically important and relatively wide space filled with cerebrospinal fluid separating the arachnoid from the pia mater surrounding the spinal cord. Together the arachnoid and pia are called the leptomeninges.

LONGITUDINAL DIVISIONS

The spinal cord is incompletely divided into 2 halves by a deep anterior median fissure and a shallow posterior median sulcus (**Fig. 4**). The anterior median fissure contains a double fold of pia mater, and its floor is the anterior (ventral) white commissure. More laterally is the anterolateral sulcus, marking the exit of the ventral roots. The posterior median sulcus is a shallow septum, on either side of which lies the posterolateral sulcus, the site of the posterior nerve roots entry. Three funiculi divide the white matter of the cord. The posterior funiculus lies between the posterior median sulcus

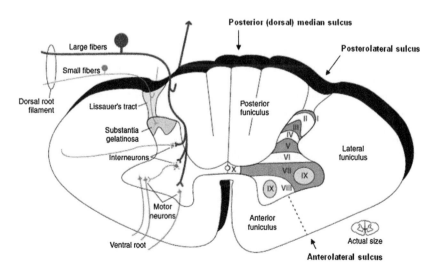

Fig. 4. The spinal cord at the eighth cervical segmental level indicating external landmarks of spinal cord, funiculi, dorsal root fiber somatotopic organization at the root entry zone, and Rexed's laminae. (*Adapted from* Nolte JK, Angevine JB. The human brain in photographs and diagrams. St Louis, MO: Mosby; 2005. p. 11; with permission.)

and the dorsal roots. The lateral funiculus lies between the dorsal and ventral roots and the anterior funiculus lies between the anterior median fissure and the ventral roots (see **Fig. 4**).

SPINAL ROOTS AND NERVES

The dorsal roots consist of several types of afferent fibers somatotopically organized such that the largest diameter fibers are medial to the smaller ones (see **Fig. 4**). These largest afferent fibers (Ia and Ib) are heavily myelinated fibers that conduct the afferent limb of muscle stretch reflexes and carry information from muscle spindles and Golgi tendon organs. Medium-sized fibers (A-beta) convey impulses from mechanoreceptors in skin and joints. Small, thinly myelinated A-delta and C-type unmyelinated fibers convey noxious and thermal sensation.

The anterior root bundles constitute the motor output from the spinal cord. These anterior root bundles are large-diameter alpha motor neuron axons to the extrafusal striated muscle fibers, and gamma motor neuron axons, which supply the intrafusal striated muscle spindles as well as preganglionic autonomic motor fibers. After the posterior and anterior roots join to form spinal nerves, they divide into a smaller primary dorsal ramus and a larger primary ventral ramus (see **Fig. 2**B). The dorsal ramus consists of a medial sensory branch and a lateral motor branch to supply the skin and paraspinous muscle at the segmental level. The ventral ramus is much larger and contributes to the brachial and lumbosacral plexuses as well as to segmental branches such as intercostal nerves.

INTERNAL ANATOMY OF THE SPINAL CORD: GRAY MATTER

The gray matter of the spinal cord is an H-shaped structure in the transverse section of the spinal cord with 2 symmetric halves connected by a narrow bridge or commissure composed of gray and white matter through which runs the central canal (see **Fig. 4**). The central canal is a continuation of the fourth ventricle. Lined with ciliated columnar epithelium, it is filled with cerebrospinal fluid. Encircling the columnar epithelium is a band of neuroglia, the substantia gliosa. The ratio of gray substance to white substance varies markedly at different levels of spinal cord. In the thoracic levels the amount of gray matter is less than that in the cervical and lumbosacral enlargements.

An imaginary coronal line through the central canal divides the gray matter into anterior and posterior columns (or anterior and posterior horns). The anterior horn contains alpha and gamma motor neurons. In the thoracic region, the posterolateral portion of the anterior column is called the lateral (intermediolateral) column. This lateral column contains preganglionic cells for the autonomic nervous system in the thoracic and upper lumbar areas. From T1 to L2 spinal segments, preganglionic sympathetic neurons within the intermediolateral gray column give rise to sympathetic axons, which leave the spinal cord through the anterior roots and travel to the adjacent sympathetic ganglia through white rami comminucantes. All spinal nerves contain gray rami communicantes; however, white rami communicantes are only found from the T1 to L2 levels. Parasympathetic preganglionic neurons arise from the spinal segments S2, S3, and S4 within the intermediolateral gray column. These neurons also leave the spinal cord through ventral roots and, after projecting to the viscera, synapse on postganglionic parasympathetic ganglia. The posterior column or horn is directed posterolaterally and is separated from the posterolateral sulcus by an important thin layer of white matter, the tract of Lissauer.

ARCHITECTURAL LAMINATION OF THE SPINAL CORD GRAY MATTER

Rexed's cytoarchitectural studies of the spinal cord gray matter are the basis of the conventional gray matter division into the 10 eponymic laminae enumerated as Rexed's laminae I to X. Laminae I to IX are arranged from dorsal to ventral, whereas Lamina X consists of a circle of cells around the central canal (see **Fig. 4**, also diagrammed in **Fig. 5**). Some of the laminae correspond to specific cell types with functional significance. Thus, Lamina II corresponds to the substantia gelatinosa and plays an important part in transmission of fibers subserving thermal and painful sensations. Lamina VII occupies the intermediate gray zone and contains Clarke's nucleus. Lamina IX contains the largest spinal cord cells, the alpha motor neurons that supply skeletal extrafusal muscle fibers.

THE SPINAL CORD WHITE MATTER
Descending Fiber Systems

The corticospinal tract, arising from the precentral motor cortex, is the largest and most significant descending tract of the human spinal cord (**Fig. 6**).[1] Almost 90% of the corticospinal tract fibers decussate in the lower medulla to form the lateral corticospinal tract, whereas 8% of the nondecussating descending fibers form the anterior corticospinal tract and 2% of noncrossing fibers generate the uncrossed lateral cortico spinal tract. The uncrossed fibers of the anterior corticospinal tract may cross to the contralateral side via the anterior white commissure to project to interneurons and lower motor neurons of the contralateral side. These fibers provide synaptic input to neurons responsible for the control of axial body and proximal limb movements. There are also fibers in the corticospinal tract that project to the dorsal gray column and function as modulators of sensory afferent information, allowing the brain to process pain stimuli selectively.

The rubrospinal tract consists of fibers that originate from the contralateral red nucleus in the brainstem and descend just anterior to the corticospinal tract, projecting to interneurons that modulate proximal, largely flexor movements of the upper limb (**Fig. 7**).

Fig. 7 also shows several other ventral descending tracts that work together to modulate responses to changes in body posture and position. The vestibulospinal fasciculus consists of lateral and medial tracts, both of which arise from brainstem vestibular nuclei and, via interneurons that project to alpha motor neurons, provide excitatory input for extensor and antigravity muscles to control tone and posture. Reticulospinal tracts also arise from extensor-biased upper motor neurons and modulate muscle spindles. The tectospinal tract, derived from the contralateral superior colliculus in the midbrain tectum, crosses to the opposite side and descends in the contralateral ventral longitudinal bundle, providing neural input to ventral gray interneurons. This anatomic tract mediates reflex head turning movements in reaction to sudden auditory, visual, and tactile stimuli.

Ascending Fiber Systems

All afferent axons have their primary neurons in the dorsal root ganglia. The level of decussation varies among ascending systems. However, as a general rule, the ascending axons synapse before decussating to the contralateral side.

The dorsal column tract is responsible for the transmission of sensations of vibration, proprioception (position sense), and 2-point discrimination from the skin and joints.[2] The fasciculus gracilis is located medially and transmits sensation from the lower half of the body, whereas the fasciculus cuneatus, which is

Somatotopic Organization of Ascending and Descending Spinal Cord Tracts and Nuclei

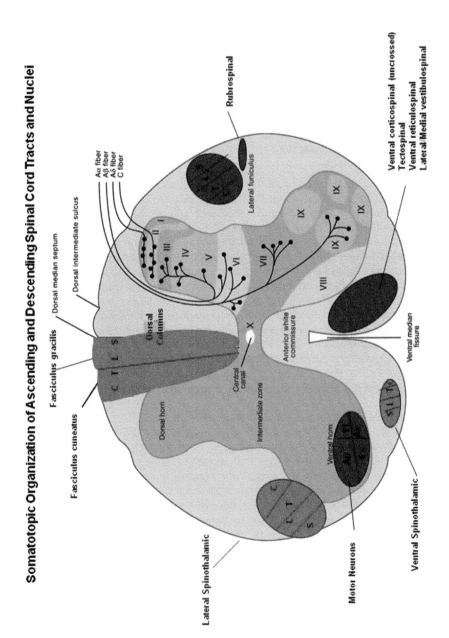

located more laterally at levels rostral to T5, carries proprioceptive input from the upper thorax through the back of the head. The gracile and cuneate fasciculi terminate in the gracile and cuneate nuclei of the lower medulla. The axons of these second-order neurons decussate as the internal arcuate fibers and travel rostrally as the medial lemniscus to the ventral posterolateral thalamic nucleus (**Fig. 7**A).

The spinothalamic tract mediates sensation of pain and temperature.[3] These sensory modalities are transmitted by small-diameter axons, which, after entering the cord via the dorsal root entry zone, divide into short ascending and descending branches that run longitudinally in Lissauer's tract for 1 to 2 segments and then synapse in the dorsal horn. The postsynaptic fibers cross to the opposite side of the spinal cord anterior to the central canal in the ventral white commissure and continue rostrally within the anterolateral funiculus (see **Fig. 7**B). The spinothalamic tract consists of a ventral tract that conveys light touch sensation, and a lateral tract that conveys pain and temperature sensation. Somatotopic organization of the spino-thalamic tracts is the opposite of the dorsal column tracts: rostral (upper limb) regions are represented medially, whereas more caudal regions are in the lateral aspect of the spinothalamic tract. The spinothalamic tract projects to ventral posterolateral and intralaminar thalamic nuclei.

The spinoreticular tract courses ipsilaterally without decussating within the ventro-lateral portion of the spinal cord ending in the reticular formation of the brainstem from which it projects to intralaminar thalamic nuclei and then to the limbic system. This tract has a regulatory role in the sensation of pain, especially deep, chronic pain as well as the emotional reaction to and memory of painful stimuli. The difficult treatment problem of chronic pain from myelopathic disease processes may derive from dysfunction of these (and other) afferent fibers.

The spinocerebellar pathway provides cerebellar inputs via 2 spinocerebellar systems that terminate on the ipsilateral cerebellum, the dorsal spinocerebellar tract arising from Clarke's nucleus at levels T1-L2 and its upper body equivalent, the ventral spinocerebellar (or cuneocerebellar) tract. These tracts convey unconscious proprio-ceptive information from Golgi tendon organs and muscle spindles to coordinate smooth execution of movements.

Fig. 5. The somatotopic organization of the spinal cord, as depicted here schematically at a cervical level, explains clinical syndromes, such as (1) the hemicord (Brown-Sequard) syndrome; (2) isolated tractopathies or preferential loss of specific sensory modalities; (3) extramedullary compressive lesions causing ascending symptoms caused by the superficial location of more caudal pathways; (4) intramedullary lesions producing descending sensory symptoms often with sacral sparing; (5) early central cord syndromes affecting the spinotha-lamic tract fibers crossing through the anterior commissure, giving "suspended" pain and temperature sensory loss. Gray matter is divided into groups of neurons that form layers in dorsal and ventral horns. Termination of large and small afferent axons in the cord varies by depth and the 2 groups enter the cord separately with little overlap. The 4 medial motor systems, represented schematically in the figure, terminate largely on interneurons that project bilaterally controlling movements that involve multiple segments. Thus unilateral lesions of the medial motor systems, unlike those of the lateral corticospinal tract, do not produce obvious clinical deficits. Ap, Appendicular; Ax, axial; C, cervical; Ex, extensor; Fl, flexor; L, lumbar; S, sacral; T, thoracic. (*Adapted and modified from* Squire LR, Bloom FE, McConnell SK, et al. Fundamental neuroscience. 2nd edition. San Diego: Academic Press; 2003. p. 681; with permission. Copyright © 2002, Elsevier Science (USA), All rights reserved.)

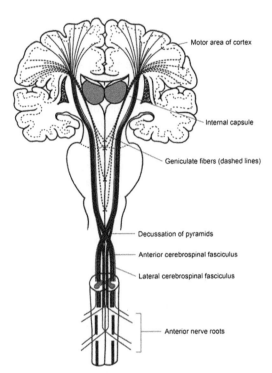

Motor area of cortex

Internal capsule

Geniculate fibers (dashed lines)

Decussation of pyramids

Anterior cerebrospinal fasciculus

Lateral cerebrospinal fasciculus

Anterior nerve roots

Fig. 6. Corticospinal tract (Drawing by Ms Lorry Tubbs).

CLINICAL APPROACH TO PATIENT WITH SPINAL CORD PROBLEM

The anatomic organization of ascending and descending pathways in the spinal cord described earlier often allows precise longitudinal and transverse localization of the pathologic process. Such localization not only directs diagnostic imaging procedures efficiently to the appropriate site but also offers early etiologic clues because many disease processes preferentially produce specific patterns of spinal cord dysfunction. For example, "tractopathies" such as dorsal column dysfunction occurs with syphilis and B12 or copper deficiency, whereas isolated spinothalamic tract dysfunction raises the suspicion of a paraneoplastic disorder. However, localization is infrequently entirely etiologically specific. Thus, Brown-Sequard syndrome can occur after trauma, or in the setting of tumor, demyelinating disease, and other intrinsic cord processes. At times, falsely localizing or misleading signs and symptoms may distract the clinician from the appropriate area of the cord. For example, isolated lower limb vibratory sense loss can be caused by an exclusively cervical process such as demyelination that involves fasciculus gracilis selectively.

The practical 5-step approach to spinal cord localization and triage outlined below takes advantage of neuroanatomic features to exclude the most emergent situations of compressive myelopathy.

STEP 1: Do symptoms and signs suggest the disease in the spinal cord?

Certain configurations classically suggest spinal cord pathologic abnormalities, but, as depicted in **Fig. 8**, there are a large number of signs and symptoms that, while possibly localizable to the spinal cord, could reflect disease in other parts of the nervous system as well. Perhaps the most confusing are paresthesias that present roughly symmetrically. These paresthesias could reflect polyneuropathy or dorsal

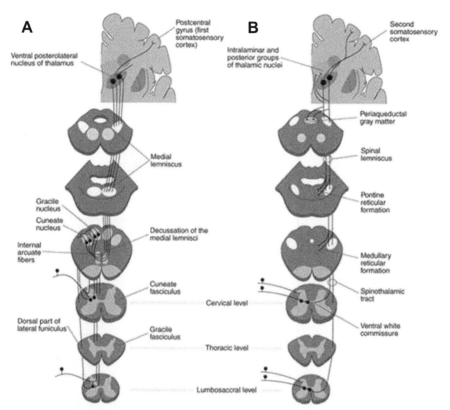

Fig. 7. Anatomic pathways of the sensory system (*A*) Dorsal column tract; (*B*) Lateral spinothalamic tract. (*Adapted and modified from* Squire LR, Bloom FE, McConnell SK, et al. Fundamental neuroscience. 2nd edition. San Diego: Academic Press/Elsevier Science; 2003. p. 682; with permission.)

column pathologic abnormalities. Lower limb paraparesis without sensory signs could be a sign of a parasagittal meningioma.

STEP 2: Is the problem a compressive myelopathy?

Although all spinal cord problems are in a sense emergencies capable of causing irreparable damage to critical structures, some myelopathies dictate more rapid intervention than others. The most important early clinical distinction involves compressive versus noncompressive syndromes. Most compressive syndromes will reveal abnormalities on magnetic resonance imaging of the spinal cord/column.

Compressive Myelopathies

Compressive myelopathies may stem from extradural or intradural processes. Tumors and trauma are major causes of compressive myelopathies. In general, extradural neoplasms are more aggressive malignancies such as metastatic disease, whereas intradural neoplasms are more indolent tumors such as meningiomas or neurofibromas. Clinical clues to the presence of compressive myelopathies include the following:

1. Radicular and vertebral pain
2. Early upper motor neuron (UMN) signs, rare lower motor neuron (LMN) signs except possible root involvement at level of compression

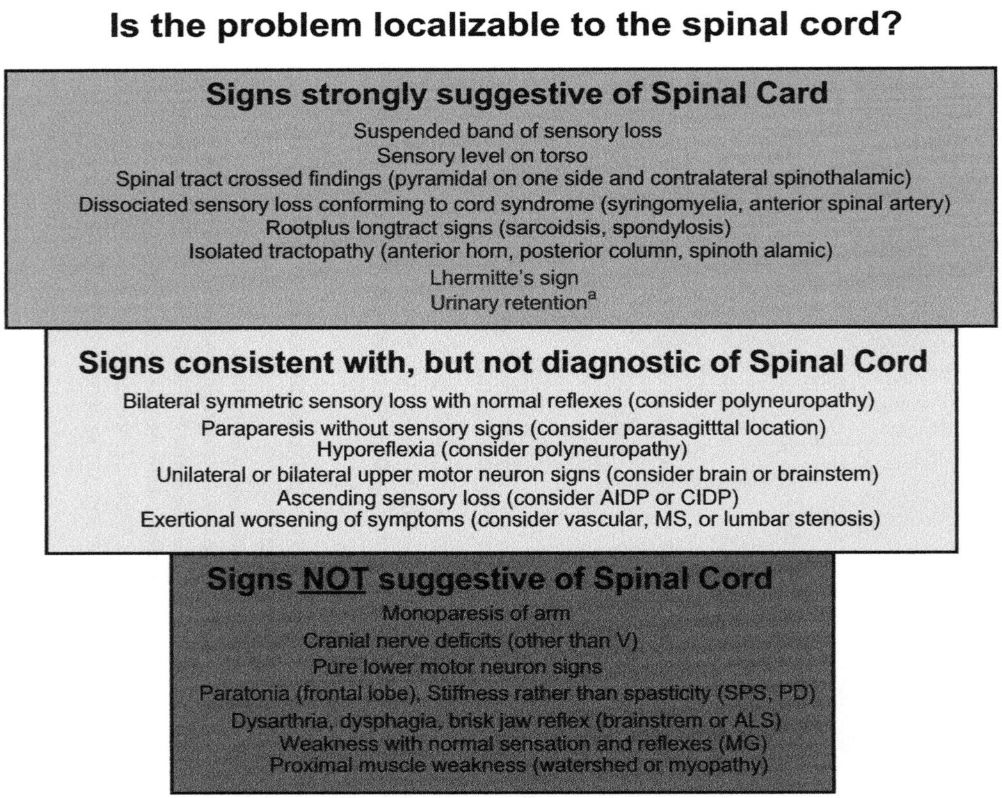

Is the problem localizable to the spinal cord?

Signs strongly suggestive of Spinal Cord

Suspended band of sensory loss
Sensory level on torso
Spinal tract crossed findings (pyramidal on one side and contralateral spinothalamic)
Dissociated sensory loss conforming to cord syndrome (syringomyelia, anterior spinal artery)
Rootplus longtract signs (sarcoidsis, spondylosis)
Isolated tractopathy (anterior horn, posterior column, spinoth alamic)
Lhermitte's sign
Urinary retention[a]

Signs consistent with, but not diagnostic of Spinal Cord

Bilateral symmetric sensory loss with normal reflexes (consider polyneuropathy)
Paraparesis without sensory signs (consider parasagitttal location)
Hyporeflexia (consider polyneuropathy)
Unilateral or bilateral upper motor neuron signs (consider brain or brainstem)
Ascending sensory loss (consider AIDP or CIDP)
Exertional worsening of symptoms (consider vascular, MS, or lumbar stenosis)

Signs NOT suggestive of Spinal Cord

Monoparesis of arm
Cranial nerve deficits (other than V)
Pure lower motor neuron signs
Paratonia (frontal lobe). Stiffness rather than spasticity (SPS, PD)
Dysarthria, dysphagia, brisk jaw reflex (brainstrem or ALS)
Weakness with normal sensation and reflexes (MG)
Proximal muscle weakness (watershed or myopathy)

Fig. 8. General diagnostic guidelines to localize the lesion to spinal cord. [a] Isolated urinary retention would be an unusual initial spinal cord symptom and also raises consideration of bifrontal pathologic abnormality or mechanical or pharmacologic obstruction, such as prostatic hypertrophy or anticholinergic toxicity. AIDP, acute inflammatory demyelinating neuropathy; ALS, amyotrophic lateral sclerosis; CIDP, chronic inflammatory demyelinating polyneuropathy; MG, myasthenia gravis; MS, multiple sclerosis; PD, Parkinson disease; SPS, stiff person syndrome. (*Modified from* Squire LR, Bloom FE, McConnell SK, et al. Fundamental neuroscience. 2nd edition. New York: Academic Press/Elsevier; 2003. p. 38; with permission.)

3. *Ascending* paresthesias (because the caudal-most dermatomes are represented superficially in the cord, see **Fig. 7**)
4. Brown-Sequard syndrome

NONCOMPRESSIVE MYELOPATHIES

Noncompressive myelopathies include most neuropathologies that initiate in the intra-medullary compartment although noncompressive and intramedullary are not synon-ymous terms, as significant inflammatory or infectious conditions can expand the cord.[4]

Clinical clues of a noncompressive myelopathy include the following:

1. Radicular and bone pain uncommon
2. Dysesthetic pain: the patient will use words to describe associated paresthesias, such as burning, tingling, or tightness
3. Late UMN with diffuse LMN at level of process
4. Dissociated sensory loss (spinothalamic dysfunction with spared dorsal columns or vice versa)
5. *Descending* sensory loss with sacral sparing because of the somatotopic organiza-tion of spinothalamic fibers (see **Fig. 7**)
6. Brown-Sequard syndrome is less common than in compressive myelopathy, but can be seen with varicella zoster virus infection[5] or multiple sclerosis (MS)
7. Early sphincter involvement in conus medullaris lesions with saddle anesthesia

STEP 3: If the lesion is likely to be in the spinal cord, longitudinal localization will be based primarily on dermatomal levels.

Fig. 3 shows anterior and posterior views of the dermatomes. Because spinothala-mic fibers ascend over 2 cord levels crossing in the anterior commissure, lesions are often located several levels above the rostral-most clinical signs. Key localizing signs at various longitudinal levels are shown in **Fig. 9**.

As described earlier in this article, disproportion between the length of the spinal cord and the length of the bony spinal vertebral column gives rise to longitudinal local-ization discrepancies. In the adult, the spinal cord ends at L1 level, but the roots descend in the cauda equina so that the L4 anterior root emerges from the 4th spinal lumbar segment opposite the vertebral level T12 and exits between the L4 and L5 vertebrae. Neoplastic or other disorders such as arachnoiditis that involve both the conus and the cauda equina produce a sometimes confusing set of signs that suggest pathologic abnormalities lower than the actual process. Any process below the L1 vertebral body will not impinge on the cord. Thus compressive lesions at the vertebral L4 level do not always dictate the same degree of urgency as similar pathologic processes such as a disc or tumor at T4.

The C1-C7 roots exist *above* their respective vertebral bodies. The C8 root is "extra" and exits between C7 and T1. Therefore, starting at the T1-T2 level, the remaining roots exit below the like-numbered vertebral body (see **Fig. 9**). At the lumbar level, however, the root affected also may be the next lower one. For example, an L4-L5 disc may impinge on the L5 root if it protrudes midline and on the L4 root if the disc emerges more laterally. There are no discs between the sacral spinal segments.

STEP 4: Once the longitudinal level is localized, transverse cord localization may help with the etiologic diagnosis.

Fig. 7 illustrates a composite diagram of tracts and nuclei at a cervical cord level and explains the occurrence of specific spinal cord syndromes. These syndromes and representative etiologies are summarized in **Table 1**.

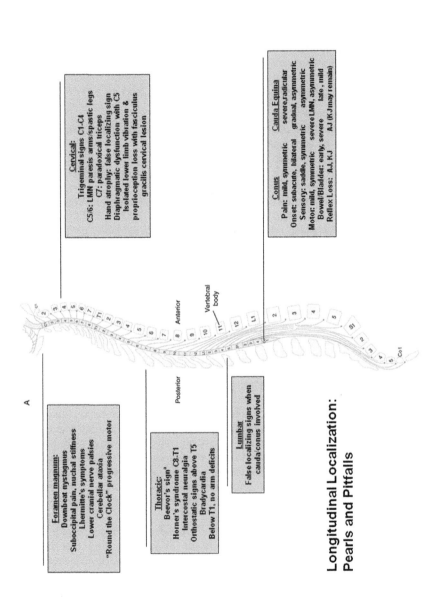

Fig. 9. In addition to dermatomal sensory motor and reflex changes, some specific signs of localizing value can help to concentrate attention on a specific level of the spinal cord. AJ, KJ, ankle and knee jerk (muscle stretch reflex); LMN, lower motor neuron. [a] Beevor's Sign: Upward retraction of abdomen when abdominal wall is stroked occurs when upper abdominal reflexes are present (T6-9) but lower reflexes (T9-11) are lost with lesion at approximately T10. (*Modified from* Squire LR, Bloom FE, McConnell SK, et al. Fundamental neuroscience. 2nd edition. New York: Academic Press/Elsevier; 2003. p. 38; with permission.)

Table 1 Localization: cord syndromes		
Syndrome	**Signs**	**Representative Conditions**
Complete cord	All function lost 1–2 levels below lesion	Transverse myelitis Multiple sclerosis, traumatic injury
Brown-Sequard	Ipsilateral motor and vibration loss; contralateral pain/temperature loss	Traumatic injury, epidural tumor, varicella zoster virus infection, multiple sclerosis
Central		
Small	Suspended sensory loss	Contusion, tumor, syrinx
Large	Dissociated sensory loss involving lateral spinothalamic tract and sparing dorsal column, anterior horn cell at level of lesion UMN signs below level of lesion	Syringomyelia, tumor neuromyelitis optica
Posterior column	Proprioception and vibration loss Deep tendon reflexes may be normal	Ischemic stroke Syphilis, multiple sclerosis B12 and copper deficiency
Anterior horn	Sensation normal, fasciculations, LMN weakness	Poliomyelitis, West Nile virus encephalomyelitis
Anterior spinal artery	Weakness Dissociated sensory loss, sparing dorsal columns	Ischemic stroke
Spinothalamic	Symmetric, longitudinally extensive, isolated pain and temperature loss	Paraneoplastic syndrome
Root + cord	One or more roots plus cord	Spondylosis, sarcoidosis, Lyme disease
Myeloneuropathy	Myelopathy plus polyneuropathy	B12 deficiency, vitamin E deficiency, sarcoidosis, genetic syndromes

Complete Transverse Cord Involvement

All sensory and motor as well as autonomic pathways are interrupted. There is diminished sensation in all dermatomes 1 or 2 levels below the area of structural damage. A period of areflexia with spinal shock may occur immediately after disease onset. Common causes include transverse myelitis, MS, and trauma.

Hemicord (Brown-Sequard) Syndrome

Injury to the lateral corticospinal tract causes ipsilateral weakness, and ipsilateral loss of vibration sense causes posterior column damage. Contralateral spinothalamic signs are present.

Central Cord Syndrome

Small lesions damaging spinothalamic fibers crossing in the ventral commissure cause bilateral "suspended" sensory loss to pain and temperature often involving the lateral aspect of upper limbs. Sacral sparing occurs until late because these fibers are laterally represented in the cord. A larger central lesion produces pain and temperature loss in a cape distribution. Damaged anterior horn cells produced lower motor neuron deficits at the level of the lesion with upper motor neuron signs, as listed below. Dorsal column function may be spared. Common causes include cord contusion hyperextension neck injuries, neuromyelitis optica, syringomyelia, and intrinsic cord tumors such astrocytoma or ependymoma.

Posterior Cord Syndrome

Loss of vibration and proprioception below the level of the lesion are hallmarks of this syndrome. If the lesion is confined to posterior columns, tendon reflexes and strength may be normal. The somatotopic organization of the dorsal columns makes it mandatory to scan the entire cord because localized fasciculus gracilis lesions may give rise to the potentially misleading finding of isolated lower limb sensory disturbance. Conditions producing selective dorsal column pathologic abnormalities include MS, B12 and copper deficiency, chemotherapy toxicities, paraneoplastic sensory neuronopathy (anti-Hu), and tabes dorsalis. In addition to sensory ataxia, trophic changes and Charcot joints may be observed.

Anterior Cord Syndrome

Pain and temperature loss occur 2 levels below the lesion, and LMN signs are seen at the level of the lesion. Weakness is prominent. Atrophy and fasciculations may be seen in longer duration disease. Dorsal columns may be spared, particularly with anterior spinal artery syndrome. Common causes are anterior spinal artery infarction, trauma (disc herniation), spinal muscular atrophy, MS, poliomyelitis, and West Nile virus.

Anterior Horn Cell and Pyramidal Tract Disease

A combination of UMN and LMN signs is seen. There is sparing of sensation and sphincter function. Additional signs and symptoms may include muscle cramping, bulbar involvement, and pseudobulbar involvement. Amyotrophic lateral sclerosis and variants are the likely causes.

Myeloneuropathy

Myelopathic signs as well as signs of a polyneuropathy are found. There is a wide variety of possible etiologies, including deficiency states such as B12, copper, and vitamin E, sarcoidosis, Sjogren syndrome, and infections such as human immunodeficiency virus and human T-lymphotropic virus infections as well as numerous genetic conditions including adrenomyeloneuropathy, metachromatic leukodystrophy, and mitochondrial disorders.[6]

STEP 5: Once having satisfactorily localized the problem to the cord in both longitudinal and transverse dimensions, the clinician should return to consider further the possibility of falsely localizing signs and problematic presentations. Five potentially misleading sets of symptoms are summarized below.

Exertional Symptoms

Both spinal cord and noncord etiologies may give rise to exertional limb symptoms. For example, lumbar stenosis and claudication on a vascular basis may cause worsening of back and lower limb pain. Exertional symptoms also occur in the setting of dural fistulas, producing venous congestion of the cord. Heat-related exacerbation of symptoms in demyelinating disease could also be construed an exertion-related spinal cord syndrome.

Ipsilateral Shoulder Weakness and Lower Cranial Nerve Problems with Spasticity

Lesions in the foramen magnum interrupt decussating pyramidal tracts to the legs, which cross below those of the arms. Crural paresis or weakness of the lower limbs may be an early sign of foramen magnum pathologic abnormality or the syndrome, which is often accompanied by suboccipital and shoulder pain, may begin with ipsilateral shoulder and arm weakness followed by leg weakness and then contralateral arm involvement in a "round-the-clock" pattern. The weakness can begin in any limb.

Cranial Nerves and Spinal Cord Syndromes

Because the descending tract of the trigeminal subserving pain descends as far as C4, lesions in the upper cord may be accompanied by facial symptoms. At the foramen magnum, lower cranial nerves IX-XII may be involved along with spinal cord structures.

Referred Pain

Visceral afferent fibers to cell bodies from T1 to L2 or L3 in dorsal root ganglia accompany sympathetic efferents in spinal nerves. Most of these afferents carry information about visceral function (distortion or inflammation of organs) that may be interpreted as pain. Visceral pain, in contrast to somatic pain, is usually poorly localized and referred to an area of the body surface corresponding to the dermatome innervated by that spinal segment. Thus, arm pain may reflect cardiac ischemia or, conversely, a sense of tightness in the chest in an MS patient may suggest acute pulmonary disease but reflect active demyelination at a thoracic spinal cord segment. Typical patterns of dermatomal distribution of referred pain are summarized in **Table 2**.

Ascending Sensory Symptoms

As discussed earlier, compressive lesions may cause ascending sensory deficits. Sensory symptoms of acute inflammatory demyelinating polyneuropathy can ascend as well, however. Clear-cut UMN signs exclude acute inflammatory demyelinating polyneuropathy, but in the early "spinal shock" phase of a spinal cord process, these may

Table 2 Symptoms are predominantly pain, deep, aching unless otherwise indicated	
Referred Symptom Patterns	
Diaphragm	C3–C4
Heart	T1–T4
Lungs	T3–T10
Stomach	T6–T9
Gallbladder	T7–T8
Duodenum	T9–T10
Appendix	T10
Reproductive organs	T10–T12
Kidney and ureter	L1–L2

Visceral pain differs from somatic pain in that it is poorly localized and referred to an area of the body surface. Visceral afferents and somatic pain fibers at specific cord levels converge on the same spinothalamic tract pathways, sometimes giving rise to diagnostic confusion.

Data from Nolte J. The human brain: an introduction to its functional anatomy. 4th edition. St Louis: Mosby; 1999.

not be present. When localization is in doubt but a spinal cord process is possible, full spinal cord imaging is always a prudent investigative approach.

REFERENCES

1. Nathan PW, Smith MC. Long descending tracts in man. I. Review of present knowledge. Brain 1955;78(2):248–303.
2. Kaas JH, Qi HX, Burish MJ, et al. Cortical and subcortical plasticity in the brains of humans, primates, and rats after damage to sensory afferents in the dorsal columns of the spinal cord. Exp Neurol 2008;209(2):407–16.
3. Hodge CJ Jr, Apkarian AV. The spinothalamic tract. Crit Rev Neurobiol 1990;5(4): 363–97.
4. Debette S, deSeze J, Pruvo JP, et al. Long term outcome of acute and subacute myelopathies. J Neurol 2009;25:980–8.
5. Mathews MS, Sorkin GC, Brant-Zawadzki M. Varicella zoster infection of the brainstem followed by brown-séquard syndrome. Neurology 2009;72(21):1874.
6. Schmalstieg WF, Weinshenker BG. Approach to acute or subacute myelopathy. Neurology 2010;75(Suppl 1):S2–8.

Spinal Cord Infections

Megan B. Richie, MD, Amy A. Pruitt, MD*

KEYWORDS

- Epidural abscess • HIV/AIDS-related myelopathy • Myelitis • Potts disease
- Varicella zoster virus • West Nile virus

KEY POINTS

- Spinal cord infections remain a significant source of morbidity for immunocompromised patients. A growing body of travelers and patients with health care contacts contributes to increasing at-risk population groups, although exposure to pathogens may be temporally remote from the patients' presentation.
- Spinal cord infections may be associated with normal magnetic resonance imaging but selective involvement of bone, roots, and specific spinal tracts may narrow diagnostic considerations.
- Empiric treatment before definitive diagnosis with steroids and/or acyclovir should be discussed with infectious disease consultants based on demographic, cerebrospinal fluid (CSF), and radiologic data.
- Neurosurgical consultation should be obtained early for patients with compressive myelopathies caused by pyogenic or granulomatous masses.
- Acellular CSF does not eliminate the possibility of a central nervous system infection, particularly in patients who are immunocompromised.

INTRODUCTION

Patients with potential spinal cord infection confront the clinician with neurologic emergencies for which timely diagnosis and intervention can mean the difference between restored neurologic function and profound disability or death. Unfortunately, infectious and noninfectious conditions involving the spinal cord may have very similar presentations but decidedly different treatments. This article outlines a clinical and laboratory approach to spinal cord infections. Selected important pathogens and their management are described. For purposes of this discussion, the authors define spinal cord infections as infectious processes whose major symptoms involve the intramedullary spinal cord parenchyma, the epidural and intradural spaces, or the spinal nerve roots. The authors do not discuss meningitis or meningoencephalitis without specific spinal cord signs and symptoms, recognizing that encephalopathy may dominate the presentation, obscuring spinal cord symptoms, and that myelitis and evolving meningoencephalitis often coexist.

Department of Neurology, University of Pennsylvania, 3400 Spruce Street, Philadelphia, PA 19104, USA
* Corresponding author.
E-mail address: pruitt@mail.med.upenn.edu

Neurol Clin 31 (2013) 19–53
http://dx.doi.org/10.1016/j.ncl.2012.09.006   neurologic.theclinics.com

Approach to Potential Spinal Cord Infections[a]

Historical Clues: travel/residence in endemic areas, tick/mosquito exposure, HIV, IVDA, STDs recent hospitalization/health care exposure (dialysis, IV lines,craniotomy, PCA pumps), cancer medication use: corticosteroids, chemotherapy, TNFα inhibitors, rituximab, recent vaccination[b]

Clinical Clues: Nonneurologic: pharynx (EBV) lung (Aspergillus, Cryptococcus, TB), liver (HTLV1, Hepatitis C) genital (HSV2), retina (CMV), blood (bacterial, fungal)
skin: dermatomal vesicles (VZV), buccal/hands/feet (Enterovirus), decubiti splinter hemorrhages (bacterial/fungal endocarditis), furuncles (S aureus) erythema migrans (Lyme), macules/petechiae: ankles, wrists (Rickettsia)

Neurologic: meningoencephalitis: fever, headache, encephalopathy (viral, bacterial, fungal) vertebral or muscular pain (M. tuberculosis, Brucella, S aureus)

Laboratory Screens[c]: **MRI Spine (Brain as indicated)**
Blood: CBC, cultures, VDRL, Lyme, HIV, toxoplasmosis   **Chest X ray**
CSF: WBC, protein, glucose, oligoclonal bands, VDRL, cryptococcal antigen, PCR: VZV, CMV, HSV1,2, EBV   seasonally: WNV, enterovirus

Pathogens in At-Risk Patient Groups

Travel, Residence In Endemic Area
TB
Brucella
Lyme
RMSF
Neurocysticercosis
Schistosomiasis
WNV
VZV

Barrier Breakdown:
Recent Hospitalization, Surgery
Bacteria: S aureus, S epidermidis
      Acinetobacter
      Gram negative rods

HIV/AIDS
Syphilis
HTLV1
HSV1,2
VZV
CMV
TB
EBV (PCNSL)
Hepatitis C
Vacuolar myelopathy

Transplant Recipients, Chemotherapy/steroids
HHV 7
CMV
VZV
HSV
EBV (B cell lymphoma)
JC virus (PML)
Aspergillus species
C. neoformans
Unusually severe: WNV, enterovirus

Empiric Treatment of Infectious Myelopathies

Neurosurgical consultation for compressive myelopathy/hydrocephalus

High suspicion bacterial infection?

No → **Rapidly progressive infectious/inflammatory signs**
Consider: IV methylprednisolone 1000 mg daily X5 days
Possible viral myelitis: consider Acyclovir

Yes → **Antibiotics**
ID consultation for local resistance trends

SUSPECTING SPINAL CORD INFECTION: A DIAGNOSTIC APPROACH

The clinician approaching patients with a potential spinal cord infection should follow a systematic strategy to optimize efficient choice of diagnostic and therapeutic options. One such strategy is suggested in **Fig. 1** and expanded with the following points:

Demographic Clues

Demographic clues help to generate a first approximation of possible pathogens in several vulnerable patient populations. However, the relevant infectious risk factors, such as blood transfusion, international residence, or travel exposure, may have occurred well before the spinal cord presentation.

Pace of Illness

Pace of illness in spinal cord infections is acute, subacute, or chronically progressive but usually not episodic or fluctuating, with exceptions such as cases of recurrent herpes simplex virus type 2 (HSV2) myelitis or subarachnoid neurocysticercosis. Compressive myelopathies such as those associated with tuberculosis (TB) or pyogenic epidural abscess may appear to have rapid onset, but further historical inquiry discloses a more indolent pain syndrome antedating neurologic deterioration. Chronic presentations are characteristic of a dauntingly wide range of infections, including human immunodeficiency virus (HIV), human T-lymphotropic virus 1 (HTLV-1), syphilis, hepatitis C, and some parasites. The list of organisms causing acute (onset sudden or evolving over less than 1 day) flaccid paralysis includes poliovirus 1/2/3; Coxsackie A and B; echoviruses; enteroviruses 70, 71, 93, and 94; West Nile virus (WNV); varicella-zoster virus (VZV); and syphilitic arteritis-related spinal stroke, although these all can also produce more subacute presentations.

Unfortunately, it is often the rapidly progressive cases that cause the greatest clinical and radiographic confusion among both infectious and noninfectious causes. Infection should be considered in all cases of acute myelitis. **Fig. 2** contrasts 2 patients with late-summer presentations of longitudinally extensive cord abnormalities and brainstem signs whose magnetic resonance imaging (MRI) scans were similar but who had, respectively, neuromyelitis optica (NMO) and WNV differentiated by NMO serology, cerebrospinal fluid (CSF) studies, and electromyography.[1]

Fig. 1. Approach to potential spinal cord infections. [a] The chart is a general guide to the differential diagnostic process and is not meant to be inclusive of all potential pathogens. Although several at-risk patient groups are highlighted, immunologically normal patients can develop many different spinal cord infections. [b] Potential vaccine-associated myelitis: hepatitis B, influenza, polio, rabies, rubella, VZV. [c] Although clinical presentation and demographics will refine diagnostic tests, these tests are reasonable basic screens for treatable infectious myelopathies. Color code: red, immunocompromised patient populations; lavender, may occur in either normal hosts or patients who are immunocompromised; blue, normal host populations. CBC, complete blood count; CMV, cytomegalovirus; EBV, Epstein-Barr virus; HHV, human herpesvirus; HIV, human immunodeficiency virus; HSV, herpes simplex virus; HTLV1, human T-cell lymphotropic virus type 1; ID, infectious disease; IVDA, intravenous drug abuse; MRI, magnetic resonance imaging; PCA, patient-controlled analgesia; PCNSL, primary central nervous system lymphoma; PML, progressive multifocal leukoencephalopathy; RMSF, Rocky Mountain spotted fever; STD, sexually transmitted diseases; TB, tuberculosis; TNFα, tumor necrosis factor α; VZV, varicella-zoster virus; WNV, West Nile virus.

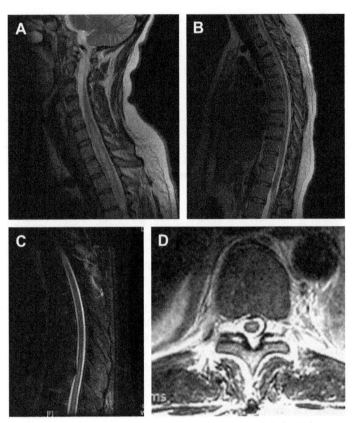

Fig. 2. WNV or not? Longitudinally extensive transverse myelitis (LTEM) suggests several infectious diagnoses but is not specific. This Fig. contrasts 2 patients with LTEM and brainstem signs. (*A, B*) A longitudinally extensive intramedullary cord signal abnormality on magnetic resonance imaging (MRI) sagittal T2-weighted images throughout the cervical and thoracic cord. Patient presented with progressive quadriparesis and central right-sided facial weakness. Signal abnormality continued rostrally, primarily on the left, into the brainstem and thalamus (not shown). WNV immunoglobulin M was negative, and the decision was made to give corticosteroids while waiting for these results. The patient had neuromyelitis optica and responded well to prolonged corticosteroids and plasmapheresis. Sagittal (*C*) and axial (*D*) MRI T2-weighted images show a similarly extensive signal abnormality, primarily in the anterior horn. The patient presented with ascending quadriparesis, downbeat nystagmus, tongue fasciculations, and lower motor neuron facial diplegia caused by WNV.

Physical Examination

The physical examination should be directed to dermatologic, pulmonary, hepatic, and cerebral manifestations of systemic infection that prompt investigations for an infectious cause. Although no specific cord syndrome predicts the cause unequivocally, some infections are strongly suggested by the clinical signs. For example, cauda equina syndrome in patients infected with HIV raises the strong possibility of cytomegalovirus (CMV) and selective anterior horn cell disease suggests poliovirus or WNV.

Diagnostic Imaging

The first confirmatory tests for any possible spinal cord infection usually will be MRI.

- *Normal* spinal MRI is often seen with many viral myelitides, including HSV, hepatitis C–associated myelopathy, Epstein-Barr virus (EBV)–associated syndromes, and AIDS vacuolar myelopathy.[2]
- *Abnormal* MRI is almost always seen in spinal cord neurocysticercosis, schistosomiasis, *Aspergillus*, TB, and pyogenic epidural abscess.
- *Either normal or abnormal neuroimaging* is consistent with many pathogens: *Cryptococcus*, VZV, HSV, EBV, CMV, HTLV-1, and WNV.

Serum and CSF Diagnostic Testing

Table 1, provides a detailed summary of serologic, CSF, and MRI diagnostic tools for spinal cord infections, indicating specifically treatable entities. Polymerase chain reaction (PCR) technology now allows the identification of minute quantities of unique nucleic acid sequences for specific organisms. It has found its greatest utility in the identification of viral infections, such as HSV2, as the etiologic agent of recurrent, usually self-limited lymphocytic meningitis known as Mollaret meningitis.[3] The increasing availability of quantitative CSF PCR now enables tracking of therapeutic responses. Knowledge of the sensitivity and specificity of PCR is necessary to interpret results accurately and to inform clinical decision making. Two important caveats about PCR are

- PCR does *not* require replicating the virus for detection so that a positive PCR does not necessarily mean ongoing infection or contribute to etiologic diagnosis in the postinfectious recovery phase of patients whose pathologic diagnosis remains obscure.
- PCR does *not* obviate microbial culture, which remains necessary to determine antimicrobial sensitivity.

In most cases of potential spinal cord infections, several principles help guide testing:

- In general, the presence of pleocytosis greater than 50 leukocytes per microliter raises suspicion of a possible infection. Although a predominantly neutrophilic CSF pleocytosis enhances suspicion of infection, this feature can occur in noninfectious myelitis such as that associated with neuromyelitis optica (NMO).[4] *The absence white blood cells in CSF does not exclude infection.*
- The sensitivity of CSF tests depends on proper test choice with respect to the onset of the illness. Thus, PCR may become negative in WNV neuroinvasive disease before the onset of neurologic symptoms, at which time CSF immunoglobulin (Ig) M is a better test.
- Serologic testing alone is insufficient to prove a causal association with a spinal cord infection. Thus, IgG in serum may only indicate past exposure, and increasing titers (usually between 2 weeks and 3 months) provide better evidence of recent infection. Nevertheless, in cases of transverse myelitis, it is important to seek serologic evidence of infection with pathogens capable of producing myelopathy both to identify treatable infections and also to obviate future unnecessary diagnostic testing for potentially relapsing inflammatory and demyelinating conditions.
- A reasonable broad-spectrum screen includes CSF PCR testing for CMV, VZV, HSV-1 and 2, and cryptococcal antigen and *blood* testing for HIV, syphilis, and Lyme, reserving other tests, such as CSF WNV and enteroviruses, for appropriate seasons and CSF EBV, JCV PCR, and CSF and serum galactomannan for *Aspergillus* for at-risk patient populations (see later discussion).

Table 1
Diagnostic Tests for Spinal Cord Infections

Disease	Blood Tests	CSF Tests[a]	Spinal MRI Special Features[b]	Other Useful Clues	References
Epidural abscess[c] (less common: *intramedullary or subdural abscess*)	Blood culture × 2 (60%–70% sensitive)	Avoid LP if possible to prevent spreading infection Culture (5%–30% sensitive) Routine studies: WBC 0–3000+ (PMNs or mononuclear) Often elevated lactate	>90% sensitive & specific Epidural space-occupying lesion T/L > C > CE, usually 3–4 segments Posterior > anterior T1 isointense or hypointense, T2 hyperintense ± enhancement or diffusion restriction Anterior: bilobed, ± osteomyelitis	Abscess culture (90% sensitive) High: ESR, CRP, WBC, ALP Low: platelets TTE/TEE for endocarditis	47–50,52–57, 119,120
			Fig. 4		
Lyme disease[c]	IgM, IgG ELISA or IFA, confirmatory WB	IgM ELISA or IFA with confirmatory WB CXCL13 DNA PCR (<40% sensitive) Routine studies: WBC <1000 (mononuclear)	May be normal Transverse myelitis, radiculomyelitis ± enhancement of parenchyma, leptomeninges, roots, CE	EMG to confirm radiculopathy Erythema migrans (60%–80%) Cardiac conduction abnormalities	24,75–79, 121–123
			Fig. 6		
Mycoplasma pneumoniae	IgM, IgG, IgA CF, ELISA, IFA	IgG, IgM CF or IFA PCR (low sensitivity) Culture (very low sensitivity) Routine studies: WBC 0–500 (mononuclear > PMN)	May be normal	IgM cold agglutinins (50%–60% sensitive) Nasopharyngeal aspirate culture, PCR Commonly have CNS coinfections (herpesviruses)	124,125

Organism	Blood/serologic tests	CSF studies	Imaging/findings	Other tests	References
TB[c] *Mycobacterium tuberculosis*	Quantiferon gold	AFB smear and culture; Sensitivity improves with larger CSF volume; PCR (60%–90% sensitive); Routine studies in radiculomyelitis: Moderately high WBCs (<1000, mononuclear); Markedly high protein if CSF block present; Glucose often ≤40% blood level	Usually abnormal; Often associated discitis, spondylitis/osteomyelitis	PPD; Sputum AFB; Hyponatremia (45%); EMG in setting of radiculitis; Chest radiograph, spine radiograph	21–23,58–70, 72–74, 126–129
			Fig. 5		
Syphilis[c] (*Treponema pallidum*)	VDRL: usually >1:32; MHA-ATP; FTA-ABS	VDRL; Routine studies: WBC 0–200 (mononuclear)	May be normal; Pachymeningitis, gummas; Infarction; Late atrophy	Optic atrophy; Dementia	80,81
VZV[c]	IgM; ELISA, IFA	DNA PCR; IgG/IgM index; ELISA, immunofixation, IFA; Routine studies: WBCs 0–1000 (mononuclear); May show elevated RBCs	Usually abnormal; Transverse myelitis, tract myelitis, polyradiculoneuritis; May be isolated to posterior columns or other tracts	EMG, SSEP, MEP to suggest myelitis; Brain MRI: small and large vessel strokes; Skin lesion biopsy	34,35, 94–105, 130–133
			Fig. 7		

(continued on next page)

Table 1
(continued)

Disease	Blood Tests	CSF Tests[a]	Spinal MRI Special Features[b]	Other Useful Clues	References
WNV	IgM, IgG ELISA, hemagglutination, plaque reduction neutralization assay	IgM, IgG ELISA or plaque reduction neutralization assay May not be positive early in course RNA PCR usually negative before neurologic onset Routine studies: WBCs <3000 (PMNs early, mononuclear late)	Often normal (better prognosis) Tract myelitis, transverse myelitis Anterior horn > CE, roots, conus medullaris T1 isointense, T2 patchy hyperintensity Often enhance	Hyponatremia Elevated CK EMG: Decr CMAPs, preserved SNAPs Brain MRI: basal ganglia Stiff person syndrome Movement disorders Seizures Fig. 2	1,82–84, 134–138
HTLV-1	IgG ELISA, particle agglutination, radioimmunoprecipitation assay Confirmatory WB PCR: higher titer associated with neurologic disease	IgG ELISA, confirmatory WB Routine studies: WBCs 0–100 (mononuclear); may be higher in acute or extensive cases	Often normal Chronic tractopathy: T > C Nonenhancing; volume loss/atrophy (20%–70%) Acute tract myelitis T1 isointense, T2 hyperintense ± enhancement, edema	CK EMG: neurogenic or myopathic, may mimic ALS, polyneuropathy (axonal ± demyelinative) Geography: southern Japan, Caribbean, South America, central Africa Fig. 3	38–40, 139–143

Organism	Serologic tests	Other tests	Imaging (MRI)	Clinical features	References
Cytomegalovirus[c]	PCR IgM, IgM ELISA, CF CMV pp65 antigen	DNA PCR (in HIV: 80% sensitive, 90% specific) IgG/IgM: low specificity (ELISA, CF) Viral culture (18% sensitive 100% specific) pp67 late gene transcripts (84% sensitive, 100% specific) Cytology for cytomegalic cells Routine studies: WBC 0–3000+ (PMN > mononuclear) Low glucose	Often normal (40%–50%) Polyradiculomyelitis: Thickened CE Enhancement: leptomeningeal, CE, and/or dorsal root Space-occupying: ring enhancement, edema Infarction caused by vasculitis	Retinitis Brain MRI: ventriculitis Listeria, HHV6 coinfection Transplant rejection Drug rash eosinophilia systemic symptoms	30,32,34, 144–148
EBV[c] *Primary infection* *Parainfectious syndromes* *PTLD/CNS lymphoma*	IgM VCA or IgG-VCA but no IgG-EBNA Serology proves recent infection, not CNS disease	PCR (may be negative) Cytomorphology Flow cytometry IgH heavy chain rearrangement Routine studies: WBC 0–200 (mononuclear); higher with primary encephalomyelitis	Usually abnormal Transverse myelitis Enhancing intramedullary masses, roots, and/or leptomeninges	Mononucleosis Ocular: vitritis Rare extra-CNS lymphoma	106–108, 149,150, 15–20
Enteroviruses: Vaccine-associated polio *(Poliovirus 1, 2, 3)* Nonpolio enteroviruses *(Coxsackievirus, enterovirus, echovirus)*	IgG ELISA, neutralizing antibody titer	IgG ELISA, neutralizing antibody titer RNA RT-PCR (nonpolio enteroviruses) Viral culture (low sensitivity) Routine studies: WBC 0–200 (mononuclear) Nonpolio EV may have concurrent meningitis with higher WBC counts and low glucose	Often normal Transverse myelitis: anterior horn cell predilection	Stool virus detection Culture, PCR (send 2–3 samples) May be chronically excreted Geography: Middle East, Africa, South/Southeast Asia, South America, Finland, Israel	85–88, 151–153, 89–93

(continued on next page)

Table 1
(continued)

Disease	Blood Tests	CSF Tests[a]	Spinal MRI Special Features[b]	Other Useful Clues	References
AIDS-associated vacuolar myelopathy[c]	IgM, IgG ELISA, antibody capture radioimmunoassay Confirmatory WB Viral load	IgM, IgG ELISA, antibody capture radioimmunoassay Confirmatory WB Routine studies: WBC: usually normal	Often normal Posterior and lateral tractopathy: T > C T1 isointense, T2 iso- or rarely hyperintense Nonenhancing, frequent atrophy Pyramidal tracts, posterior column predilection	Leukopenia Cognitive dysfunction Brain MRI: atrophy	29,36,37
Hepatitis C[c] *Hepatitis A, B*	IgG ELISA, IFA Confirmatory WB RNA viral load	IgG ELISA, IFA with confirmatory WB RNA PCR (rarely positive) Routine studies: WBC 0–200 (mononuclear)	May be normal	Liver function abnormalities	33,154–156
HSV 1 and 2[c]	IgG, IgM ELISA, IFA, CF IgM may increase even in reactivation	DNA PCR IgG, IgM ELISA CSF/serum antibody ratio 2 wk to 3 mo after symptom onset Viral culture (low sensitivity) Routine studies: WBC 0–200 (mononuclear)	Usually abnormal HSV-1: more localized lesions HSV-2: more extensive & continuous	Skin lesions Encephalitis HSV-1 >2 Brain MRI: temporal lobe Seizures	2–4,32, 34,35, 157–161

				113–118, 162–171
Cysticercosis^c	IgG Antibodies	Scolex: pathognomonic	Eosinophilia	
IgG	ELISA (sensitive 87% specific 97%), EITB, CF, IFA, WB	General cyst evolution:	Rectal biopsy or stool specimen	
ELISA (sensitive 50% specific 70%),	Sensitivity worse if intramedullary	Vesicular: No edema; eccentric scolex	CT of spine revealing during calcified stages	
EITB	Routine studies:	T1 hypointense cyst, hyperintense scolex;	Geography: Brazil, Peru, Mexico, Korea, India, Southeast Asia;	
Specificity worsens in endemic areas	Arachnoiditis (subarachnoid cyst)	T2 hyperintense cyst, hypointense scolex	Incubation period may be long (>10 y)	
	Markedly high WBCs up to 1000s	Colloidal: Thickened wall, enhancement, edema, but no scolex seen (T1 hyperintense)		
	Low to undetectable glucose	Capsule: T1 hyperintense, T2 hypointense		
	Intramedullary or intradural-extramedullary cyst	Granulonodular: calcium, enhancement		
	WBC 0–200 (mononuclear, rare eosinophils)	Involution: small calcified nodule only seen on CT; no enhancement		
	Very high protein if CSF block	Subarachnoid cyst: if rupture → arachnoiditis		

(continued on next page)

Table 1
(continued)

Disease	Blood Tests	CSF Tests[a]	Spinal MRI Special Features[b]	Other Useful Clues	References
Schistosomiasis S mansoni S haematobium rarely S japonicum	IgG > IgM, IgE Against soluble egg antigen or adult antigens ELISA, WB, CF, IFA, agglutinin	IgG > IgM, IgE Against soluble egg antigen or adult antigens ELISA (50% sensitive 95% specific), IFA, CF, hemagglutinin, WB CSF-specific IgG index or ratios between egg and worm antigen help differentiate infection from exposed Circulating cathodic antigen Routine studies: WBC <1000 (mononuclear, eosinophils in 30%–50%) Normal CSF in <10%	Abnormal in >90%, may see 2+ manifestations in combination: Transverse myelitis: Usually T9 or below Little to no mass effect Nodular granulomatous: Usually T9 or below Enhancement: heterogeneous, nodular, arborized, or linear Mass effect, may mimic tumor Vasculitis: anterior spinal artery infarction	Stool (× 3) or urine for eggs <50% sensitive Kato-Katz vs sedimentation Rectal biopsy (80%–95% sensitive) Hypogammaglobulinemia Low: hemoglobin, albumin High: Eosinophils, BUN/Cr Geography: North and Central Africa, Arabian Peninsula, Brazil, Caribbean, Indonesia, China, Japan, Philippines, Thailand	108–112, 172–179
Toxoplasmosis (*Toxoplasma gondii*)	IgG, IgM, IgA ELISA	IgG, IgM ELISA PCR: Highly specific; sensitivity 60%–80% off prophylaxis but 20%–25% on prophylaxis Routine studies: WBC 0–500 (mononuclear or PMNs)	Usually abnormal Transverse myelitis Arachnoiditis Mass lesion, cavitary lesion Homogenous contrast enhancement	Evidence of immunodeficiency (lymphopenia, low immunoglobulin, low CD3/4/8, and so forth)	31,180–183

Echinococcus	IgG, IgE CF, ELISA, or agglutination with confirmatory WB Low sensitivity (25%–60%)	Not usually performed because most are removed surgically and diagnosed by pathology	Usually abnormal Homogenous cystic mass: T > L > C, sacral Flattened sausage, 2 dome-shaped ends, no debris in lumen, thin nonseptated walls May be epidural, subdural (extramedullary), or intramedullary, with variable bony involvement Arachnoiditis if cyst rupture	Casoni test: 95% sensitivity but has low specificity Eosinophilia Geography: Mediterranean, Africa, South America, Eastern and Southern Europe, India, China, Australia, New Zealand; case reports in United States [184–186]

Abbreviations: AFB, Acid-fast bacilli; ALS, amyotrophic lateral sclerosis; BUN, serum urea nitrogen; C, cervical; CK, creatine kinase; CMAP, compound motor action potential; CNS, central nervous system; CE, contrast enhancing; CF, complement fixation; Cr, creatinine; CT, computed tomography; Decr, decreased; EBNA, Epstein Barr nuclear antigen; ELISA, enzyme-linked immunosorbent assay; EMG, electromyogram; ESR, erythrocyte sedimentation rate; FTA-ABS, fluorescent treponemal antibody absorption test; IFA, immunofluorescent antibody; Ig, immunoglobulin; L, lumbar; LP, lumbar punctur; PCR, polymerase chain reaction; PMN, polymorphonuclear leukocytes; PPD, purifed protein derivatibe; PTLD, Posttransplantation lymphoproliferative disorder; SNAP, sensory nerve action potential; SSEP, somatosensory evoked potentials; T, thoracic; TEE, transesopahgeal echocardiogram; TTE, transtorhaoci echocardiogram; WB, Western blot; WBC, white blood cell.

[a] Spinal cord infections have wide ranges of protein elevation that are not particularly helpful diagnostically. This table cites noteworthy alterations in protein and infections associated with glucose less than 50% concomitant blood glucose in patients who are euglycemic. The preferred diagnostic blood and CSF tests are in boldface. In general, pleocytosis and abnormal glucose and protein occur when infections produce arachnoiditis, although intramedullary infections from the same pathogen are less likely to evoke a brisk CSF inflammatory response (cysticercosis, TB).

[b] Many spinal cord infections have MRI abnormalities resembling transverse myelitis:T1 isointensities/hypointensities. T2 hyperintensities. ± cord edema. ± parenchymal enhancement. Radiculomyelitis with enhancement leptomeninges, roots, cauda equina occurs in a more restricted group of infections, such as TB, Lyme, CMV.

[c] Spinal cord infection with specific treatment.

Empiric Treatment

Given the potential catastrophic complications of spinal cord infection, what should the clinician recommend while waiting for diagnostic results?

In a recent series, 28.8% of patients presenting with acute noncompressive myelopathy still had no definitive cause for the myelopathy after 6 years of follow-up.[5] Thus, treatment to preserve function often must begin without diagnostic confirmation.

- The acute administration of high-dose corticosteroids for myelopathies of unknown cause (1 g of intravenous [IV] methylprednisolone daily for 5 days) has been recommended, and possible recent viral infection does not preclude corticosteroid treatment.[4] However, this strategy could potentially interfere with the diagnostic confirmation of possible EBV-associated B-cell lymphoma and should be withheld until CSF cytology is obtained in such situations.
- *Check a CD4 count* in the presence of a diagnostic puzzle in apparently immunocompetent patients.
- *Consider empiric acyclovir* if there is a strong suspicion for herpesvirus infection and the patients' renal function is normal. One of the most common treatable causes of myelitis, HSV2 infection, may cause urinary retention, genital paresthesias, and radiculopathies in patients unaware of herpetic eruptions caused by this recurrent and preventable infection.
- *Call neurosurgical consultants* early in such emergent situations as suspected epidural pyogenic or granulomatous abscess, compressive myelopathy of unknown cause, and neurocysticercosis with basal cisternal involvement and incipient hydrocephalus.

SPINAL CORD INFECTIOUS CONSIDERATIONS IN AT-RISK PATIENT POPULATIONS
Infectious Myelopathies in Patients with Cancer

Cancer and its treatment pose a host of noninfectious differential diagnostic concerns that complicate the evaluation for potential spinal cord infection. These concerns include (1) *recurrence of disease* or spread to epidural space from boney metastases; (2) *treatment-related myelopathies* that mimic infection, such as radiation myelitis or superficial siderosis, and toxicity from chemotherapeutic agents, such as cytarabine, methotrexate, thiotepa, carmustine, bevacizumab, and cisplatin[6,7]; and (3) *paraneoplastic myelopathies* with selective dorsal column or spinothalamic tract dysfunction, sometimes called tractopathies.[8]

Hematopoietic cell transplant (HCT)– and solid-organ transplant (SOT)–associated infections include transverse myelitis caused by HHV7, VZV, nosocomial infections, such as complications of IV lines, bacterial abscess, endocarditis, neutropenia-related invasive fungal infections (Aspergillus, Candida), and pathogens affecting the spinal cord that are acquired from donated organ or tissue (CMV, WNV, HTLV-1). After more than 3 months following HCT or SOT, progressive multifocal leukoencephalopathy becomes a concern, although the spinal cord infrequently is the sole site of John Cunningham virus infection.[9,10] Occurring more than several months after transplantation and often in the setting of graft-versus-host disease are immune-mediated conditions with syndromes mimicking demyelinating disease or acute disseminated encephalomyelitis (ADEM).[11–13] Heavily treated patients with cancer and others with acquired or congenital immune deficiency may be vulnerable to much more serious consequences of common infections (enterovirus), uncommon infections (WNV), or vaccine-preventable disease (poliomyelitis).[14]

Posttransplantation lymphoproliferative disorder (PTLD) in HCT and SOT recipients results from EBV-induced proliferation of engrafted donor B lymphocytes because of the exogenous T-cell suppression necessary to preserve the graft. Cerebral and spinal or leptomeningeal manifestations of PTLD range from a mononucleosislike picture to fulminant lymphoma with multiple ring-enhancing mass lesions.[15,16] Serum and CSF PCR for EBV may be negative.[17] Treatment strategies are directed at suppressing neoplastic proliferations with methotrexate or with preemptive management by infusion of EBV virus–specific donor T cells.[18–20]

HIV/AIDS

Patients with HIV are susceptible to a host of spinal cord pathogens. Clinical challenges include the following:

1. Atypical CSF cell counts: Patients with low CD4+ counts may not be able to mount an appropriate CSF pleocytosis, and spinal fluid may show a reduction in expected magnitude, unusual differential count, or total absence of cells.[21–23]
2. Insensitive serologic titers caused by impaired humoral response: Both false-negative and false-positive results occur with greater frequency.[24,25] In contrast, culture results may be more sensitive to infection in patients with HIV because of the reduced clearance and the greater likelihood of dissemination outside the CNS, offering potential biopsy sites. For example, recognition of CMV retinitis could offer substantial evidence that a radicular spinal syndrome was caused by that herpesvirus.[26]
3. Neuroimaging can prove difficult to interpret because patients with HIV have a higher risk for CNS neoplasms, including lymphoma and metastatic disease or rarely Kaposi sarcoma, plasmacytoma, or astrocytoma.[27]

Spinal cord pathogens and HIV

It may be clinically useful to classify infection in patients with HIV based on the CD4 count, although considerable flexibility is required because there is overlap in CD4 counts for any particular pathogen.

Infections that can occur with any CD4 count

Notable bacterial pathogens in the HIV population are epidural abscesses, tuberculosis, and syphilis,[28,29] whereas viral possibilities include HSV and VZV.[29]

Infections with low CD4 count

CMV occurs primarily in patients with a CD4 count less than 100.[30] CMV polyradiculitis may be fulminant with neutrophilic CSF pleocytosis and clinical clues of areflexia, urinary retention, and sacral paresthesias. CMV DNA is detected by CSF PCR, and prompt therapy with ganciclovir or foscarnet or both affects rapid improvement.

Patients with HIV are also more susceptible to fungal causes of spinal infection, which can manifest in conjunction with cryptococcal meningitis (CD4 <200) or as an epidural abscess (any CD4 count). Patients with HIV with a CD4 count less than 200 are at risk for parasitic infection with *Toxoplasma gondii*, which can rarely affect the spinal cord in isolation.[31] EBV-associated lymphoma also occurs at a time of significant immunologic impairment.

Coinfections

It is important to remember the possibility of multiple infections. Concurrent CMV and HSV2 myelitis has been observed in patients with HIV and may have a synergistic effect in producing spinal cord disease.[32] Hepatitis C virus has been associated with both progressive and recurrent myelopathy.[33] Serologic evidence alone is often insufficient to prove causal infection because positive serologies against organisms, such as the herpesviruses or *Toxoplasma*, may only indicate past exposure. Instead, techniques, such as PCR or serial antibody titers, must be used to support active disease.[34,35] Pursuing further workup for multiple infections is especially important when patients do not respond to initial antibiotic therapy.

Primary HIV myelopathy

Primary HIV myelopathy can only be definitively diagnosed by biopsy and, therefore, is often a diagnosis of exclusion.[36] Spinal cord disease was present in about 10% of patients with AIDS in the pre–highly active antiretroviral therapy era but is currently much less common. Up to 90% of patients with HIV-associated vacuolar myelopathy have cognitive impairment.[37] Although this type of myelopathy may respond to antiretroviral drugs, painful dysesthesias and dorsal column dysfunction with pure sensory ataxia do not.

HTLV-1

HTLV-1-associated myelopathy may occur with or without HIV. A primary risk factor for HTLV-1 is IV drug abuse. Both HTLV-1 and HIV are retroviruses that can produce similar chronic myelopathy syndromes but have different effects on the host immune response. It can be difficult to determine which virus is primarily responsible for myelopathic symptoms. One clinical clue is that HIV myelopathy is more likely than HTLV to have associated cognitive symptoms or dementia. HTLV-1, the agent of tropical spastic paraparesis and endemic to southern Japan, the Caribbean, South America, and Central Africa, may show a nonenhancing longitudinally extensive central cord lesion on MRI (**Fig. 3**). Coinfection with HIV and HTLV has been shown to increase the risk of neurologic disease caused by either virus, suggesting that the two may act synergistically.[38] There is evidence to suggest that HTLV can induce T-cell proliferation and, thus patients with HIV whose CD4 counts are stable but show continued clinical progression of their HIV should be tested for HTLV if they have the appropriate behavioral or geographic exposure.[39–41]

Immune reconstitution inflammatory syndrome

Immune reconstitution inflammatory syndrome (IRIS) is characterized by a paradoxic clinical worsening in patients with a CD4 count less than 200 in the setting of institution of antiretroviral therapy. IRIS has been associated with several infections that affect the spinal cord, including syphilis, cryptococcosis, VZV, toxoplasmosis, and TB (see later discussion). Evidence suggests that patients with a lower CSF pleocytosis in the setting of infection (thus, presumably those with the greatest initial immune impairment) are at an increased risk for IRIS with HIV treatment than those with more pronounced pleocytosis.[42,43] IRIS should, therefore, always be considered in any patient with HIV newly receiving antiretroviral therapy who shows clinical deterioration despite appropriate antibiotic treatment of a spinal cord infection. Consideration should be given to the temporary use of corticosteroids to reduce counterproductive inflammation that may damage the spinal cord.

Travel and/or Residence in Endemic Areas

It would be impossible to list all the potential considerations of unusual (in North America) conditions seen in patients who arrive on US shores to be seen by clinicians who may not have encountered any prior cases of these diseases. That list would likely need to be updated annually as emerging infections challenge clinicians' diagnostic skills.[44] Similarly, relative risks for such infections as WNV and Lyme differ within domestic US regions each year. General considerations include the fact that the

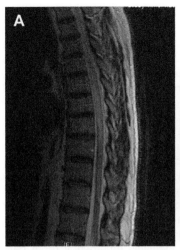
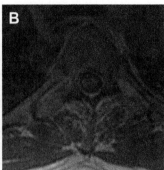

Fig. 3. This 52-year-old HIV-negative patient with a history of remote hepatitis C and intravenous drug abuse in Vietnam had at least 2 years of insidiously progressive numbness and paraparesis. The patient is HTLV positive. CSF showed multiple oligoclonal bands and an elevated IgG synthesis rate. NMO IgG antibody is negative. Sagittal (A) and axial (B) T2 thoracic MRIs show longitudinally extensive intramedullary signal abnormality that is not confined to a particular spinal tract and that on gadolinium images (not shown) did not enhance. The differential diagnosis of intramedullary cord signal abnormality extending over greater than 3 spinal cord segments includes primary spinal cord neoplasm (astrocytoma/ependymoma), WNV, NMO, ischemia (dural fistula), toxic and deficiency B12 and copper, ADEM, posterior reversible encephalopathy syndrome, systemic lupus erythematosus–associated myelitis, sarcoidosis, and, as here, indolent infection.

exposure to the relevant pathogen may have occurred many months or even years previously (neurocysticercosis, brucellosis, schistosomiasis, TB).

Nosocomial Risks

Recent residence in a US hospital may have infectious consequences as portentous as international travel. Indeed, the distinction between nosocomial and community-acquired infections has increasingly become blurred, particularly for methicillin-resistant *Staphylococcus aureus* (MRSA)–related infections, because many patients have health care contacts through dialysis centers, home health visits, and residential nursing facilities.[45] Specific concerns about recent hospitalization should lead to inquiry about instrumentation: dialysis, indwelling IV lines, intrathecal catheters for pain or spasticity management, transfusions, decubitus care, and recent antibiotic courses.

SELECTED SPINAL INFECTIONS

The following section discusses 4 bacterial, 3 viral, and 2 parasitic spinal cord conditions that have specific treatments and are likely to be encountered in neurologic practice. Although general antimicrobial guidelines are provided, clinicians designing therapy should consult their infectious disease colleagues for local nosocomial trends and resistance patterns. Initial empiric coverage for emergent CNS infections has been reviewed recently in *Neurologic Clinics of North America*.[46]

Bacterial Infections

Spinal epidural bacterial abscess

Spinal epidural abscess (SEA) is a medical and sometimes surgical emergency. Risk factors include recent barrier breach, such as IV drug abuse, spinal surgery, intrathecal pumps, and skin and soft tissue infections, and systemic conditions, such as diabetes mellitus, renal failure, alcoholism, and bacteremia/endocarditis. The main routes of infection are hematogenous dissemination or contiguous spread from osteomyelitis or muscle or soft tissue abscess.[47,48]

Clinical presentation includes back pain that usually only lasts a few days but may be more indolent.[49] There is often fever and elevated white blood count, C-reactive protein (CRP) and erythrocyte sedimentation rate (ESR). A cautionary note about pyomyositis is appropriate when considering SEA. This severe muscle infection, most often caused by S aureus or Escherichia coli, can present with pain and weakness that initially may suggest a spinal cord process. Cramping and localized tenderness and edema of the thigh muscles may be a crucial clue to septicemia.[50,51]

A treatment guideline from Duke University Medical Center combines risk factor assessment, ESR, and CRP testing and identifies emergency room patients with back pain with SEA with high sensitivity, an important distinction, because once weakness appears, neurologic deterioration may be very rapid.[52] Lumbar puncture is suggested only if there are clinical signs raising the possibility of meningitis, and the level chosen should minimize the risk of passage of the needle through the infected area or below an area of obstruction. MRI is the critical diagnostic procedure (**Fig. 4**). MRI may also help differentiate tumor from infection in that disc or facet infection may be revealed with engorgement of epidural plexus and prominent dural contrast enhancement.[53] Diffusion-weighted imaging can be helpful in differentiating far less common intramedullary pyogenic abscesses from other mass lesions.[54]

Common organisms are S aureus, gram-negative rods, streptococci, and Mycobacterium tuberculosis. Antibiotic coverage should target gram-positive organisms with vancomycin and gram-negative bacilli with piperacillin-tazobactam, cefotaxime, and meropenem. For patients with beta-lactam sensitivity, levofloxacin or aztreonam may be used. Prognosis is guarded, with mortality still 5% to 20% in modern series and complete neurologic recovery in only 45% of survivors.[55] Negative prognostic features include MRSA infection, motor deficits, age older than 50 years, cervical and thoracic level involvement, concurrent sepsis, delayed diagnosis, diabetes, and prior spinal surgery.[56] Surgical consultation should occur early, yet the role of emergent decompressive surgery remains controversial. In a recent retrospective Duke series of 104 patients with SEA, 61.5% underwent computed tomography (CT)–guided aspiration or antibiotics alone, whereas 38.5% had surgical decompression. Distinction between ventral or dorsal SEA seemed important; the latter caused compression earlier and warranted surgical intervention, whereas ventral abscesses responded to conservative antibiotic management.[57]

TB of the spine

Potts disease, or tuberculous spondylitis, is the most common skeletal manifestation of TB. Estimated to occur to some degree in 1.7% of the world's population, Potts disease prevalence recently is increasing in developed countries due to a combination of immigration from endemic areas, development of drug-resistant strains, and HIV infection.[58] Tuberculous spondylitis can cause neurologic symptoms via direct extension from the vertebrae to the spinal cord.[59–61] The case study in this article illustrates typical demographic, clinical, and radiographic findings (**Fig. 5**) in spinal TB. Included in the differential diagnosis of tuberculous spondylitis are other infections producing

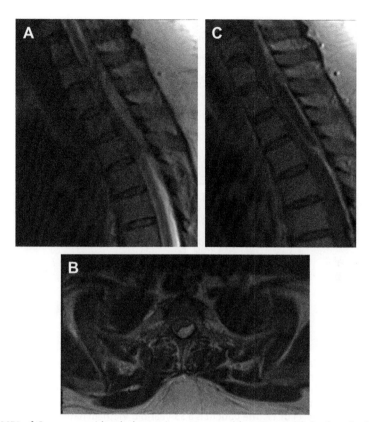

Fig. 4. MRI of *S aureus* epidural abscess in a 41-year-old patient with back pain, bilateral lower limb paralysis, an L1 sensory level and urinary retention. There are no MRI findings suggestive of discitis or osteomyelitis. (*A*) A sagittal T2 image showing a dorsal extradural mass, which on axial view (*B*) displaces the cord to the right. Gadolinium-enhanced sagittal view (*C*) shows the peripherally enhancing dorsal epidural collection from C6 to T5. There is no definite intrinsic cord signal abnormality.

the often quite indolent symptoms of granulomatous infection. Brucellosis is a zoonosis endemic to Saudi Arabia and other parts of the Middle East. This gram-negative bacillus is acquired by ingestion of raw meat or unpasteurized dairy products from animals, such as sheep, goats, or camels. Diskitis, osteomyelitis, paraspinous inflammation, bacteremia, and endocarditis all have been described with *Brucella melitensis.*[62]

In the absence of skeletal lesions, TB can appear as simultaneous spinal cord and root inflammation and spinal tuberculomas, which in turn may be extradural, intradural extramedullary, or intramedullary.[63,64] Tuberculous radiculomyelitis or spinal arachnoiditis is the most common primary cord manifestation of TB. Typically, the CSF is highly inflammatory with parameters in the range of tuberculous meningitis (see **Table 1**). Hypoglycorrhachia, with CSF sugar less than 50% of concomitant blood sugar, is a hallmark; protein levels may increase to a level causing blockage of CSF flow.[65] MRI shows thickened, clumped nerve roots that extensively enhance.[66] Inflammation may lead to arterial compromise and ischemia, and syringomyelia may be a late complication.[67,68] Spinal tuberculomas infrequently show CSF abnormalities and may cause confusion with spinal cord neoplasm.[69,70]

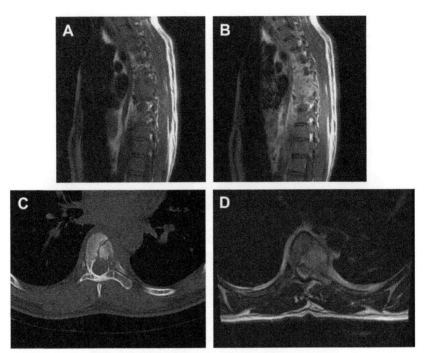

Fig. 5. Case study. Sagittal T1 without (*A*) and with (*B*) gadolinium contrast show a homogeneously enhancing mass centered at the left T7 vertebral body. (*C*) Axial noncontrast images demonstrate a pathologic fracture of the T7 vertebral body. (*D*) T2 axial images show that the mass extends into the paravertebral soft tissues and left epidural space and is compressing the cord at the level of T7. The patient is a 33-year-old Vietnam native who was found to have a tuberculous abscess (Potts disease). See the case study in the text.

A clinical phenomenon characteristic of spinal tuberculosis as well as other spinal infections, such as toxoplasmosis, is the therapeutic paradox.[71] Some patients become symptomatic from spinal cord disease only after tuberculous therapy is initiated for extraspinal disease or there may be paradoxic growth of known spinal tuberculomas after treatment initiation. This phenomenon reflects the recovery of patients' delayed hypersensitivity response and increased immune system activity directed at mycobacterial antigens liberated with antimicrobial treatment. As such, it is a version of IRIS, and the vigorous inflammatory response may be detrimental to patients' neurologic recovery. In these cases, corticosteroids have been use as adjuvant treatment with considerable ongoing debate about when to institute antiretroviral therapy in HIV patients with active TB.[72–74]

Neuroborreliosis (Lyme disease)

Like its fellow spirochete *Treponema pallidum*, the etiologic agent of syphilis, Lyme disease is a great imitator, producing neurologic syndromes that can suggest everything from multiple sclerosis or lymphoma to radiculopathy or poliomyelitis.[75] With greater recognition of the telltale erythema migrans rash and with increasingly sophisticated MRI studies that show pial and spinal root enhancement, the diagnosis can be made earlier. Thus, the occurrence of brain and spinal cord parenchymal disease seems to be declining. The CNS is likely seeded within days of infection; the immune response has a strong B-cell component, somewhat like neurosyphilis. A B-cell the chemokine CXCL13 increases in the CSF before it does so in the blood and may be a sensitive marker for untreated neuroborreliosis in the early stages of the disease before the antibody index is positive.[76,77]

Meningitis, cranial neuritis (particularly cranial nerve VII), and multifocal radiculitis are early manifestations of CNS Lyme disease. Very painful, sometimes migratory radiculitis can be confusing and lead to testing for structural problems only to be (fortunately rarely) complicated over a period of hours to days by the rapid development of spinal cord signs and symptoms. Spastic paraparesis, usually at the midthoracic level, is the most common syndrome. CSF oligoclonal bands and elevated IgG synthesis may be present, but Lyme myelitis may be present before antibody titers in CSF begin to increase. MRI may be tract specific and, therefore, suggest WNV (see later discussion) or may resemble a longitudinally extensive transverse myelitis, raising the possibility of NMO.[78] Avid root enhancement should favor neuroborreliosis (**Fig. 6**).[79] One should also consider other summer time catastrophic paralytic conditions: poliomyelitis and some other enteroviruses, and WNV (see next section).

Syphilis (Treponema pallidum)
Although *Treponema pallidum* invasion of the CNS occurs in many untreated patients within the first year after infection, only about 5% will develop clinical neurosyphilis. Even in the AIDS era, syphilitic spinal cord disease is uncommon. Berger[29] has classified the forms of spinal cord disease as follows:

Meningovascular
This form is currently more common than parenchymatous, occurring 6 years (on average) after primary infection. Thickened, inflamed meninges and Heubner endarteritis are seen. The clinical presentation may be nonspecific mimicking viral myelitis with genital and sacral numbness, central cord abnormalities on MRI, and a lymphocytic pleocytosis. The myelitic form of syphilis is more likely to respond to treatment than spinal ischemia syphilis.[80] A serum rapid plasma regain of 1:32 or greater increases the likelihood of neurosyphilis and dictates CSF examination.[81]

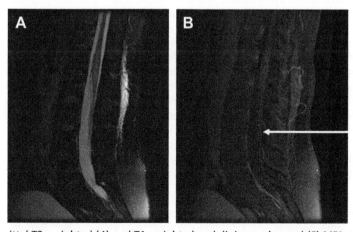

Fig. 6. Sagittal T2-weighted (*A*) and T1-weighted gadolinium-enhanced (*B*) MRIs of patient who developed rapid paraparesis and radicular pain and was found to have Lyme disease. There is both intramedullary contrast-enhancing signal abnormality at the conus and avid enhancement of nerve roots (*arrow*). A similar picture is seen with other infections, such as VZV; but the combination of cord signal abnormality and prominent root enhancement is most suggestive of *Borrelia burgdorferi* infection.

Parenchymatous

Cord compression may be caused by gummas within the cord, hypertrophic pachy-meningitis, or vertebral osteitis. Tabes dorsalis with its hallmark lancinating painful crises and later ataxia is seen with a latency of 10 to 15 years after primary infection, although the time to symptoms in patients with HIV/AIDS may be much less. A final form of parenchymatous disease is spinal cord infarction from syphilitic vasculitis.

Treatment remains 12 to 24 million units aqueous penicillin daily in divided doses every 4 hours for 14 days. Corticosteroids may be added to reduce cord edema and prevent Jarisch-Herxheimer reactions.

Viral Infections

WNV

WNV is a flavivirus that has been recognized as a cause of seasonal paralytic disease in the United States since 1999. Only one in 150 immunocompetent patients infected with WNV develops neuroinvasive disease; but the incidence of CNS disease has been estimated as high as 40% in patients who are immunocompromised, such as transplant recipients.[82] Such patients receive immune suppressants that act by inhibiting T-lymphocyte function to block rejection, but more recent identification of B-cell–mediated transplant rejection has dictated use of rituximab, a monoclonal antibody directed against the B-cell–specific antigen CD20. Transplant recipients who receive rituximab may be vulnerable to rapidly progressive fatal WNV meningoencephalitis. Myelitis at all levels of the spinal cord, brainstem, proximal ventral roots, hippocampi, and cerebral white matter may be seen, yet such patients fail to generate any CSF or serum WNV IgM and IgG.[83]

The most common neuromuscular syndrome of WNV is a poliomyelitis with asymmetric paralysis with or without brainstem involvement and respiratory failure. The acute flaccid paralysis may occur without any fever or signs of meningoencephalitis. Although anterior horn cells and brainstem motor neurons are the major areas affected, there may be myelitis and also Guillain-Barré syndrome. Autonomic instability indicates spinal sympathetic neuron dysfunction.[84] Electromyography can be helpful in clarifying the anterior horn cell nature of the process (see second case in **Fig. 2**). Unfortunately, there is no specific treatment of WNV.

Poliovirus poliomyelitis should be considered in the differential diagnosis in previously unvaccinated patients or immunodeficient patients[14,85] Particular vigilance is appropriate when there is a history of residence in or travel to India, Afghanistan, Nigeria, or Pakistan where wild-type poliomyelitis is still reported. The World Health Organization has recommended the use of inactivated polio vaccine in countries where wild-type poliovirus has been eradicated, but oral polio vaccine continues to be used in many countries. As recently as 2011, vaccine-associated paralytic poliomyelitis was reported in Japan, and occurrence of cases imported to the US mandates continued vigilance.[86–88] Nonpolio enteroviruses of the RNA picornavirus family continue to cause paralytic disease outside the United States.[89–93]

VZV

VZV produces a wide range of neurologic complications both in immunocompetent, (usually elderly), patients and in immunocompromised individuals.[94] Primary infection with VZV causes chickenpox, which, particularly in older patients, may be associated with serious complications, such as meningoencephalitis and pneumonia. VZV remains in dorsal root ganglia from which it can reactivate primarily because of an age-related decline in cell-mediated immunity. Patients at risk for VZV reactivation include those receiving chronic corticosteroid therapy, fingolimod multiple sclerosis treatment, and tumor necrosis factor α (TNF-α) inhibitors as disease-modifying anti-rheumatic drugs. Randomized controlled trials have established an increased risk of bacterial infection in patients receiving TNF-α inhibitors (level A), and strong observational cohort studies (level B) suggest also increased susceptibility to VZV infection.[95–97]

Among *immunocompetent patients*, dermatomal rash in 1 to 3 dermatomes (shingles) is the most common manifestation. Recommendations that stipulate the use of the well-tolerated and highly effective varicella zoster vaccine in immunocompetent adults have been followed suboptimally, resulting in a large population of older individuals at risk for shingles and postherpetic neuralgia.[98] Zoster sine herpete (active VZV infection without rash) is seen in patients who are both immunocompetent and immunocompromised.

Segmental motor weakness, recurrent myelopathy, transverse myelitis, polyradiculitis, and a Brown-Séquard syndrome are all potential presentations of VZV.[99–102] MRI may demonstrate both intramedullary and extramedullary intradural manifestations of infection (**Fig. 7**). **Table 1** details the diagnostic approach to VZV in serum and CSF; it should be emphasized that many patients will have *no* CSF pleocytosis at the time of significant CNS VZV disease, making aggressive search for VZV antibody mandatory.[103] Reports of Brown-Séquard syndrome after an episode of geniculate zoster and of protracted zoster sine herpete over multiple dermatomes distinct temporally and physically from initial thoracic zoster indicate that simultaneous reactivation of VZV can occur in multiple sensory ganglia with or without rash.[104] Simultaneous detection of CSF VZV DNA and IgG antibody illustrates that chronic active VZV ganglionitis is yet another manifestation of VZV infection. An important observation is that, in such cases, prolonged pain can be responsive to intravenous acyclovir.[105]

EBV

EBV infection produces infectious mononucleosis as well as nasopharyngeal carcinoma, Burkitt lymphoma, Hodgkin disease, and lymphoproliferative diseases in patients who are immunocompromised. *Primary EBV infection* can be associated with direct viral infection with CSF pleocytosis-associated encephalomyelitis and acute myeloradiculitis with or without encephalitic features. A *parainfectious immune response* produces cerebellar dysfunction, Guillain Barré syndrome, myelopathy, cranial neuritis, and encephalopathy.[106] Serology revealing an IgM antibody response to viral capsid antigen or IgG response against VCA but no IgG response to EB nuclear antigen suggests recent infection and provides evidence, but not proof, that the neurologic syndrome is associated with EBV active infection. CSF EBV PCR testing is still required. Nevertheless, the pathogenic significance of EBV in CSF in normal hosts and its association with acute or indolent neurologic disease remains controversial. Peripheral blood mononuclear cells contain EBV DNA, and CSF blood contamination can lead to false positives. Detailed CSF analysis to determine copy number of EBV DNA in CSF versus peripheral blood may help to clarify.[107] CSR EBV PCR is very useful in AIDS and transplant patients for whom its presence is highly sensitive for *lymphoma*, although negative PCR does not exclude lymphoma (see earlier discussion of PTLD).

Parasitic Infections

Schistosomiasis

Schistosomiasis, a helminthic infection, is one of the most widespread parasitic diseases, infecting some 200 million people worldwide and causing symptoms in at least 60% of these.[108] *Schistosoma mansoni* and *Schistosoma haematobium* are

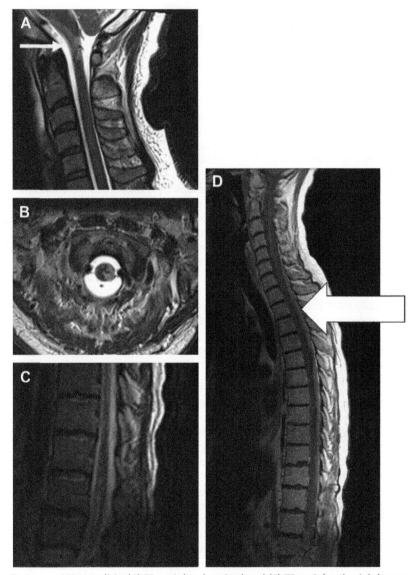

Fig. 7. Aspects VZV myelitis: (*A*) T2-weighted sagittal and (*B*) T2-weighted axial show a cervicomedullary junction signal abnormality (*arrow, A*) resulting in a left Brown-Séquard syndrome with dysphagia in patient who is HIV positive with CD4 count 20. He had no skin rash. CSF had more than 1000 white blood cells, half of which were polymorphonuclear leucocytes. In the series reported by Nagel,[103] rash was present in 63% but the average time from rash to neurologic symptoms was 4 months; CSF had pleocytosis in 67%, but positive PCR in only 30%, whereas 93% had anti-VZV IgG antibody in CSF with reduced serum/CSF radio of VZV IgG confirming intrathecal synthesis.[90] Sagittal T2-weighted (*C*) and sagittal (T1-weighted with gadolinium) (*D*) images of a different patient who had acute lympho-blastic leukemia and an L2–3 dermatomal rash and iliopsoas weakness followed by progressive generalized weakness and encephalopathy. There is conus medullaris signal abnormality (*C*) and a longitudinally extensive contrast-enhancing subdural collection (*arrow, D*), presumably a reaction to the infectious processes. The VZV infection was fatal in both patients.

the usual cause of myelopathy, whereas *Schistosoma japonicum* causes encephalitic disease. Travel-related cases and population migration have led to increasing numbers of cases recognized in North America. Spinal cord schistosomiasis is more common in children, adolescents, and young adults in endemic areas than in older patients. About one-quarter have hepatomegaly, but most have no symptoms outside the CNS.

The presentation is usually acute or subacute with pain in the lower back and a chronic or rarely fluctuating progression for several months. The spinal cord level is usually below T6. There can be a predominance of medullary spinal cord involvement or it can be combined with radicular symptoms. Cauda equina/conus syndrome is also seen with a more indolent evolution.[109] MRI is very sensitive, often raising the differential diagnosis of spinal cord neoplasm.[110] Rectal biopsy allows *S mansoni* egg identification. Laminectomy should be avoided for diagnostic purposes. Praziquantel is the treatment of choice for all *Schistosoma* species.[111] Corticosteroid treatment is started immediately for patients strongly suspected of having spinal cord schistosomiasis, with praziquantel beginning after confirmation of diagnosis. Recommended corticosteroid doses and preparations vary.[112]

Cysticercosis

Neurocysticercosis (NCC) denotes brain or, less commonly, spinal infection with the cystic larval form of the tapeworm, *Taenia solium*. Its major public health significance is as a prime cause of adult-onset epilepsy in endemic regions caused by intraparenchymal brain cysts, the most common form of NCC.[113] Spinal subarachnoid NCC causes subarachnoid and ventricular disease leading to hydrocephalus. Patients with basal subarachnoid NCC are also at high risk for spinal subarachnoid space involvement. In a recent series, 61% of patients with basal subarachnoid NCC had spinal cysts, most commonly in the lumbosacral regions; and *MRI of the spine should be performed in all NCC cases with basal subarachnoid disease*.[114]

Spinal meningitic forms of NCC with extramedullary intradural cysts or intramedullary masses are uncommon in the United States but can be expected to be seen with increasing frequency because of travel and immigration.[115] Cysts and associated arachnoiditis (pachymeningitis) can affect multiple cranial and spinal nerve roots leading to nerve entrapments, hydrocephalus, gait disorders, chronic meningitis, vasculitis, and spinal or cerebral stroke. Rupture of cysts produces recurrent lymphocytic meningitis, and migratory radicular pain indicates the ongoing inflammatory reaction to the infection.[116] Long courses of albendazole with judicious use of glucocorticoids to control inflammation are indicated.[117] Surgical resection of the lesions that cluster near the fourth ventricle is required because of obstructive hydrocephalus. Increasing proficiency with endoscopic surgery has improved the prognosis of such patients.[118]

Case study: chronic back pain

History

A 33-year-old Vietnamese man who had moved to this country 3 years earlier presented with back pain. He had no significant past medical history but had a 5-lb weight loss recently. He was a nonsmoker, and he denied IV drug abuse. His wife had received one year of treatment for TB 6 years ago. He presented 2 months before admission with a month of back pain radiating from the midthoracic level to the left costochondral junction. Chest radiograph and plain radiographs of his thoracic spine were negative at that time. There was no history of trauma and no complaint of cough, bowel or bladder problems, fever, night sweats, or rash. He was still complaining of focal midthoracic back pain 1 month later when he was seen by an orthopedist who found normal strength and reflexes.

MRI of the thoracic spine showed a pathologic fracture at T7 and an enhancing mass encroaching on the spinal canal (see **Fig. 5**).

On admission he was mildly anemic with hemoglobin 12.2, hematocrit 33, mean corpuscular volume 66; the white blood count and liver functions were normal. He was HIV negative.

Case Formulation

A Vietnamese man with no history of trauma has a chronic (3-month) presentation with focal back pain, anemia, and mild weight loss. He has an abnormal MRI with a pathologic fracture and an enhancing, aggressive lesion. Fortunately, he has no neurologic signs (yet). The case illustrates the use of the diagnostic approach discussed in this article: consider the country of origin of this presumably immunocompetent patient and his wife's history, the pace of the illness, systemic symptoms, the nature of the neurologic localizing findings, and the laboratory data. The differential diagnosis is as follows:

1. Infection (Potts disease, other granulomatous or pyogenic abscess, such as brucellosis, actinomycosis, blastomycosis, candidiasis, cryptococcosis, histoplasmosis)

2. Malignancy (metastatic or primary tumor, multiple myeloma, angiolipoma)

Follow-up

The laboratory studies were as follows: blood cultures negative, purified protein derivative positive, and serum Quantiferon gold positive.

After a CT-guided biopsy by interventional neuroradiology was inconclusive with negative cultures, open biopsy with bone biopsy, T7 laminectomy, and resection of the mass with T5-T9 screw fixation was performed. Tissue was sent for pathologic examination and cultures, which were positive for *M tuberculosis*.

Still neurologically normal and with pain improved, he was started on a 4-drug therapy plus pyridoxine (ethambutal, rifampin, isoniazid, pyrazinamide), with at least 1 year of treatment planned.

ACKNOWLEDGMENTS

The authors thank Dr Hugo Aparicio for supplying the clinical information and MRI scans for the case of tuberculous spondylosis.

REFERENCES

1. Prasad S, Brown MJ, Galetta SL. Transient downbeat nystagmus from West Nile virus encephalomyelitis. Neurology 2006;66(2):1599–600.
2. Wong SH, Boggild M, Enevoldson TP, et al. Myelopathy but normal MRI: where next? Pract Neurol 2008;8:90–102.
3. O'Sullivan CE, Aksamit AJ, Harrington JR, et al. Clinical spectrum and laboratory characteristics associated with detection of herpes simplex virus DNA in cerebrospinal fluid. Mayo Clin Proc 2003;78:1347–52.
4. Schmalstieg WF, Weinshenker BG. Approach to acute or subacute myelopathy. Neurology 2010;75(Suppl 1):S2–8.
5. Debette S, de Seze J, Pruvo JP, et al. Long-term outcomes of acute and subacute myelopathies. J Neurol 2009;256:980–8.
6. Graber JJ, Nolan CP. Myelopathies in patients with cancer. Arch Neurol 2010; 67(3):298–304.

7. Kumar N. Superficial siderosis: associations and therapeutic implications. Arch Neurol 2007;64:491–6.
8. Flanagan EP, McKeon A, Lennon VA, et al. Paraneoplastic isolated myelopathy: clinical course and neuroimaging clues. Neurology 2011;76(24):2089–95.
9. Bernal-Caso F, Joseph JT, Koralnik IJ. Spinal cord lesions of progressive multifocal leukoencephalopathy in an acquired immune deficiency syndrome patient. J Neurovirol 2007;13:474–6.
10. Takeda S, Yamazaki K, Miyakaawa T, et al. Progressive multifocal leukoencephalopathy showing extensive spinal cord involvement in a patient with lymphocytopenia. Neuropathology 2009;29:485–93.
11. Sakai M, Ohashi K, Ohta K, et al. Immune-mediated myelopathy following allogeneic stem cell transplantation. Int J Hematol 2006;84(3):272–5.
12. Matsuo Y, Kamezaki K, Takeishi S, et al. Encephalomyelitis mimicking multiple sclerosis associated with chronic graft-versus-host disease after allogeneic bone marrow transplantation. Intern Med 2009;48(16):1453–6.
13. Armstrong RJ, Elston JS, Hatton CS, et al. De novo relapsing-remitting multiple sclerosis following autologous stem cell transplantation. Neurology 2010;75(1): 89–91.
14. Devries AS, Harper J, Murray A, et al. Vaccine-derived poliomyelitis 12 years after infection in Minnesota. N Engl J Med 2011;364(24):2316–23.
15. Buell JF, Gross TG, Hanaway MJ, et al. Posttransplant lymphoproliferative disorder: significance of central nervous system involvement. Transplant Proc 2005;37:954–5.
16. Cavaliere R, Petroni G, Lopes MB, et al. Primary central nervous system posttransplantation lymphoproliferative disorder: an International Primary Central Nervous System Lymphoma Collaborative Group Report. Cancer 2010;116: 863–70.
17. Hamadani M, Mratin LK, Benson DM, et al. Central nervous systems posttransplant lymphoproliferative disorder despite negative serum and spinal fluid Epstein-Barr virus DNA PCR. Bone Marrow Transplant 2007;39:249–51.
18. Nabors LB, Palmer CA, Julian BA, et al. Isolated central nervous system posttransplant lymphoproliferative disorder treated with high-dose intravenous methotrexate. Am J Transplant 2009;9:1243–8.
19. Ahmad I, Cau NV, Kwan J, et al. Preemptive management of Epstein-Barr virus reactivation after hematopoietic stem-cell transplantation. Transplantation 2009; 87:1240–5.
20. Evens AM, Roy R, Sterrenberg D, et al. Post-transplantation lymphoproliferative disorders: diagnosis, prognosis, and current approaches to therapy. Curr Oncol Rep 2010;12:383–94.
21. Bandyopadhyay SK, Bandyopdhyay R, Dutta A. Profile of tuberculous meningitis with or without HIV infection and the predictors of adverse outcome. West Indian Med J 2009;58(6):589–92.
22. Vinnard C, Macgregor RR. Tuberculous meningitis in HIV-infected individuals. Curr HIV/AIDS Rep 2009;6(3):139–45.
23. Cecchini D, Ambrosioni J, Brezzo C, et al. Tuberculous meningitis in HIV-infected and non-infected patients: comparison of cerebrospinal fluid findings. Int J Tuberc Lung Dis 2009;13(2):269–71.
24. Cerny R, Machla L, Bojar M, et al. Neuroborreliosis in an HIV-1 positive patient. Infection 2006;34(2):100–2.
25. Nissapatorn V, Sawangjaroen N. Parasitic infections in HIV infected individuals: diagnostic and therapeutic challenges. Indian J Med Res 2011;134(6):878–97.

26. Thurnher MM, Post MJ, Jinkis JR. MRI of infections and neoplasms of the spine and spinal cord in 55 patients with AIDS. Neuroradiology 2000;42(8):551–63.
27. Hogan C, Wilkins E. Neurological complications in HIV. Clin Med 2011;11(6): 571–5.
28. Taber KH, Hayman LA, Shandera WX, et al. Spinal disease in neurologically symptomatic HIV-positive patients. Neuroradiology 1999;41(5):360–8.
29. Berger JR. Infectious myelopathies. Continuum (Minneap Minn) 2011;17(4): 761–75.
30. Guiot HM, Pita-Garcia IL, Bertran–Pasarell J, et al. Cytomegalovirus polyradiculomyelopathy in AIDS: a case report and review of the literature. P R Health Sci J 2006;25(4):359–62.
31. Vyas R, Ebright JR. Toxoplasmosis of the spinal cord in a patient with AIDS: case report and review. Clin Infect Dis 1996;23(5):1061–5.
32. Pinto A, Santos E, Correa DF, et al. CMV and HSV-2 myeloradiculitis in an HIV infected patient. Rev Inst Med Trop Sao Paulo 2011;53(3):173–5.
33. Aktipi KM, Ravaglia S, Ceroni M, et al. Severe recurrent myelitis in patients with hepatitis C infection. Neurology 2007;68(6):468–9.
34. Cinque P, Bossolasco S, Lundkvist A. Molecular analysis of cerebrospinal fluid in viral diseases of the central nervous system. J Clin Virol 2003;26(1):1–28.
35. Boivin G. Diagnosis of herpesvirus infections of the central nervous system. Herpes 2004;11(Suppl 2):48A–56A.
36. DiRocco A, Simpson DM. AIDS-associated vacuolar myelopathy. AIDS Patient Care STDS 1998;12(6):457–61.
37. Fauci AS, Lane HC. HIV neurology. In: Hauser SL, Josephson SA, editors. Harrison's neurology in clinical medicine. 2nd edition. New York: McGraw Hill; 2010. p. 493–506.
38. Silva MT, Neves ES, Grinsztejn B, et al. Neurological manifestations of coinfection with HIV and human T-lymphotropic virus type 1. AIDS 2012;26:521–2.
39. Casseb J, de Oliveria AC, Vergara MP, et al. Presence of tropical spastic paraparesis/human T-cell lymphotropic virus type 1-associated myelopathy (TSP/HAM-like) among HIV-1-infected patients. J Med Virol 2008;80(3):392–8.
40. Tulius Silva M, De Melo Espindola O, Bezerra Leit AC, et al. Neurological aspects of human T lymphotropic virus coinfection. AIDS Rev 2009;11(2):71–8.
41. Boulware DR, Bonham SC, Meya DB, et al. Paucity of initial cerebrospinal fluid inflammation in cryptococcal meningitis is associated with subsequent immune reconstitution inflammatory syndrome. J Infect Dis 2010;202(6):962–70.
42. Clark BM, Krueger RG, Price P, et al. Compartmentalization of the immune response in varicella zoster virus immune restoration disease causing transverse myelitis. AIDS 2004;18(8):1218–21.
43. Tahir M, Sinha S, Sharma SK, et al. Immune reconstitution inflammatory syndrome manifesting as disseminated tuberculosis, deep venous thrombosis, encephalopathy and myelopathy. Indian J Chest Dis Allied Sci 2008;50(4):363–4.
44. Tyler KL. Emerging viral infections of the CNS: parts I and II. Arch Neurol 2009; 66:939–58, 1065–74.
45. Moellering RC Jr. The growing menace of community acquired methicillin resistant Staphylococcus aureus. Ann Intern Med 2006;144:368–70.
46. Pruitt AA. Neurologic infectious disease emergencies. Neurol Clin 2012;30(1): 129–60.
47. Darouiche RO. Spinal epidural abscess. N Engl J Med 2006;35:2012–20.
48. Pradilla G, Nagahama Y, Spivak AM, et al. Spinal epidural abscess: current diagnosis and management. Curr Infect Dis Rep 2010;12:484–91.

49. Huang PY, Chen SF, Chang WN, et al. Spinal epidural abscess in adults caused by Staphylococcus aureus: clinical characteristics and prognostic factors. Clin Neurol Neurosurg 2012;114:572–6.

50. Moellering RC Jr, Abbott GF, Ferraro MJ. Case records of the MGH. Case 2-2011: a 30-year-old woman with shock after treatment of a furuncle. N Engl J Med 2011;364:266–75.

51. Vigil KJ, Johnson JR, Johnston BD, et al. E coli pyomyositis: an emerging infectious disease among patients with hematologic malignancies. Clin Infect Dis 2010;50:374–80.

52. Davis DP, Salazar A, Chan TC, et al. Prospective evaluation of a clinical decision guideline to diagnose spinal epidural abscess in patients who present to the emergency department with spine pain. J Neurosurg Spine 2011;14:765–70.

53. Diehn FE. Imaging of spine infection. Radiol Clin North Am 2012;50:777–98.

54. Dörflinger-Hejlek E, Kirsch EC, Reiter H, et al. Diffusion-weighted MR imaging of intramedullary spinal cord abscess. AJNR Am J Neuroradiol 2010;31:1651–2.

55. Reihsaus E, Waldaur H, Seeling W. Spinal epidural abscess: a meta-analysis of 915 patients. Neurosurg Rev 2000;23:175–204.

56. Pradilla G, Ardila GP, Hsu W, et al. Epidural abscesses of the CNS. Lancet Neurol 2009;8:292–300.

57. Karikari IO, Powers CJ, Reynolds RM, et al. Management of a spontaneous spinal epidural abscess: a single-center 10-year experience. Neurosurgery 2009;65:919–24.

58. Skaf GS, Kanafani ZA, Araj GF, et al. Non-pyogenic infections of the spine. Int J Antimicrob Agents 2010;36(2):99–105.

59. Garcia-Monco JC. Central nervous system tuberculosis. Neurol Clin 1999;17(4): 737–59.

60. Ferrer M, Gutieerez Torres L, Ayala Ramirez O, et al. Tuberculosis of the spine. A systematic review of case series. Int Orthop 2010;36(2):221–31.

61. Sree Harsha CK, Shetty AP, Rajasekaran S. Intradural spinal tuberculosis in the absence of vertebral or meningeal tuberculosis: a case repot. J Orthop Surg 2006;14(1):71–5.

62. Drapkin MS, Kamath RS, Kim JY. Case 26-2012: a 70-year-old woman with fever and back pain. N Engl J Med 2012;367:754–62.

63. Luo L, Pino J. An intradural extramedullary tuberculoma of the spinal cord in a non-HIV-infected patient: case report and review of the literature. Lung 2006;184(3):187–93.

64. Dastur HM. Diagnosis and neurosurgical treatment of tuberculous disease of the CNS. Neurosurg Rev 1983;6(3):111–7.

65. Thwaites G, Fisher M, Hemingway C, et al. British Infection Society guidelines for the diagnosis and treatment of tuberculosis of the central nervous system in adults and children. J Infect 2009;59(3):167–87.

66. Wasay M, Arif H, Khealani B, et al. Neuroimaging of tuberculous myelitis: analysis of ten cases and review of literature. J Neuroimaging 2006;16(3):197–205.

67. Kaynar MY, Kocer N, Gencosmanoglu BE, et al. Syringomyelia as a late complication of tuberculous meningitis. Acta Neurochir (Wien) 2000;142(8):935–8 [discussion: 938–9].

68. Muthukumar N, Sureshkumar V. Concurrent syringomyelia and intradural extramedullary tuberculoma as late complications of tuberculous meningitis. J Clin Neurosci 2007;14(12):1225–30.

69. Roca B. Intradural extramedullary tuberculoma of the spinal cord; a review of reported cases. J Infect 2005;50(5):425–31.

70. Mohit AA, Santiago P, Rostomily R. Intramedullary tuberculoma mimicking primary CNS lymphoma. J Neurol Neurosurg Psychiatry 2004;75(11):1636–8.
71. Kung DH, Hubenthal EA, Kwan JY, et al. Toxoplasmosis myelopathy and myopathy in an AIDS patient: a case of immune reconstitution inflammatory syndrome? Neurologist 2011;17(1):49–51.
72. Hernandez-Albujar S, Arribas JR, Royo A, et al. Tuberculous radiculomyelitis complicating tuberculous meningitis: case report and review. Clin Infect Dis 2000;30(6):915–21.
73. Kayaoglu CR, Tuzun Y, Boga Z, et al. Intramedullary spinal tuberculoma: a case report. Spine 2000;25(17):2265–8.
74. Sinha S, Shekhar RC, Singh G, et al. Early versus delayed initiation of antiretroviral therapy for Indian HIV-infected individuals with tuberculosis on antituberculosis treatment. BMC Infect Dis 2012;12(1):168.
75. Charles V, Duprez TP, Kabamba B, et al. Poliomyelitis-like syndrome with matching magnetic resonance features in a case of Lyme neuroborreliosis. J Neurol Neurosurg Psychiatry 2007;78(10):1160–1.
76. Halperin JJ. Neurologic manifestations of Lyme disease. Curr Infect Dis Rep 2011;13:360–6.
77. Schmidt C, Plate A, Angele B, et al. A prospective study on the role of CXCL13 in Lyme neuroborreliosis. Neurology 2011;76(12):1051–8.
78. Bigi S, Aebi C, Nauer C, et al. Acute transverse myelitis in Lyme neuroborreliosis. Infection 2010;38(5):413–6.
79. Hattingen E, Weidauer S, Kieslich M, et al. MR imaging in neuroborreliosis of the cervical spinal cord. Eur Radiol 2004;14(11):2072–5.
80. Chilver-Stainer L, Fischer U, Hauf M, et al. Syphilitic myelitis: rare, nonspecific, but treatable. Neurology 2009;72:673–5.
81. Marra CM, Maxwell CL, Smith SL, et al. Cerebrospinal fluid abnormalities in patients with syphilis: association with clinical and laboratory features. J Infect Dis 2004;189:369–76.
82. Kumar D, Drebot MA, Wong SJ, et al. A seroprevalence study of West Nile virus infection in solid organ transplant recipients. Am J Transplant 2004;4:1883.
83. Levi ME, Quan D, Ho JT, et al. Impact of rituximab–associated B-cell defects on West Nile virus meningoencephalitis in solid organ transplant recipients. Clin Transplant 2010;24:223–38.
84. Leis AA, Stokic DS. Neuromuscular manifestations of West Nile virus infection. Front Neurol 2012;3:1–16.
85. Khetsuriani N, Prevots DR, Quick L, et al. Persistence of vaccine-derived poliovirus among immunodeficient persons with vaccine-associated paralytic poliomyelitis. J infect Dis 2003;188(12):1845–52.
86. Hosada M, Inoue H, Miyazawa Y. Vaccine associated paralytic poliomyelitis in Japan. Lancet 2012;379:520.
87. Aylward B, Yamad T. The polio endgame. N Engl J Med 2011;364(24):2273–5.
88. Centers for Disease Control and Prevention (CDC). Update on vaccine-derived polioviruses-worldwide, July 2009-March 2011. MMWR Morb Mortal Wkly Rep 2011;60(25):846–50.
89. Saeed M, Zaidi SZ, Naeem A, et al. Epidemiology and clinical findings associated with enteroviral acute flaccid paralysis in Pakistan. BMC Infect Dis 2007;7:6.
90. Rahimi P, Tabatabaie H, Gouya MM, et al. Direct identification of non-polio enteroviruses in residual paralysis cases by analysis of VP1sequences. J Clin Virol 2009;45(2):139–41.

91. Yang TT, Huang LM, Lu CY, et al. Clinical features and factors of unfavorable outcomes for non-polio enterovirus infection of the central nervous system in northern Taiwan, 1994-2003. J Microbiol Immunol Infect 2005;38(6):417–24.

92. Gharbi J, Jaidane H, Ben M'hadheb M, et al. Epidemiological study of non-polio enterovirus neurological infections in children in the region of Monastir, Tunisia. Diagn Microbiol Infect Dis 2006;54(1):31–6.

93. Junttila N, Leveque N, Kabue JP, et al. New enteroviruses, EV-93 and EV-94, associated with acute flaccid paralysis in the Democratic Republic of the Congo. J Med Virol 2007;79(4):393–400.

94. Nagel MA, Gilden DH. The protean neurologic manifestations of varicella-zoster virus infection. Cleve Clin J Med 2007;74:489–94.

95. Curtis JR, Patkar N, Xie A, et al. Risk of serious bacterial infections among rheumatoid arthritis patients exposed to tumor necrosis factor alpha antagonists. Arthritis Rheum 2007;56(4):1125–33.

96. Brassard P, Kezouh A, Suissa S. Antirheumatic drugs and the risk of tuberculosis. Clin Infect Dis 2006;43(6):717–22.

97. Strangfeld A, Listing J, Herzer P, et al. Risk of herpes zoster in patients with rheumatoid arthritis treated with anti-TNF-α agents. JAMA 2009;301(7):737–44.

98. Javed S, Javed SA, Tyring SK. Varicella vaccines. Curr Opin Infect Dis 2012;25: 135–40.

99. Gilden D, Cohrs RJ, Mahalingam R, et al. Varicella zoster virus vasculopathies: diverse clinical manifestations, laboratory features, pathogenesis, and treatment. Lancet Neurol 2009;8:731–40.

100. Gilden D, Nagel MA, Ransooff RM, et al. Recurrent varicella zoster virus myelopathy. J Neurol Sci 2009;276(1–2):196–8.

101. Cortese A, Tavazzi E, Delbue S, et al. Varicella zoster virus-associated polyradiculoneuritis. Neurology 2009;73(16):1334–5.

102. Mathews MS, Sorkin GC, Brant-Zawadzki M, et al. Varicella zoster infection of the brainstem followed by Brown-Sequard syndrome. Neurology 2009;72(21): 1874.

103. Nagel MA, Cohrs RJ, Mahalingam R, et al. The varicella zoster virus vasculopathies: clinical, CSF, imaging and virologic features. Neurology 2008;70:853–60.

104. Young-Barbee C, Hall DA, LoPresti JJ. Brown Sequard syndrome after herpes zoster. Neurology 2009;72:670–1.

105. Wolf J, Nagel MA, Mahalingam R, et al. Chronic active varicella zoster virus infection. Neurology 2012;79:828–9.

106. Majid A, Galetta SL, Sweeney CJ, et al. Epstein-Barr virus myeloradiculitis and encephalomyeloradiculitis. Brain 2002;125:159–65.

107. Sanefuji M, Ohga S, Kira R, et al. Epstein Barr virus-associated meningoencephalomyelitis; intrathecal reactivation of the virus in an immunocompetent child. J Child Neurol 2008;23(9):1072–7.

108. Ross AG, Bartley PB, Adrian CS, et al. Schistosomiasis. N Engl J Med 2002;346: 1212–20.

109. Ferrari TC, Moreira PR. Neuroschistosomiasis: clinical symptoms and pathogenesis. Lancet Neurol 2011;10:853–64.

110. Camargos ST, Dantas FR, Teixeira AL. Schistosomal myelopathy mimicking spinal cord neoplasm. Scand J Infect Dis 2005;37(5):365–7.

111. Ross AG, Vickers D, Olds GR, et al. Katayama syndrome. Lancet Infect Dis 2007;7:218–24.

112. Ross AG, McManus DP, Farrar J, et al. Neuroschistosomiasis. J Neurol 2012; 259(1):22–32.

113. Garcia HH, Del Brutto OH. Neurocysticercosis: updated concepts about an old disease. Lancet Neurol 2005;4:653–61.
114. Callacondo D, Garcia HH, Gonzales I, et al. High frequency of spinal involvement in patients with basal subarachnoid neurocysticercosis. Neurology 2012; 78:1394–400.
115. Lambertucci JR, Vale TC, Pereira AC, et al. Isolated cervical spinal cord cysticercosis. Neurology 2011;77(23):e138.
116. Boulos MI, Aviv RI, Lee L. Spinal neurocysticercosis manifesting as recurrent aseptic meningitis. Can J Neurol Sci 2010;37:878–80.
117. Venna N, Coyle CM, Gonzalez RG, et al. Case 25-2012: a 48 year old woman with diplopia, headaches, and papilledema. N Engl J Med 2012;366:1924–34.
118. Proano JH, Torres-Corzo J, Rodriguez-DellaVecchia R, et al. Intraventricular and subarachnoid basal cisterns neurocysticercosis: a comparative study between traditional treatment versus neuroendoscopic surgery. Childs Nerv Syst 2009; 25:1467–75.
119. Ersahin Y. Spinal epidural abscess: a meta-analysis of 915 patients. Neurosurg Rev 2001;24(2–3):156.
120. Lury K, Smith JK, Castillo M. Imaging of spinal infections. Semin Roentgenol 2006;41(4):363–79.
121. Mantieene C, Albucher JF, Catalaa I, et al. MRI in Lyme disease of the spinal cord. Neuroradiology 2001;43(6):485–8.
122. Meurs L, Labeye D, Declercq I, et al. Acute transverse myelitis as a main manifestation of early stage II neuroborreliosis in two patients. Eur Neurol 2004;52(3): 186–8.
123. Chang BL, Shih CM, Ro LS, et al. Acute neuroborreliosis with involvement of the central nervous system. J Neurol Sci 2012;295(1–2):10–5.
124. Tsiodras S, Kelesidis I, Kelesidis T, et al. Central nervous system manifestations of Mycoplasma pneumoniae infections. J Infect 2005;51(5):343–54.
125. Tsiodras S, Kelesidis T, Kelesidis I, et al. Mycoplasma pneumoniae-associated myelitis: a comprehensive review. Eur J Neurol 2006;13(2):112–24.
126. Moghtaderi A, Alavi-Naini R. Tuberculous radiculomyelitis: review and presentation of five patients. Int J Tuberc Lung Dis 2003;7(12):1186–90.
127. Suda S, Ueda M, Komaba Y, et al. Tuberculous myelitis diagnosed by elevated adenosine deaminase activity in cerebrospinal fluid. Clin Neurosci 2008;15(9): 1068–9.
128. Arora S, Kumar R. Tubercular spinal epidural abscess involving the dorsal-lumbar region without osseous involvement. J Infect Dev Ctries 2011;5(7): 544–9.
129. Centers for Disease Control. Updated guidelines for the sue of nucleic acid amplification tests in the diagnosis of tuberculosis. MMWR Morb Mortal Wkly Rep 2009;58:7–10.
130. Toledano R, Lopez-Sendon J, Gilo F, et al. Posterior horn varicella-zoster virus myelitis. J Neurol 2007;254(3):400–1.
131. Tavazzi E, Minoli L, Ferrante P, et al. Varicella zoster virus meningo-encephalo-myelitis in an immunocompetent patient. Neurol Sci 2008;29(4):279–83.
132. Haug A, Mahalingam R, Cohrs RJ, et al. Recurrent polymorphonuclear pleocytosis with increased red blood cells caused by varicella zoster virus infection of the central nervous system. Case report and review of the literature. J Neurol Sci 2010;292(1–2):85–8.
133. Lee CC, Wu JC, Huang WC, et al. Herpes zoster cervical myelitis in a young adult. J Chin Med Assoc 2010;73(11):605–10.

134. Sejvar JJ, Leiss AA, Stokic DS, et al. Acute flaccid paralysis and West Nile virus infection. Emerg Infect Dis 2003;9(7):788–93.

135. Jeha LE, Sila CA, Lederman RJ, et al. West Nile virus infection: a new acute paralytic illness. Neurology 2003;61(1):55–9.

136. Li J, Loeb JA, Shy ME, et al. Asymmetric flaccid paralysis: a neuromuscular presentation of West Nile virus infection. Ann Neurol 2003;53(6):703–10.

137. Kleinschmidt-DeMasters BK, Marder BA, Levi ME, et al. Naturally acquired West Nile virus encephalomyelitis in transplant recipients. Arch Neurol 2004;61(8):1210–20.

138. Ali M, Safriel Y, Sohi J, et al. West Nile virus infection: MR imaging findings in the nervous system. AJNR AM J Neuroradiol 2005;26(2):289–97.

139. Lenzi ME, Cuzzi-Maya T, Oliveira AL, et al. Dermatological findings of human T lymphotropic virus type 1 (HTLV-I)-associated myelopathy/tropical spastic paraparesis. Clin Infect Dis 2003;36(4):507–13.

140. Grindstaff P, Gruener G. The peripheral nervous system complications of HTLV-1 myelopathy (HAM/TSP) syndromes. Semin Neurol 2005;25(3):315–27.

141. Bagnato F, Butman JA, Mora CA, et al. Conventional magnetic resonance imaging features in patients with tropical spastic paraparesis. J Neurovirol 2005;11(6):525–34.

142. Umehara F, Nose H, Saito M, et al. Abnormalities of spinal magnetic resonance images implicate clinical variability in human T-cell lymphotropic virus type I-associated myelopathy. J Neurovirol 2007;13(3):260–7.

143. Delgado SR, Sheremata WA, Brown AD, et al. Human T-lymphotropic virus type I or II (HTLV-I/II) associated with recurrent longitudinally extensive transverse myelitis (LETM): two case reports. J Neurovirol 2010;16(3):249–53.

144. Whiteman ML, Dandapani BK, Shebert RT, et al. MRI of AIDS-related polyradiculomyelitis. J Comput Assist Tomogr 1994;18(1):7–11.

145. Giobbia M, Carniato A, Scotton PG, et al. Cytomegalovirus-associated transverse myelitis in a non-immunocompromised patient. Infection 1999;27(3):228–30.

146. Maschke M, Kastrup O, Diener HC. CNS manifestations of cytomegalovirus infections: diagnosis and treatment. CNS Drugs 2002;16(5):303–15.

147. Fux CA, Pfister S, Nohl F, et al. Cytomegalovirus-associated acute transverse myelitis in immunocompetent adults. Clin Microbiol Infect 2003;9(12):1187–90.

148. Rigamonti A, Usai S, Ciusani E, et al. Atypical transverse myelitis due to cytomegalovirus in an immunocompetent patient. Neurol Sci 2005;26(5):351–4.

149. Wong M, Connolly AM, Noetzel MJ. Poliomyelitis-like syndrome associated with Epstein-Barr virus infection. Pediatr Neurol 1999;20(3):235–7.

150. Muhlau M, Bulow S, Stimmer H, et al. Seronegative Epstein-Barr virus myeloradiculitis in an immunocompetent 72-year-old woman. Neurology 2005;65(8):1329–30.

151. Paz JA, Vallada MG, Marques SN, et al. Vaccine-associated paralytic poliomyelitis: a case report of domiciliary transmission. Rev Hosp Clin Fac Med Sao Paulo 2000;55(3):101–4.

152. Asahina N, Matsunami Y, Sueda K, et al. Vaccine-associated paralytic poliomyelitis in a non-immunocompromised infant. Pediatr Int 2010;52(5):838–41.

153. Ferraz-Filho JR, dos Santos Torres U, de Oliveira EP, et al. MRI findings in an infant with vaccine-associated paralytic poliomyelitis. Pediatr Radiol 2010;40(Suppl 1):S138–40.

154. Grewal AK, Lopes MB, Berg CL, et al. Recurrent demyelinating myelitis associated with hepatitis C viral infection. J Neurol Sci 2004;224(1–2):101–6.

155. Acharya JN, Pacheco VH. Neurologic complications of hepatitis C. Neurology 2008;14(3):151–6.

156. Stubgen JP. Immune-mediated myelitis associated with hepatitis virus infections. J Neuroimmunol 2011;239(1–2):21–7.

157. Shyu WC, Lin JC, Chang BC, et al. Recurrent ascending myelitis: an unusual presentation of herpes simplex virus type 1 infection. Ann Neurol 1993;34(4):625–7.

158. Nakajima H, Furutama D, Kimura F, et al. Herpes simplex virus myelitis: clinical manifestations and diagnosis by the polymerase chain reaction method. Eur Neurol 1998;39(3):163–7.

159. Azuma K, Yoshimoto M, Nishimura Y, et al. Herpes simplex virus type 1 myelitis with a favorable outcome. Intern Med 2001;40(10):1068–9.

160. Gobbi C, Tosi C, Stadler C, et al. Recurrent myelitis associated with herpes simplex virus type 2. Eur Neurol 2001;46(4):215–8.

161. Eberhardt O, Kuker W, Dichgans J, et al. HSV-2 sacral radiculitis (Elsberg syndrome). Neurology 2004;63(4):758–9.

162. Mohanty A, Venkatrama SK, Das S, et al. Spinal intramedullary cysticercosis. Neurosurgery 1997;40(1):82–7.

163. Leite CC, Jinkins JR, Escobar BE, et al. MR imaging of intramedullary and intradural-extramedullary spinal cysticercosis. AJR Am J Roentgenol 1997; 169(6):1713–7.

164. Mohanty A, Das S, Kolluri VR, et al. Spinal extradural cysticercosis: a case report. Spinal Cord 1998;36(4):285–7.

165. Gaur V, Gupta RK, Dev R, et al. MR imaging of intramedullary spinal cysticercosis: a report of two cases. Clin Radiol 2000;55(4):311–4.

166. Parmar H, Shah J, Patwardhan V, et al. MR imaging in intramedullary cysticercosis. Neuroradiology 2001;43(11):961–7.

167. Sheehan JP, Sheehan J, Lopes MB, et al. Intramedullary spinal cysticercosis. Case report and review of the literature. Neurosurg Focus 2002;12(6):e10.

168. Alsina GA, Johnson JP, McBride DQ, et al. Spinal neurocysticercosis. Neurosurg Focus 2002;12(6):e8.

169. Paterakis KN, Kapsalaki E, Hadjigeorgiou GM, et al. Primary spinal intradural extramedullary cysticercosis. Surg Neurol 2007;68(3):309–11 [discussion: 312].

170. Goncalves FG, Neves PO, Jovem CL, et al. Chronic myelopathy associated to intramedullary cysticercosis. Spine 2010;35(5):E159–62.

171. Del Brutto OH. Neurocysticercosis: a review. ScientificWorldJournal 2012;2012: 159821.

172. Junker J, Eckardt L, Husstedt I. Cervical intramedullar schistosomiasis as a rare cause of acute tetraparesis. Clin Neurol Neurosurg 2001;103(1):39–42.

173. Moreno-Carvalho OA, Nascimento-Carvalho CM, Bacelar AL, et al. Clinical and cerebrospinal fluid (CSF) profile and CSF criteria for the diagnosis of spinal cord schistosomiasis. Arq Neuropsiquiatr 2003;61(2B):353–8.

174. Carod Artal FJ, Vargas AP, Horan TA, et al. Schistosoma mansoni myelopathy: clinical and pathologic findings. Neurology 2004;63(2):388–91.

175. Saleem S, Belal AI, el-Ghandour NM. Spinal cord schistosomiasis: MR imaging appearance with surgical and pathologic correlation. AJNR Am J Neuroradiol 2005;26(7):1646–54.

176. Nascimento-Carvalho CM, Moreno-Carvalho OA. Neuroschistosomiasis due to Schistosoma mansoni: a review of pathogenesis, clinical syndromes and diagnostic approaches. Rev Inst Med Trop Sao Paulo 2005;47(4):179–84.

177. Carod-Artal FJ. Neurological complications of Schistosoma infection. Trans R Soc Trop Med Hyg 2008;102(2):107–16.

178. Jiang YG, Zhang MM, Xiang J. Spinal cord schistosomiasis japonica: a report of 4 cases. Surg Neurol 2008;69(4):392–7.

179. de Jongste AH, Tilanus AM, Bax H, et al. New insights in diagnosing Schistosoma myelopathy. J Infect 2010;60(3):244–7.
180. Poon TP, Tchertkoff V, Pares GF, et al. Spinal cord toxoplasma lesion in AIDS: MR findings. J Comput Assist Tomogr 1992;16(5):817–9.
181. Lortholary O, Lisovoski F, Brechot JM, et al. Myelitis due to Toxoplasma gondii in a patient with AIDS. Clin Infect Dis 1994;19(6):1167–8.
182. Cosan TE, Kabukcuoglu S, Arslantas A, et al. Spinal toxoplasmic arachnoiditis associated with osteoid formation: a rare presentation of toxoplasmosis. Spine 2001;26(15):1726–8.
183. Straathof CS, Kortbeek LM, Roerdink H, et al. A solitary spinal cord toxoplasma lesion after peripheral stem-cell transplantation. J Neurol 2001;248(9):814–5.
184. Schnepper GD, Johnson WD. Recurrent spinal hydatidosis in North America. Case report and review of the literature. Neurosurg Focus 2004;17(6):E8.
185. Sapkas GS, Machinis TG, Chloros GD, et al. Spinal hydatid disease, a rare but existent pathological entity: case report and review of the literature. South Med J 2006;99(2):178–83.
186. Midyat L, Gokce S, Onder A, et al. A very rare cause of childhood paraparesis: primary intradural extramedullary spinal hydatid cyst. Pediatr Infect Dis J 2009; 28(8):754–5.

Multiple Sclerosis and the Spinal Cord

William Sheremata, MD, FRCP(C)*, Leticia Tornes, MD

KEYWORDS

- Multiple sclerosis • Clinically isolated syndrome • Spinal cord syndromes
- MS treatment • MRI • Useless hand syndrome • Suspended sensory loss
- Disability

KEY POINTS

- Multiple sclerosis (MS) may present as an acute or subacute myelopathy. Of the population identified as having transverse myelitis (TM), a large proportion is subsequently diagnosed with clinically definite MS. Thus:
- Keeping MS in the differential diagnosis of all patients recognized to have spinal cord disease is crucial.
- If the TM occurs in the absence of prior neurologic disease, it is termed a clinically isolated syndrome (CIS).
- The importance of identifying CIS is that there is now overwhelming evidence that there is consistently better response to therapy at this stage of MS.
- Therapy at this stage has been proved to delay clinical attacks and decrease radiological burden of disease, which in turn may lessen future disability.

INTRODUCTION

Multiple sclerosis (MS) is a central nervous system (CNS) inflammatory disorder characterized by relapses of disease affecting different parts of the white matter of brain and spinal cord over time.[1] Onset typically occurs between the ages of 18 and 50 years and is twice as common in women as in men. The clinical manifestations of disease typically are disseminated in both time and space but vary greatly. Visual symptoms and brain stem manifestations are ordinarily recognized with ease by the neurologist. Although signs of spinal involvement are common, they are often mistakenly attributed to cerebral involvement in MS.

In his foreword to the August 1983 *Multiple Sclerosis* volume of the *Neurologic Clinics*, and again in 1995, Antel[2,3] succinctly described the onset of MS. It typically occurs in a young adult with relapsing-remitting (RR) episodes of multifocal neurologic

Department of Neurology, Multiple Sclerosis Center of Excellence, University of Miami Miller School of Medicine, Clinical Research Building, 13th Floor, 1120 Northwest 14th Street, Miami, FL 33136, USA
* Corresponding author.
E-mail address: wsherema@med.miami.edu

Neurol Clin 31 (2013) 55–77
http://dx.doi.org/10.1016/j.ncl.2012.09.007   neurologic.theclinics.com
0733-8619/13/$ – see front matter © 2013 Elsevier Inc. All rights reserved.

dysfunction, related to (inflammatory) lesions of the CNS white matter, with accumulation of disability with recurrences. This definition applies to about 70% to 85% of the population of patients with MS but approximately 15% to 30% show a progressive spinal cord disease from the outset of their illness.[4–6] It was Charcot,[7] the first professor of neurology, who first characterized MS as a CNS disease in nineteenth century Paris.

In his book *Diseases of the Nervous System* Charcot[7] attributed the original observation of "sclerose en plaques" (disseminated sclerosis; ie, MS) to Jean Cruveilhier, Professor of Anatomy at the University of Paris. He referred the attendees at his lectures on MS to the chapters on "Paraplegia" in Cruveilier's 1829 to 1842 *Atlas on Anatomic Pathology*.[8] In his introduction to MS as a clinical illness in that book, Charcot[7] commented, "There is a more or less marked decline of the motor power of the limbs, which is frequently manifested at the very outset of the disease, and which is not usually connected with any notable disturbance of sensibility. Generally one of the lower limbs is first and solely affected.[7]" Although he attributed manifestations of MS to the brain and spinal cord, Charcot's[7] description of the histopathology of MS was drawn primarily from study of spinal cord specimens. Although he described relapses and remissions with progression of illness as features of MS, he also described the progressive spinal form of illness, the incomplete form of MS, now known as primary progressive MS (PPMS). The reader is referred to the 1983 and 1995 *Neurologic Clinics* regarding evolving basic concepts of MS.[2,3] Also, a more recent general review of MS has been published.[6]

MS may present with a wide range of clinical manifestations, ranging from visual to gait problems.[1–3,5,6] Illness usually comprises acute attacks of neurologic deficits followed by periods of remission. Subsequent attacks consist of either new neurologic deficits or relapses of a previous problem. To establish a diagnosis of MS, lesions in the CNS must be separated both in time and space. With the advent of modern neuroimaging, visualization of white matter changes on brain magnetic resonance imaging (MRI) is now easily available.[9] MS is typically regarded as a brain disorder; however, most hemispheric lesions in MS are clinically silent, whereas the cardinal clinical signs and symptoms of MS typically result from spinal cord involvement.[1–4,6–8]

Poser and colleagues[10] in 1966 reviewed the clinical characteristics of 111 autopsy-proved American, English, and Norwegian MS cases. Although a great variety of presentations were documented in their series, the investigators reported that weakness was the first symptom in 42% of cases and difficulty in walking was commonly seen at the onset of MS. Almost all cases had evidence of spasticity and weakness recorded by the time of death. The Kurtzke Extended Disability Status Scale (EDSS), now universally used for assessing impairment and rating disability, is depends largely on gait.[11]

PATHOLOGY

Charcot[7] characterized MS as disseminated sclerosis or widespread scarring affecting the CNS.[7] The affected platelike areas of glial scar, the plaques (ie, sclerose en plaques), also showed evidence of inflammation and myelin breakdown (demyelization) with relative sparing of axons (**Fig. 1**). More modern observations have shown that perivascular mononuclear cell infiltration, principally macrophages with smaller numbers of small lymphocytes, is seen in early active plaques (**Fig. 2**).[1,6,12] Demyelination is present, but there is also less obvious loss of axons in the plaques. Macrophages can be seen to contain lipid and myelin fragments.[1,12–15] Later, inflammatory cells diminish and gliosis becomes increasingly apparent (**Fig. 3**). These lesions are randomly scattered through the CNS with different stages of activity. Trapp and colleagues[15] have now shown that axonal loss is more marked than had been generally acknowledged.

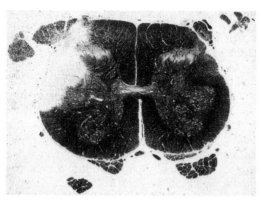

Fig. 1. Sharp, well-circumscibed area of demyelination in lumbar cord.

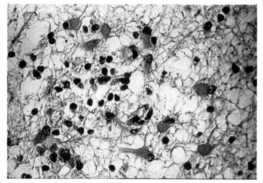

Fig. 2. Peri-venous lymphocytic infiltrate in area of demyelination in a relatively new/evolving plaque.

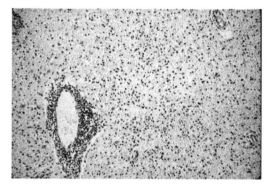

Fig. 3. Chronic MS plaques with reactive astrocytes (cells with lots of pink cytoplasm) and isolated dark nuclei consisting of lymphocytes.

PATHOPHYSIOLOGY OF MS

Implications in the use of this term have changed or evolved over the last 4 decades.[1,16,17] Until the early 1980s, this involved discussions of the impact of the loss of (nodes) of myelin and the impact on salutatory conduction, explaining the impact of temperature on transmission failure that had been documented 3 decades earlier. Transmission failure was equated with loss of nodes of myelin interfering with salutatory conduction and the failure to meet a markedly increased energy cost for neurotransmission.[17] Inflammatory mediators have been also investigated in relation to transmission failure.[6] The recognition of the role of demyelination uncovering fast-conducting potassium channels led to the investigation of 4-aminopyridine (dalfampridine).[18] Trapp and colleagues[15] suggested that axonal loss is the underlying explanation for progression of disability, apart from the acute consequences of inflammation.[15] At present, considerations in the pathophysiology of MS include include genetic factors, mechanisms of viral infection, and the role of immune mechanisms in mediating tissue damage.[1,6,14,16]

DIAGNOSIS

The diagnosis of MS rests primarily on evidence that the CNS lesions are disseminated both in time and space. Using the Schumacher and colleagues[19] (1965) criteria, the clinician established the anatomic localization of the CNS (brain and/or spinal cord) lesions by deduction from the clinical symptoms and neurologic signs found on examination. Later, the finding of cerebrospinal fluid (CSF) immunoglobulin abnormalities was used to support the diagnosis. These criteria were subsequently modified by Poser and colleagues[20] in establishing the Poser (1983) Diagnostic Criteria. The Poser criteria embraced additional paraclinical evidence of disease. For the first time, electrophysiologic findings, primarily visual evoked responses, and MRI were incorporated to support a diagnosis of MS, which were major to the dependence on prolonged clinical follow-up and the CSF examination. More recently, the 2000 McDonald criteria (McDonald and colleagues[21]), with 2005[22] and 2010[23] revisions (**Table 1**),[23] have replaced these with a simpler, clearer, and more specific iteration of MRI requirements to establish the diagnosis of a clinically isolated syndrome (CIS) identifying MS with high probability at its first clinical manifestation. The diagnosis of MS rests on ruling out other disorders that may have similar clinical presentations.

DIFFERENTIAL DIAGNOSIS OF MS

Because MS presents with symptoms and signs of spinal cord involvement in a large proportion of cases, the whole spectrum of spinal cord disease must be considered in the differential diagnosis.[1,16,24,25] One of the most important in the differential diagnosis is acute disseminated encephalomyelitis (ADEM), an acute demyelinating disease that most commonly follows banal respiratory illness or immunization.[1,16,24] The interval between the initial infection or immunization may be several weeks and may even have been forgotten by the patient. A relapse of neurologic disease, ordinarily signifying clinically definite MS, occurs in 25% to 35% of cases.[1,24] Active infection of the spinal cord must be considered based on history of exposure (ie, genital or labial herpes[16,24]).

Neuromyelitis optica (NMO), although less common, is always in the differential diagnosis.[16,26] The clinical presentation is often more dramatic and may be associated with striking pain.[26–28] The pain may arise before overt changes in the MRI of the affected segments of the spinal cord. The evolution of the clinical picture extends

Table 1
The 2010 McDonald criteria for diagnosis of MS clinical presentation and additional data needed for MS diagnosis

Clinical Presentation	Additional Data Needed for MS Diagnosis
≥2 attacks[a]; objective clinical evidence of ≥2 lesions or objective clinical evidence of 1 lesion with reasonable historical evidence of a prior attack[b]	None[c]
≥2 attacks[a]; objective clinical evidence of 1 lesion	Dissemination in space, shown by ≥1 T2 lesion in at least 2 of 4 MS-typical regions of the CNS (periventricular, juxtacortical, infratentorial, or spinal cord)[d]; or await a further clinical attack[a] implicating a different CNS site
1 attack[a]; objective clinical evidence of ≥2 lesions	Dissemination in time, shown by simultaneous presence of asymptomatic gadolinium-enhancing and nonenhancing lesions at any time; or A new T2 and/or gadolinium-enhancing lesion(s) on follow-up MRI, irrespective of its timing relative to a baseline scan; or Await a second clinical attack[a]
1 attack[a]; objective clinical evidence of 1 lesion (clinically isolated syndrome)	Dissemination in space and time, shown by, for DIS: ≥1 T2 lesion in at least 2 of 4 MS-typical regions of the CNS (periventricular, juxtacortical, infratentorial, or spinal cord)[d]; or await a second clinical attack[a] implicating a different CNS site; and, for DIT: Simultaneous presence of asymptomatic gadolinium-enhancing and nonenhancing lesions at any time; or A new T2 and/or gadolinium-enhancing lesion(s) on follow-up MRI, irrespective of its timing relative to a baseline scan; or Await a second clinical attack[a]
Insidious neurologic progression suggesting MS (PPMS)	1 y of disease progression (retrospectively or prospectively determined) plus 2 of 3 of the following criteria[d]: 1. Evidence for DIS in the brain based on ≥1 T2 lesions in the MS-characteristic (periventricular, juxtacortical, or infratentorial) regions 2. Evidence for DIS in the spinal cord based on ≥2 T2 lesions in the cord 3. Positive CSF (isoelectric focusing evidence of oligoclonal bands and/or increased IgG index)

If the criteria are fulfilled and there is no better explanation for the clinical presentation, the diagnosis is MS; if suspicious, but the criteria are not completely met, the diagnosis is possible MS; if another diagnosis arises during the evaluation that better explains the clinical presentation, then the diagnosis is not MS.

Abbreviations: DIT, dissemination in time; DIS, dissemination in space; IgG, immunoglobulin G.

[a] An attack (relapse; exacerbation) is defined as patient-reported or objectively observed events typical of an acute inflammatory demyelinating event in the CNS, current or historical, with duration of at least 24 hours, in the absence of fever or infection. It should be documented by contemporaneous neurologic examination, but some historical events with symptoms and evolution characteristic for MS, but for which no objective neurologic findings are documented, can provide reasonable evidence of a prior demyelinating event. However, reports of paroxysmal symptoms (historical or current) should consist of multiple episodes occurring over not less than 24 hours. Before a definite diagnosis of MS can be made, at least 1 attack must be corroborated by findings on neurologic examination, visual evoked potential response in patients reporting prior visual disturbance, or MRI consistent with demyelination in the area of the CNS implicated in the historical report of neurologic symptoms.

[b] Clinical diagnosis based on objective clinical findings for 2 attacks is most secure. Reasonable historical evidence for 1 past attack, in the absence of documented objective neurologic findings, can include historical events with symptoms and evolution characteristics for a prior inflammatory demyelinating event; however, at least 1 attack must be supported by objective findings.

[c] No additional tests are required. However, it is desirable that any diagnosis of MS be made with access to imaging based on these criteria. If imaging or other tests (for instance, CSF) are undertaken and are negative, extreme caution needs to be taken before making a diagnosis of MS, and alternative diagnoses must be considered. There must be no better explanation for the clinical presentation, and objective evidence must be present to support a diagnosis of MS.

[d] Gadolinium-enhancing lesions are not required; symptomatic lesions are excluded from consideration in patients with brainstem or spinal cord syndromes.

over longer periods of time than a typical MS attack. The abnormal T2 signal in the cord typically extends 3 or more vertebral lengths.[26] The abnormal signal is most often in the central portion of the cord but may seem to involve the posterior columns in some. A word of caution: an appearance of flow artifacts within the cord may arise before increased T2 signal within the cord; in addition, movement artifacts in distressed patients may make visualizing the abnormal cord difficult. Recovery of function is generally viewed as less favorable than in MS, but, after the use of rituximab, that has improved slightly.[27,28]

Sarcoidosis may mimic MS and must also be considered in the differential diagnosis.[1,6,16,29] Most patients with sarcoidosis have concomitant pulmonary involvement. Neurosarcoid classically involves the meninges and produces cranial and spinal neuropathies. Intraparenchymal involvement occurs in the brain, but is less likely to occur in the spinal cord. Increase of angiotensin-converting enzyme (ACE) and chest radiograph are minimum investigations. A computed tomography scan of the chest may be used to identify pulmonary and mediastinal involvement. Radioisotope scans are often overinterpreted and must be considered in context. For those without pulmonary or mediastinal involvement, the old gold standard of finding granulomas in at least 2 biopsies of muscle or other organs is the most reliable test.[29]

Collagen vascular disease is also a consideration and, in MS, antinuclear and anti–double-stranded DNA antibodies are detected in about half of patients, albeit in low titer.[1,6,22] The 2 rarely coexist. In our experience, spinal cord involvement in systemic lupus erythematosus and in polyarteritis tends to be severe and resembles NMO more than MS. Infectious causes, such as human T-lymphotropic virus (HTLV) –I/II and human immunodeficiency virus (HIV) retroviruses, as well as other infectious and biochemical disorders, must be distinguished from MS.[30,31] Sjögren disease may present with a myelopathy and must also be considered in the context of the differential diagnosis of MS as well as NMO.[1,25]

THE ROLE OF MRI IN THE DIAGNOSIS OF MS

Early use of brain MRI in MS revealed distinctive white matter lesions with increased T2 signal in brains of most, but not, all patients.[9] Imaging obtained at that time lacked spatial resolution and had other technological limitations. Despite the challenge, in 1982, we began imaging the spinal cord as part of a prospective brain MRI study of patients with MS.[32] We did this because of the high frequency of clinical signs pointing to spinal cord involvement in MS. Studies of 77 patients with MS yielded usable images of both brain and spinal cord and, of those imaged within 36 months of their first symptoms of MS, despite the presence of diagnostic CSF changes, half did not exhibit typical T2-bright plaques.[33] However, more than half of those without plaques in their cerebral white matter showed spinal cord lesions. With increasing duration of illness, the proportion of cases with plaques identified in their brains also increased, peaking at 9 to 12 years of illness, and 90% showed brain white matter involvement.

Additional studies have supported and extended the observations that a proportion of patients with MS, particularly early in their illness, may not have brain involvement evident by brain MRI.[34] Absence of brain lesions is a more frequent observation in patients with a progressive myelopathy (ie, PPMS).

CLINICAL PRESENTATION OF MS AS A MYELOPATHY

Patients with MS presenting for the first time with multiple neurologic deficits are less of a diagnostic predicament than those who are monosymptomatic.[1,6] However, a significant proportion of the MS population is found among those presenting with a spinal cord syndrome (ie, an acute myelopathy).[1,6,35–39] Such patients more often present with a subacute monosymptomatic motor and/or sensory syndrome principally involving their lower extremities. The population of patients with MS often has a less severe presentation than patients with a cord syndrome secondary to systemic disease or NMO.[35,39] Investigation after initial presentation should include brain imaging, even in the absence of symptoms or signs of any brain involvement. In this article, patients presenting with signs of a myelopathy with motor and sensory deficits are referred to as classic presentations. Separate discussions follow of some other identifiable presentations, some with an accompanied illustrative case.

Classic Presentation

In our experience, approximately half of all patients with MS initially, or in relapse, present acutely with impaired gait. Often they complain of heaviness or numbness in a lower extremity with symptoms increasing over hours and days, and at times affecting the contralateral limb. Patients may complain of a loss of energy and often frank fatigue. Some may describe the fatigue as incapacitating, despite minimal neurologic findings on examination. Motor examination may reveal a deficit without detectable sensory loss, despite subjective sensory symptoms. Follow-up examination within a few days may yield different findings. Examination may reveal either absence of abnormality or, in contrast, marked deficits may be evident. Symptoms often remit, even without treatment. In a prospective treatment trial of natalizumab in acute relapses, we found remission in response to placebo commonly occurred within 5 to 7 days.[40] However, rapid resolution of proprioceptive loss observed in the following case history is rare without treatmenvt.

Illustrative case #1

A 29-year-old, previously healthy man presented with a 3-day history of tingling in the lateral aspect and lateral 2 digits of the right foot. He had experienced transient numbness of his right hand a month earlier. MRI had been done at that time that reported a small number of non-enhancing periventricular lesions. His neurologist suggested that MS should be considered and the patient requested a second opinion. At the time of consultation he was asymptomatic except for anxiety. Examination revealed only mild loss of smooth visual pursuit on horizontal gaze and a subtle impairment of the right lower limb during walking. He had no other findings on examination. MRI of the brain and cervical spine were requested.

Impaired gait began a day following the consultation and increased progressively over the next 6 days until he became unable to walk without assistance. Reexamination, 9 days after onset, revealed a man with severe ataxia and a complete right foot drop. In contrast with the presence of mild hip flexor weakness, marked proprioceptive loss was found in all 4 extremities. His cervical cord MRI revealed a large, partially enhancing midcervical lesion (**Figs. 4–6**). Treatment with corticotrophin was followed by resolution of his symptoms and signs within 10 days.

Comment: a young man presented with minimal symptoms and a great deal of denial. He then suffered a major relapse under the supervision of the consultant neurologist. He made a rapid recovery, despite major disability, with corticotrophin therapy.

Transverse Myelitis

Transverse myelitis (TM) is not a disease but rather a clinical phenomenon. It may be best described as the subacute presentation of neurologic illness characterized by clinical signs localized to a single spinal cord level.[16,41] Although TM is a collection of disorders, primary demyelinating disease (ie, ADEM, MS, and NMO) makes up a large proportion of cases.[16,24–26,41] The clinical findings of motor and/or sensory

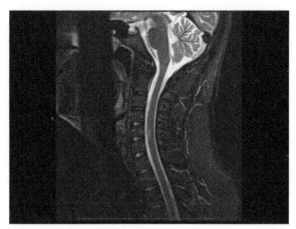

Fig. 4. Large cervical cord lesion, T2 sagittal.

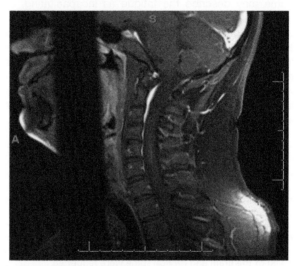

Fig. 5. Large enhancing cervical cord lesion.

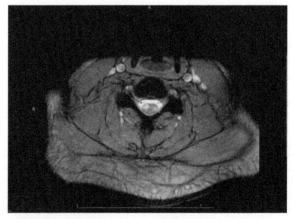

Fig. 6. Large cervical lesion, Axial T2.

abnormalities localizable to the spinal cord, often accompanied by bladder and or bowel disturbance, are the most common features of TM. Although a clear sensory level is often a tip-off to the diagnosis, the finding of a motor level may be the only clue to its localization. There are several distinctive presentations of TM that are more common in MS, such as Lhermitte phenomenon[42] and the useless hand syndrome,[43] both associated with cervical cord lesions on MRI. The use of MRI is important, not only to localize the lesion responsible for the clinical picture but also to identify other causes, including those that may need more urgent intervention, such as a compressive cord lesion or tumor.

If the TM is the first attack of MS, it is termed a CIS. Following the observations that up to 70% of patients with CIS have clinically silent brain white matter lesions and that these lesions predict subsequently developing CD MS, several long-term follow-up studies on CIS cases were performed.[35,37,39,44] In 2009, Debette and colleagues[35] reported the outcomes of 170 patients presenting with an acute myelopathy (excluding traumatic and compressive spinal cord disease) after a median 73 months of follow-up. At initial diagnosis, 101 patients were diagnosed with myelopathy of undetermined cause and, at the end of the follow-up, 46 of these patients were diagnosed with clinically definite MS.[35] In retrospect, 73.3% of the 46 patients with CD MS fulfilled 2001 McDonald criteria and 80% had oligoclonal bands in their CSF at initial presentation. Those patients with acute myelopathies that were eventually diagnosed with MS were most frequently young women with a subacute course, predominantly sensory symptoms and mild functional impairment.[35]

Fisniku and colleagues[39] reported on the London cohort of 107 patients with CIS (optic neuritis [50%], brainstem syndrome [24%], and spinal cord syndrome [28%]) followed for 20 years. During follow-up, 67 of the 107 patients (63%) were diagnosed

---

Illustrative case #2

A 43-year-old self-employed man awoke with a feeling of stiffness and an inability to move his legs 3 years before being seen at our center. His physician obtained a chest radiograph and ordered blood testing but could not find an explanation. Although he was unable to walk for 2 weeks, he fully recovered within a month. One year following this, he developed pain and weakness in his left shoulder accompanied by prominent fatigue. His physician treated him for a shoulder strain and he slowly recovered. Nine months later, he awoke with a return of stiffness and weakness of his legs, and was unable to walk. He again experienced severe fatigue and was unable to empty his bladder or defecate. An emergency MRI revealed a single enhancing spinal cord lesion at T8. Neurologic examination after the MRI revealed bilateral lower extremity weakness and a T8 sensory level to pain. Despite intravenous (IV) methylprednisolone for 5 days, full recovery required a month.

Several months later, he again awoke with marked stiffness in his legs and an inability to walk accompanied by marked fatigue. Neurologic examination once more revealed bilateral weakness accompanied by increased tone in both lower extremities, accompanied by a T8 sensory level to pain. He was again admitted and treated with IV steroids. MRI of the thoracic spine, done while on steroids, failed to show the spinal cord lesion but 2 periventricular lesions were seen in his brain. A lumbar puncture performed that day revealed 10 lymphocytes/mm³ but the immunoglobulin G index was normal. He experienced no immediate response to treatment, but subsequently slowly improved with residual deficit. An MRI of the thoracic cord performed 1 month later, which again revealed an enhancing T8 lesion in his spinal cord. On referral to our center 6 weeks after onset of his last relapse, examination revealed a spastic paraparesis with a T10 sensory level (**Fig. 7**).

Comment: the patient likely had CIS at his first or second relapse. It would have been beneficial to the patient to obtain brain imaging at that point and, if CIS criteria were met, initiation of therapy would have been warranted.

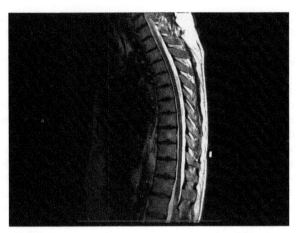

Fig. 7. TM, thoracic lesion.

with CD MS. There was a statistically significant difference in conversion rate depending on T2 lesions on brain MRI. Patients with CIS with brain lesions were more likely to develop CD MS (60 of 73 [82%]) and those without brain lesions (7 of 34 [21%]).[39] Of the patients with CIS with a spinal cord syndrome specifically, 17 out of 28 (61%) went on to develop CD MS.[39] In the patients with brain T2 lesion, on average, there was a 2-year period from CIS to CD MS diagnosis. In summary, it is clear that the likelihood of TM evolving into CD MS is at least as high as it is with optic neuritis and brainstem presentations and appropriate follow-up, both clinically and radiologically, is necesssay.[25,35–39,44,45]

Illustrative case #3

A 35-year-old woman awoke one Sunday morning unable to move her legs. Examination at a community hospital revealed frank paraplegia with only minor loss of pinprick extending below her costal margin and normal bowel and bladder function. MRI of the brain and spine did not reveal detectable abnormalities and CSF studies were reported as normal. No improvement was seen in response to IV methylprednisolone and she was discharged home as hysterical.

Reexamination at our center 2 months later revealed a paraplegic woman with a T10 motor level and a positive Beevor sign. Repeat imaging did not reveal brain or spinal cord abnormalities. One month after consultation, she developed urinary retention and was admitted to the hospital where she complained of visual impairment in her left eye, but no visual loss was found. A cervical MRI was interpreted as normal although a faint increase in T2 signal at C5 to C6 was questioned. No signal change was seen in her optic nerves. She had no clinical response to a further course of IV methylprednisolone. She returned to work, despite being wheelchair-bound, without improvement. She subsequently had recurrent episodes of pyelonephritis and complained of impaired upper extremity function and eventually stopped working. Ten years after onset, she was rereferred from a nursing home where she had been bedbound. However, she died of a fulminant infection 1 day before her appointment at our center. Her mother reluctantly agreed to necropsy, despite her conviction that her daughter had a psychiatric problem. At necropsy, classic changes of MS were found limited to the cervical and thoracic spinal cord.

Comment: although imaging at the outset of her illness failed to show abnormalities in the brain or spinal cord, a woman progressed to severe disability and death. A tissue diagnosis of MS was eventually established.

Lhermitte Sign

Lhermitte and colleagues[42] characterized the phenomenon of electrical current on neck flexion in his seminal report to the Neurologic Society of Paris in 1924, and since then has been termed Lhermitte sign. At that meeting he described a 43-year-old woman who, 1 month after onset of paresthesiae in her legs, experienced "a violent shock in the neck and a pain resembling an electric current which traveled the body from the neck to the feet." Her symptoms were recognized and accepted as a manifestation of MS on that occasion.

Illustrative case #4

A 31-year-old woman presents with 2 months of recurrent numbness and tingling in her right hand and both feet with associated painful dysesthetic sensations in her lower extremities. She later experienced what was described as an electric vibration in her legs when she flexed her neck. At consultation, examination revealed no abnormal findings and MRI showed multiple nonenhancing T2 bright white matter lesions in the cerebral hemispheres. Following the examination she was referred for cervical cord imaging, which revealed a single small enhancing lesion in the right posterior column at C4 to C5. Neurologic reexamination immediately following the study documented Lhermitte sign in the absence of other findings. Her symptoms abated without therapeutic intervention (**Figs. 8** and **9**).

Comment: a young woman presented with a classic presentation of Lhermitte phenomenon and it alerted neurologists. Note that patients' use of adjectives vary, with some describing the sensation as electrical, vibration, buzzing, or burning.

Useless Hand Syndrome

Oppenheim in 1911 postulated that a cervical cord lesion may account for the "sudden numbness and awkwardness of one arm in which the sense of posture was most seriously affected," and since then it has been referred to as the useless hand of Oppenheim.[43] Miller and colleagues[36] in1987 first reported 5 cases with a correlation between proprioceptive loss and the presence of ipsilateral cervical cord lesions visualized by MRI.

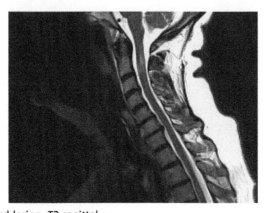

Fig. 8. Cervical cord lesion, T2 sagittal.

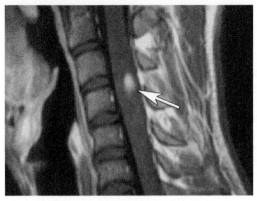

Fig. 9. Enhancing cervical cord lesion, post contrast sagittal.

Illustrative case #5

A 34-year-old woman with RR MS presented with relapse 8 months postpartum and 2 months after discontinuing breast feeding. Before her pregnancy she had experienced Lhermitte phenomenon and MRI showed 2 nonenhancing midcervical cord lesions. Ten days before presentation she developed painful dysesthesiae in her right ear, which moved down her neck to involve her right hand. She then became unable to manipulate buttons or write. However, it was only when she struck her face with a coffee cup that she sought consultation. Examination revealed a lack of arm swing, right arm drift, and pseudoathetoid movements of her right upper extremity. The patient was unable to reposition her hands without opening her eyes. A right sided C2 to C8 sensory level to pain was found with severe loss of position sense in the right upper extremity. MRI obtained 8 days later revealed an enhancing lesion within a larger area of increased T2 signal involving the right posterior column of the spinal cord opposite C1 and C2 (**Figs. 10** and **11**). Two smaller midcervical cord areas of increased T2 signal seen 2 months earlier, before initiating her interferon, did not enhance in either study. About 1 month after onset, without treatment, there was no subjective improvement, but clinical examination revealed improvement because she was able to detect the drift in her upper extremity and she was able to reposition without visual control. Position sense testing revealed only mild loss of position sense limited to her right hand; despite the improvement, she was still unable to write or type with her right hand.

Comment: this is a classic presentation of useless hand syndrome that has disabled an intelligent young woman. Although she preferred not to avail herself of treatment, she slowly improved.

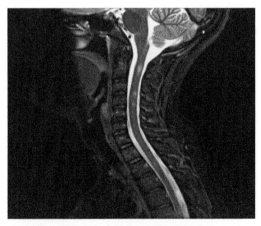

Fig. 10. C1 to C2 and smaller midcervical lesions, T2 sagittal.

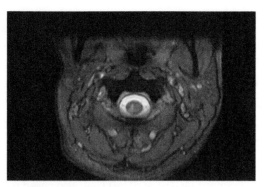

Fig. 11. Right cervical cord lesion, T2 axial.

Paroxysmal Tonic Spasms (Paroxysmal Dystonia)

Mathews[46] first described paroxysmal tonic seizures (spasms) in 1 or more limbs and their association with MS. Tonic spasms are usually brief events lasting seconds to minutes, often stimuli sensitive and at times subtle. As an alternative, the term paroxysmal dystonia may be used to describe them. Such spasms may, rarely, involve all 4 extremities as well as the truncal muscles and at times they may be prolonged and associated with pain. In NMO, the spasms are more striking and we reported them as the initial manifestation in some cases.[47,48] We have also seen the spasms in cases of human retrovirus–associated myelopathy (HAM/TSP).[31] Caution is advised, because, to the unaware, they may be regarded as evidence of a conversion reaction, especially in those patients in whom the spinal imaging may not reveal the site of spinal cord involvement. Paroxysmal tonic spasms respond well to low-dose carbamazepine, regardless of the primary disease.[47]

Illustrative case #6

A 19-year-old woman traveling with her mother arrived from England searching for her missing father. The patient presented for evaluation of new-onset gait ataxia. Examination did not reveal findings, but shortly afterwards she experienced numbness and weakness of her right arm. The patient was treated with corticotrophin and she responded well. Several months later, she developed recurrent painful tonic spasms lasting several minutes involving all 4 limbs as well as her truncal muscles. Despite their dramatic appearance and severity, the tonic spasms stopped within 48 hours of the initiation of carbamazepine at a dosage of 400 mg daily.

Comment: this is the first case that the author had seen and it was not recognized until a senior neurologist, who had studied with Mathews, immediately recognized the disorder and treated her.

THE TREATMENT OF MS
Management Goals

MS and its management has been a challenge since its original description (the management of TM is discussed in detail in elsewhere in this issue by Dr. Frohman). There are several important considerations related to early recognition of CIS as a predictor of CD MS. The major goal in the management of MS is to maintain the patients' functional independence by reducing the accumulation of disability. Once a diagnosis of MS is established, this is best accompanied by optimistically introducing disease-modifying therapy that can potentially reduce the risk of future relapse, and, more importantly, the risk of future disability. The promise of better tolerated, more convenient, and more effective therapy is an important element in the management of patients with MS.

Pharmacologic Strategies

There are 3 categories of treatment of MS: (1) management of acute relapses, (2) disease-modifying therapies, and (3) symptomatic treatments (**Box 1**).

Management of acute relapses

Exacerbations of MS abate spontaneously without pharmacologic intervention. However, abbreviating more severe attacks of MS by using drugs is an important option. Adrenocorticotrophic hormone (ACTH; ACTHAR Gel), also called corticotrophin, is the only validated treatment of relapses of MS that has been approved by the US Food and Drug Administration (FDA).[49] However, most neurologists prescribe either high-dose oral or high-dose IV steroids for exacerbations of MS. Major relapses associated with marked edema of the spinal cord, more typical of NMO, seem to respond rapidly to IV methylprednisolone (Solumedrol).[50] However, there are no adequate head-to-head studies of IV methylprednisolone compared with either ACTH or higher doses of oral steroids in MS. At times, patients with MS are on steroids chronically, but there is no scientific basis for this practice and there are many potential problems with their use. Side effects of steroid use include an increased risk of viral, bacterial, yeast, and fungal infection and parasitic infestation. Other complications of steroids include psychiatric problems, cataracts, osteoporosis, and ischemic necrosis of hips and other joints.[51]

There are some patients with MS with severe attacks that may be refractory to ACTH or steroids. In these patients, plasma exchange may be used. There was a randomized, double-blind clinical trial that was done to evaluate plasma exchange versus placebo in patients with acute CNS inflammatory demyelinating disease refractory to high-dose corticosteroids. There was a statistically significant difference and those in the treatment group were much improved compared with those in the placebo group (42.1% vs 5.9%).[52]

Disease-modifying therapy

In the last 2 decades several drugs have been approved for the management of MS (**Box 2, Table 2**). Interferon (IFN)-β-1b (Betaseron) was approved in the spring of 1993.[53,54] Soon after this, 3 additional drugs were approved: IFN-β-1a 30 μg weekly (Avonex) in 1996,[55,56] followed by glatiramer acetate (Copaxone) in 1997,[57,58] and a higher dosage form of IFN-β-1a (Rebif) in 2002.[59] Rebif was approved following a head-to-head comparison with Avonex (the EVidence for Interferon Dose-response: European North American Comparative Efficacy [EVIDENCE] study) that showed greater benefit for Rebif.[60] However, modest benefit of a similar degree was shown in all of the pivotal studies that led to marketing approval in the United States and Europe. A reduction in relapse rate of approximately 30% was obtained for each of the products. More importantly, a reduction of a sustained increase in disability for

---

Box 1
The 3 categories of MS management goals

1. Symptomatic management

2. Management of exacerbations of illness

3. Reducing the risk of exacerbation and increased disability

---

Box 2
FDA-approved disease-modifying treatments (DMT) for MS

- First line
  - Interferons
    - Interferon-β 1-a: Avonex
    - Interferon-β 1-b: Betaseron/Extavia
    - Interferon-β 1-a: Rebif
  - Glatiramer acetate: Copaxone
  - Fingolimod: Gilenya
- Second line
  - Natalizumab: Tysabri
  - Fingolimod: Gilenya
  - Mitoxantrone: Novantrone

Table 2
Symptomatic management

Symptoms	Treatment Options
Fatigue	1. Exercise 2. amantadine 100 mg 2 times daily 3. modafinil 100–400 mg daily
Weakness/ambulation	1. Physical therapy 2. dalfampridine
Spasticity	1. baclofen (oral or intrathecal) 2. tizanidine 3. clonazepam 4. dantrolene 5. gabapentin 6. botulinum toxin A
Paroxysmal symptoms	1. carbamazepine
Bladder/Erectile dysfunction	1. oxybutynin 2. intravesical botulinum toxin A 3. Intermittent catheterization
Sexual dysfunction	1. sildenafil 2. vardenafil 3. alprostadil
Mood and emotional issues	1. Therapy 2. Psychology/psychiatry 3. Antidepressants 4. Anxiolytics 5. Exercise
Pain	1. carbamazepine 2. phenytoin 3. gabapentin 4. amitriptyline 5. nortriptyline

6 months of 36% to 38% was also documented. The most attractive aspect of these medications is their long-term safety profile, established over the last 2 decades.

A recent National Institutes of Health (NIH)–sponsored trial (CombiRx [Combination Therapy in Patients With Relapsing-Remitting Multiple Sclerosis]) examining the combination of Avonex with Copaxone failed to show greater clinical effectiveness in combination, although greater efficacy in reducing the risk of new plaques was shown in MRI outcomes.[61]

The interferons and glatiramer were also studied in CIS. CIS is the first clinical presentation of RR MS and, as described earlier, usually consists of one of the following syndromes: unilateral optic neuritis, TM or a brainstem attack.[62] The trials included patients with CIS and an abnormal brain MRI, as these patients are likely to develop CD MS.[25,35,37,39] All CIS trials showed that treatment delayed both a second attack and MRI lesion activity.[63]

The Controlled High Risk Avonex in Multiple Sclerosis (CHAMPS) (Avonex) study showed that the patients on weekly intramuscular IFN-β-1-a had a 37% conversion to clinically definite MS versus 50% for those on placebo after 3 years.[64] The subcutaneous IFN-β-1a (Rebif) was studied in 2 trials, 1 with low-dose, once-weekly drug versus placebo for 2 years in Early Treatment of MS Study (ETOMS), which showed a conversion rate of 34% versus 45% in placebo.[65] The second trial for IFN β-1a, REbif FLEXible dosing in early MS (REFLEX), was multiarm, once-weekly high dose, 3-times-weekly high dose, or placebo, and showed that the 2-year cumulative probability of clinically definite MS was lower for both treated groups than for placebo.[66] The Betaseron in Newly Emerging MS for Initial Treatment (BENEFIT) trial also had a 50% conversion rate to CD MS in the placebo group and a 35% conversion in the treated group after 2 years.[67] Glatiramer acetate was studied in the Effect of glatiramer on conversion to clinically definite MS in patients with CIS (PRECISE) trial and showed a 35% conversion rate in the treated group versus 50% in the placebo group.[68]

Natalizumab (Tysabri) is a second-generation DMT for MS and is an IV drug that is given once every 4 weeks. It is a monoclonal antibody directed against the α-1-β-4-integrin, an adhesion molecule inhibitor that prevents activated T cells from crossing the blood brain-barrier.[69] In the clinical trial, natalizumab showed a 67% reduction in relapse rates over 2 years compared with placebo.[69] The drug was taken off the market after 3 cases of progressive multifocal leukoencephalopathy (PML) were discovered in 2005 and then reintroduced in 2006. The risk of developing PML while on natalizumab is increased if the patient was previously exposed to immunosuppressive therapy, if they are on drugs for over 24 months, or if the patient is JC virus antibody positive.[70,71] It is therefore crucial to inform patients who are, or will be, starting therapy of the risks and benefits and provide appropriate counseling regarding natalizumab and PML risk.[71]

Fingolimod (Gilenya) was the first oral agent approved by the FDA in 2010 for the treatment of RR MS based on its clinical and MRI efficacy shown in clinical trials.[72,73] Fingolimod is a modulator of sphingosine 1-phosphate (S1P) receptors (S1PR). The binding of the drug to $S1P_1$ on lymphocytes causes the internalization and degradation of the receptors. As a result, the receptors are depleted from the cell surface and lymphocytes cannot egress from lymph nodes into the circulation.[74] Fingolimod has been associated with adverse events such as bradycardia and atrioventricular block at treatment initiation, macular edema, hypertension, and increase in liver enzymes.[73] Dose-dependent reductions in peripheral blood lymphocyte counts after fingolimod treatment initiation have also been reported. The clinical trials reported an efficacy of 54% versus placebo,[72,73] however, it is not more effective than the injectable therapies in reducing the risk of sustained progression of disability. Other oral products are under review at the present time. Although oral drugs are more convenient, compliance with oral medications outside of monitored studies is poor.

Symptomatic treatment

The treatment of MS must also encompass symptomatic treatment. Symptomatic management not only includes the treatment of symptoms related to neurologic impairment but also includes the treatment of psychological issues such as anxiety and depression that are not covered in this article. There are a myriad of symptoms directly related to the MS disease; some include spasticity, disorders of gait, paroxysmal disorders, impairment of bladder, bowel, pain, and fatigue.

Fatigue is one of the most common and bothersome symptoms patients with MS face, often preventing them from attending to their families, careers, and education. It is estimated that up to 90% of patients with MS report fatigue at some point during their disease course.[75] Other confounders to the fatigue, such as lack of sleep and depression, must first be separated. Once those have been addressed, the fatigue may be treated with graded exercise, cooling therapies, and medications.[75] Medications that are used for fatigue include amantadine, modafinil, and armodafinil.

Bladder function is another common symptomatic issue that arises in patients with MS. The dysfunction produces symptoms of urgency, frequency, and urge incontinence and is present in up to 75% of patients with MS.[76] The dysfunction is caused by damage to the autonomic pathways. The bladder may be hypertonic, hypotonic, or both. The failure to store urine from a hypertonic bladder is caused by autonomic and corticospinal tract dysfunction from contraction of the detrusor muscle when the bladder is only partially full. This condition can be treated with anticholinergic medications, which block detrusor muscle contractions. If the cause is unclear and there may be components of both hypertonic and hypotonic bladder, there needs to be a urologic examination with formal urodynamic evaluation to characterize the problem. In the neurologist's office, a simple postvoid residual can be performed by performing an ultrasound after voiding; any amount more than 100 mL of urine is considered high and abnormal. These patients with large postvoid residual urine volumes are also at risk for urinary tract infections, which may cause of worsening of other MS symptoms. In late MS, the patient may need to perform intermittent catheterization, and a review on the subject by De Ridder and colleagues[77] recommends high fluid intake, increase mobility, use of silicone catheters, an adequate bowel program, and vitamin C and cranberry supplements. Nocturia is also a common issue in patients with MS that can be managed conservatively with limited fluids after a certain time, but, if needed, desmopressin may be used to block urine production. Patients on desmopressin must be monitored for hyponatremia.[78]

Motor weakness is common in MS, especially when there is spinal cord involvement. The weakness is upper motor neuron in nature and is associated with spasticity and hyperreflexia. Lower extremity weakness is one of the most feared complications for patients with MS, because this often leads to the use of a cane or wheelchair, which many patients see as a loss of independence. Physical therapy and combined exercise training is useful to patients when their walking is affected.[79] The consultation of a physiatrist is often helpful to determine whether any assistive device is needed and, if so, can help the patient be fitted for devices such as ankle-foot orthosis, canes, walkers, or wheelchairs.

Dalfampridine-SR (Ampyra) is now, after the completion of 2 clinical trials, approved to improve walking and walking speed in patients with MS.[18,80] The medication must be used with caution in patients with renal dysfunction and must be avoided in patients with a history of seizures.

Spasticity is a major issue that can interfere with many aspects of the life of a patient with MS life, not only walking. It can interfere with balance, sleep, dressing, and other activities of daily living. It usually affects the lower extremities more than the upper extremities and is part of the upper motor neuron symptoms that are commonly caused by spinal cord lesion burden. Spasticity is associated with stiffness, cramps, clonus, and, at times, painful spasms, and with proper therapy has been shown to improve quality of life.[81] Conservative measures are usually tried first for mild cases and include stretching and physical therapy. For more severe spasticity, medications are often needed. The most common medications used are baclofen, tizanidine, diazepam, gabapentin, and dantrolene.[81,82] In severe cases, an intrathecal baclofen pump is used to treat refractive spasticity.[81]

The paroxysmal disorders are a group of unusual manifestation occurring almost exclusively in MS. They include paroxysmal dystonia, paroxysmal akinesia, paroxysmal choreoathetosis, paroxysmal dysarthria, and brief pains, such as trigeminal neuralgia. They may occur in isolation or with other manifestations of MS. Of these, the most commonly recognized is paroxysmal dystonia, which, along with the other paroxysmal manifestations, is often misinterpreted as evidence of a conversion reaction, especially when it occurs early in the clinical course of MS. This alteration of limb posture is transient but recurring, affecting 1 or all of the limbs and lasting minutes to hours.[46,47] The trunk and limbs may rarely be involved and the picture may resemble tetanus. These episodes may be associated with severe pain. A small amount of carbamazepine works well in controlling the spasms.[47] Over the years we have seen many unfortunate patients receive inappropriate high doses of psychotropic medications without benefit for months.

SUMMARY/DISCUSSION

MS may present as an acute or subacute myelopathy. Of the population identified as TM, a large proportion is subsequently diagnosed with CD MS. Thus, keeping MS in the differential diagnosis of all patients recognized to have spinal cord disease is crucial. If the TM occurs in the absence of prior neurologic disease, it is termed a CIS. The importance of identifying CIS is that there is now overwhelming evidence that there is consistently better response to therapy at this stage of MS. Therapy at this stage has been proved to delay clinical attacks and decreases radiological burden of disease, which in turn may lessen future disability.

ACKNOWLEDGMENTS

Many thanks to Dr. Michael D. Norenberg, M.D. Professor, Department of Pathology, Biochemistry & Molecular Biology, Neurology, Neurosurgery, Member of the Neuroscience Program, and The Miami Project to Cure Paralysis (Affiliate Faculty) Director, Neuropathology and Neuropathology Research, for providing pathology slides.

REFERENCES

1. Compston A, Confavreux C, Lassmann H, et al, editors. McAlpine's multiple sclerosis. 4th edition. London: Churchill Livingston Elsevier; 2006.
2. Antel JP, editor. Multiple sclerosis, foreword. Neurol Clin, vol. 1. Philadelphia: WB Saunders; 1983.
3. Antel JP, editor. Multiple sclerosis. foreword. Neurol Clin, vol. 13. Philadelphia: WB Saunders; 1995. Number 1.

4. Weinshenker BG, Bass B, Rice GP, et al. The natural history of multiple sclerosis: a geographically based study. I. Clinical course and disability. Brain 1989;112(Pt 1): 133–46.

5. Thompson AJ, Polman CH, Miller DH, et al. Primary progressive multiple sclerosis. Brain 1997;120(Pt 6):1085–96.

6. Noseworthy JH, Lucchinetti C, Rodriguez M, et al. Multiple sclerosis. N Engl J Med 2000;343(13):938–52. http://dx.doi.org/10.1056/NEJM200009283431307.

7. Charcot JM. Lectures on the diseases of the nervous system delivered at La Salpêtrière. London: The New Sydenham Society; 1877 [Sigerson G, Trans.].

8. Cruveilhier J. Anatomie pathologique du corps humain. Paris: J. B. Bulleire; 1849. p. 1829–42.

9. Young IR, Hall AS, Pallis CA, et al. Nuclear magnetic resonance imaging of the brain in multiple sclerosis. Lancet 1981;2(8255):1063–6.

10. Poser CM, Presthus J, Hoersdal O. Clinical characteristics of autopsy-proved multiple sclerosis. Neurology 1966;16:791.

11. Kurtzke JF. Rating neurologic impairment in multiple sclerosis: an expanded disability status scale (EDSS). Neurology 1983;33(11):1444–52.

12. Lumsden C. The neuropathy of multiple sclerosis. In: Vincent P, Bruyn G, editors. Handbook of clinical neurology. New York: Elsevier; 1970. p. 277–305.

13. Powell HC, Lampert PW. Pathology of multiple sclerosis. Neurol Clin 1983;1: 631–44 WB Saunders, Philadelphia.

14. Lassmann H, Wekerle H. The pathology of multiple sclerosis. In: Compston A, Confavreux C, Lassmann H, et al, editors. McAlpine's multiple sclerosis. 4th edition. London: Churchill Livingston Elsevier; 2006. p. 567–99.

15. Trapp BD, Peterson J, Ransohoff RM, et al. Axonal transection in the lesions of multiple sclerosis. N Engl J Med 1998;338(5):278–85. http://dx.doi.org/10.1056/NEJM199801293380502.

16. Frohman EM, Wingerchuk DM. Clinical practice. Transverse myelitis. N Engl J Med 2010;363(6):564–72. http://dx.doi.org/10.1056/NEJMcp1001112.

17. Waxman SG. Membranes, myelin, and the pathophysiology of multiple sclerosis. N Engl J Med 1982;306(25):1529–33. http://dx.doi.org/10.1056/NEJM198206243062505.

18. Goodman AD, Brown TR, Edwards KR, et al. A phase 3 trial of extended release oral dalfampridine in multiple sclerosis. Ann Neurol 2010;68(4): 494–502. http://dx.doi.org/10.1002/ana.22240.

19. Schumacher GA, Beebe G, Kibler RF, et al. Problems of experimental trials of therapy in multiple sclerosis: report by the panel on the evaluation of experimental trials of therapy in multiple sclerosis. Ann N Y Acad Sci 1965;122: 552–68.

20. Poser CM, Paty DW, Scheinberg L, et al. New diagnostic criteria for multiple sclerosis: guidelines for research protocols. Ann Neurol 1983;13(3):227–31. http://dx.doi.org/10.1002/ana.410130302.

21. McDonald WI, Compston A, Edan G, et al. Recommended diagnostic criteria for multiple sclerosis: Guidelines from the international panel on the diagnosis of multiple sclerosis. Ann Neurol 2001;50(1):121–7.

22. Polman CH, Reingold SC, Edan G, et al. Diagnostic criteria for multiple sclerosis: 2005 revisions to the "McDonald criteria". Ann Neurol 2005;58(6):840–6. http://dx.doi.org/10.1002/ana.20703.

23. Polman CH, Reingold SC, Banwell B, et al. Diagnostic criteria for multiple sclerosis: 2010 revisions to the McDonald criteria. Ann Neurol 2011;69(2):292–302. http://dx.doi.org/10.1002/ana.22366.

24. Dale RC, de Sousa C, Chong WK, et al. Acute disseminated encephalomyelitis, multiphasic disseminated encephalomyelitis and multiple sclerosis in children. Brain 2000;123(Pt 12):2407–22.

25. de Seze J, Stojkovic T, Breteau G, et al. Acute myelopathies: clinical, laboratory and outcome profiles in 79 cases. Brain 2001;124(Pt 8):1509–21.

26. Wingerchuk DM, Lennon VA, Pittock SJ, et al. Revised diagnostic criteria for neuromyelitis optica. Neurology 2006;66(10):1485–9. http://dx.doi.org/10.1212/01.wnl.0000216139.44259.74.

27. Jacob A, Weinshenker BG, Violich I, et al. Treatment of neuromyelitis optica with rituximab retrospective analysis of 25 patients. Arch Neurol 2008;65:1443–8.

28. Bedi GS, Brown AD, Delgado SR, et al. Impact of rituximab on relapse rate and disability in neuromyelitis optica. Mult Scler 2011;17:1225–30.

29. Iannuzzi MC, Rybicki BA, Teinstein AS. Sarcoidosis. N Engl J Med 2007;357:2153–65.

30. Berger JR, Sheremata WA, Resnick L, et al. Multiple sclerosis like illness associated with human immunodeficiency virus infection. Neurology 1989;39:324–9.

31. Sheremata WA, Berger JR, Harrington W Jr, et al. Human lymphotropic (HTLV-1) associated myelopathy: a report of ten cases born in the United States. Arch Neurol 1992;49:1113–8.

32. Sheldon JJ, Siddarthan R, Tobias J, et al. MR imaging of multiple sclerosis: comparison with clinical, paraclinical, laboratory, and CT examinations. Am J Neuroradiol 1985;6:663–9.

33. Honig HS, Sheremata WA. Magnetic resonance imaging of spinal cord lesions in multiple sclerosis. J Neurol Neurosurg Psychiatry 1989;52:459–66.

34. Thorpe JW, Kidd D, Moseley IF, et al. Spinal MRI in patients with suspected multiple sclerosis and negative brain MRI. Brain 1996;119:709–14.

35. Debette S, de Seze J, Pruvo J-P, et al. Long-term outcome of acute and subacute myelopathies. J Neurol 2009;256:980–8.

36. Miller DH, McDonald WI, Blumhardt ID, et al. Magnetic resonance imaging in noncompressive spinal cord syndromes. Ann Neurol 1987;22:714–25.

37. O'Riordan JI, Thompson AJ, Kingsley DP, et al. The prognostic value of brain MRI in clinically isolated syndromes of the CNS. A 10-year follow-up. Brain 1998;121:495–505.

38. Brex PA, Ciccarelli O, O'Riordan R, et al. A longitudinal study of abnormalities on MRI and disability from multiple sclerosis. N Engl J Med 2002;346:158–64.

39. Fisniku LK, Brex PA, Altmann DR, et al. Disability and T2 MRI lesions: a 20 year follow-up of patients with relapse onset of multiple sclerosis. Brain 2008;131:808–17.

40. O'Connor P, Miller DH, Riester K, et al, International Natalizumab Trial Group. Relapse rates and enhancing lesions in a phase II trial of natalizumab in multiple sclerosis. Mult Scler 2005;11:565–72.

41. Scott TF, Frohman EM, De Seze J, et al. Evidence-based guideline: clinical evaluation and treatment of transverse myelitis: report of the therapeutic and technology assessment subcommittee of the American Academy of Neurology. Neurology 2011;77:2128–34.

42. Lhermitte J, Dollak I, Nicolas M. Les douleurs a type de decharge electrique consecutives a la flexion cephalique dans la sclerose en plaques. Rev Neurol 1924;31:56.

43. Coleman RJ, Russon L, Currie S. Useless hand of Oppenheim – magnetic resonance imaging findings. Postgrad Med J 1993;69:149–50.

44. Jacobs I, Kinkel DR, Kinkel WR. Silent brain lesions in patients with isolated idiopathic optic neuritis. A clinical and nuclear magnetic resonance imaging study. Arch Neurol 1986;43:452–5.
45. Ormerod IE, McDonald WI, de Boulay GH, et al. Disseminated lesions at presentation in patients with optic neuritis. J Neurol Neurosurg Psychiatry 1986;49:124–7.
46. Mathews WB. Tonic seizures in disseminated sclerosis. Brain 1958;81:193–206.
47. Usmani N, Bedi G, Lam BL, et al. Association between paroxysmal tonic spasms and neuromyelitis optica. Arch Neurol 2012;69:121–4.
48. Kim SM, Go MJ, Sung JJ, et al. Painful tonic spasm in neuromyelitis optica. Arch Neurol 2012;69(8):1026–31.
49. Rose AS, Kuzma JW, Kurtzke JF, et al. Cooperative study in the evaluation of therapy in multiple sclerosis. ACTH vs. placebo–final report. Neurology 1970;20(5):1–59.
50. Cree B. Neuromyelitis optica: diagnosis, pathogenesis and treatment. Curr Neurol Neurosci Rep 2008;8(5):427–33.
51. Stanbury RM, Graham EM. Systemic corticosteroid therapy–side effects and their management. Br J Ophthalmol 1998;82(6):704–8.
52. Weinshenker BG, O'Brien PC, Petterson TM, et al. A randomized trial of plasma exchange in acute central nervous system inflammatory demyelinating disease. Ann Neurol 1999;46(6):878–86.
53. The IFNB Multiple Sclerosis Study Group. Interferon beta-1b is effective in relapsing-remitting multiple sclerosis. 1. Clinical results of a multicenter, randomized, double-blind, placebo-controlled trial. Neurology 1993;43:655–61.
54. Paty DW, Li KD, UBC MS/MRI Group and the IFN Multiple Sclerosis Study Group. Interferon beta-1b is effective in relapsing-remitting multiple sclerosis. Neurology 1993;42:662–7.
55. Jacobs LD, Cookfair DL, Rudick RA, et al. Intramuscular interferon beta-1a for disease progression in relapsing multiple sclerosis. Ann Neurol 1996;39:285–94.
56. Rudick RA, Goodkin DE, Jacobs LD, et al. Impact of interferon beta-1a on neurologic disability in relapsing multiple sclerosis. Neurology 1997;49:358–63.
57. Johnson KP, Brooks BR, Cohen JA, et al. Copolymer 1 reduces relapse rate and improves disability in relapsing-remitting multiple sclerosis: results of a phase III multicenter, double-blind, placebo-controlled trial. Neurology 1995;45:1268–76.
58. Johnson KP, Brooks BR, Ford CC, et al. Sustained clinical benefits of glatiramer acetate in relapsing multiple sclerosis patients observed for 6 years. Mult Scler 2000;6:255–66.
59. PRISMS (Prevention of Relapses and Disability by Interferon b-1a Subcutaneously in Multiple Sclerosis) Study Group. Randomized double-blind placebo-controlled study of interferon b-1a in relapsing/remitting multiple sclerosis. Lancet 1998;352:1498–504.
60. Panitch H, Goodin DS, Francis G, et al. Randomized, comparative study of interferon β-1a treatment regimens in MS: the EVIDENCE Trial. Neurology 2002;59:1496–506.
61. Lublin F. AAN presentation of the CombiRx study. AAN abstract book. San Diego (CA); 2012.
62. Miller D, Barkhof F, Montalban X, et al. Clinically isolated syndromes suggestive of multiple sclerosis, part I: natural history, pathogenesis, diagnosis, and prognosis. Lancet Neurol 2005;4(5):281–8. http://dx.doi.org/10.1016/S1474-4422(05)70071-5.

63. Coyle PK. Early treatment of multiple sclerosis to prevent neurologic damage. Neurology 2008;71(Suppl 3):53–7.
64. Jacobs LD, Beck RW, Simon JH, et al. Intramuscular interferon beta-1a therapy initiated during a first demyelinating event in multiple sclerosis. CHAMPS study group. N Engl J Med 2000;343(13):898–904. http://dx.doi.org/10.1056/NEJM200009283431301.
65. Comi M, Filippi F, Barkhof L, et al, Hommes and the Early Treatment of MS Study Group. Effect of early interferon treatment on conversion to definite multiple sclerosis; a randomised study. Lancet 2001;357:1576–82.
66. Comi G, De Stefano N, Freedman MS, et al. Comparison of two dosing frequencies of subcutaneous interferon beta-1a in patients with a first clinical demyelinating event suggestive of multiple sclerosis (REFLEX): a phase 3 randomised controlled trial. Lancet Neurol 2012;11:33–41.
67. Kappos L, Polman CH, Freedman MS, et al, BENEFIT Study Group. Treatment with interferon beta-1b delays conversion to clinically definite and McDonald MS in patients with clinically isolated syndromes. Neurology 2006;67:1242–9.
68. Comi G, Martinelli V, Rodegher M, et al. Effect of glatiramer acetate on conversion to clinically definite multiple sclerosis in patients with clinically isolated syndrome (PreCISe study): a randomised, double-blind, placebo-controlled trial. Lancet 2009;374(9700):1503–11. http://dx.doi.org/10.1016/S0140-6736(09)61259-9.
69. Polman CH, O'Connor PW, Havrdova E, et al. A randomized, placebo-controlled trial of natalizumab for relapsing remitting multiple sclerosis. N Engl J Med 2006;334:899–910.
70. Bloomgren G, Richman S, Hotermans C, et al. Risk of natalizumab-associated progressive multifocal leukoencephalopathy. N Engl J Med 2012;366:1870–80.
71. Fox RJ, Rudick RA. Risk stratification and patient counseling in natalizumab in multiple sclerosis. Neurology 2012;78:436–7.
72. Cohen JA, Barkhof F, Comi G, et al. Oral fingolimod or intramuscular interferon for relapsing multiple sclerosis. N Engl J Med 2010;362(5):402–15. http://dx.doi.org/10.1056/NEJMoa0907839.
73. Kappos L, Radue EW, O'Connor P, et al. A placebo-controlled trial of oral fingolimod in relapsing multiple sclerosis. N Engl J Med 2010;362(5):387–401. http://dx.doi.org/10.1056/NEJMoa0909494.
74. Cohen JA, Chun J. Mechanisms of fingolimod's efficacy and adverse effects in multiple sclerosis. Ann Neurol 2011;69(5):759–77. http://dx.doi.org/10.1002/ana.22426.
75. Schwid SR, Covington M, Segal BM, et al. Fatigue in multiple sclerosis: current understanding and future directions. J Rehabil Res Dev 2002;39:211–24.
76. DasGupta R, Fowler CJ. Bladder, bowel and sexual dysfunction in multiple sclerosis: management strategies. Drugs 2003;63(2):153–66.
77. De Ridder D, Ost D, Van der Aa F, et al. Conservative bladder management in advanced multiple sclerosis. Mult Scler 2005;11(6):694–9.
78. Cvetkovic RS, Plosker GL. Desmopressin: in adults with nocturia. Drugs 2005;65(1):99–107 [discussion: 108–9].
79. Motl RW, Smith DC, Elliot J, et al. Combined training improves walking mobility in persons with significant disability from multiple sclerosis: a pilot study. J Neurol Phys Ther 2012;36:32–7.
80. Goodman AD, Brown TR, Krupp LB, et al. Sustained-release oral fampridine in multiple sclerosis: a randomised, double-blind, controlled trial. Lancet 2009;373(9665):732–8. http://dx.doi.org/10.1016/S0140-6736(09)60442-6.

81. Rizzo MA, Hadjimichael OC, Preiningerova J, et al. Prevalence and treatment of spasticity reported by multiple sclerosis patients. Mult Scler 2004;10(5):589–95.
82. Feldman RG, Kelly-Hayes M, Conomy JP, et al. Baclofen for spasticity in multiple sclerosis. Double-blind crossover and three-year study. Neurology 1978;28(11): 1094–8.

Transverse Myelitis

Shin C. Beh, MD[a], Benjamin M. Greenberg, MHS, MD[a],
Teresa Frohman, PA-C[a], Elliot M. Frohman, MD, PhD[a,b,*]

KEYWORDS

- Transverse myelitis • Longitudinally-extensive transverse myelitis • Multiple sclerosis
- Lupus myelopathy • Sjogren's myelopathy • Idiopathic transverse myelitis

KEY POINTS

- Transverse myelitis (TM) constitutes a pathobiologically heterogeneous syndrome that has significant neurologic implications and requires urgent attention.
- Magnetic resonance imaging (MRI) evaluation of the entire spinal cord axis is mandatory in all myelopathic patients.
- The length of the spinal cord lesion on MRI is an important discriminator with etiologic and prognostic significance; longitudinally extensive transverse myelitis (LETM) refers to lesions that extend over 3 or more vertebral segments.
- Early and timely identification and immunotherapy are critical to minimize, or even prevent, future disability.
- The long-term management should focus on neurorehabilitation and a multidisciplinary approach aimed at managing the various complications of spinal cord damage.

INTRODUCTION

Acute noncompressive myelopathies have been recognized since the nineteenth century.[1] The terms myelitis and myelopathy are often used interchangeably, but have different connotations. Both suggest a lesion affecting the spinal cord. Whereas myelopathy is a broad, generic term (much like neuropathy or encephalopathy) that

Disclosures & Conflicts of Interest: Dr Beh is the recipient of the Biogen Idec Clinical MS Fellowship award. Dr Greenberg has received honoraria from EMD Serono, American Academy of Neurology, Multiple Sclerosis Association of America, and National Multiple Sclerosis Society; consulting fees from Acorda, DioGenix, and Greater Good Foundation; and grants from Amplimmune, Accelerated Cure Project, and Guthy Jackson Charitable Foundation. Teresa Frohman is a consultant and speaker for Biogen Idec and Novartis. Dr Frohman has received speaker fees from Biogen Idec, Teva Neuroscience, and Acorda Pharmaceuticals, and consulting fees from Biogen Idec, Teva Neurosciences, Abbott, Acorda Therapeutics, and Novartis.
[a] Department of Neurology and Neurotherapeutics, University of Texas Southwestern Medical Center, 5323, Harry Hines Blvd, Dallas, TX 75390, USA; [b] Department of Ophthalmology, University of Texas Southwestern Medical Center, 5323, Harry Hines Blvd, Dallas, TX 75390, USA
* Corresponding author. Multiple Sclerosis Clinical Care Center, UT Southwestern Medical Center, 5323 Harry Hines Boulevard, Dallas, TX 75235.
E-mail address: elliot.frohman@utsouthwestern.edu

does not imply any particular etiology, myelitis refers to an inflammatory disease process.

Transverse myelitis (TM) includes a pathobiologically heterogeneous syndrome characterized by acute or subacute spinal cord dysfunction resulting in paresis, a sensory level, and autonomic (bladder, bowel, and sexual) impairment below the level of the lesion.[2,3] Etiologies for TM can be broadly classified as parainfectious, paraneoplastic, drug/toxin-induced, systemic autoimmune disorders (SAIDs), and acquired demyelinating diseases like multiple sclerosis (MS) or neuromyelitis optica (NMO).[3–6] Patients with isolated TM present a diagnostic dilemma, as it is common in both MS and NMO, but may also be the initial manifestation of SAIDs. Also, there are noninflammatory etiologies (eg, vascular, metabolic) that may mimic the clinical and radiologic appearance of TM. Further complicating the diagnostic process is the frequent coexistence of systemic autoantibodies in NMO and, sometimes, MS. The implications of an incorrect diagnosis can be severe, as treatment may not only be ineffective, but may exacerbate the underlying disease process. The cause of TM remains unknown despite an extensive workup in about 15% to 30%[4] of patients and is therefore referred to as "idiopathic" according to set criteria.[7] **Box 1** explains important terms related to TM.

The annual incidence of TM ranges from 1.34 to 4.60 cases per million,[8–10] but increases to 24.6 cases per million if acquired demyelinating diseases like MS are included.[11] TM can occur at any age, although a bimodal peak in incidence occurs in the second and fourth decades of life.[8–10,12] Half of patients have an antecedent infection.[10]

Case report

A 30-year-old white woman presents with 3 days of progressive paraparesis, constipation, and urinary incontinence. In addition, she reports a feeling a circumferential tightness around her abdomen (as though she was wearing a corset). Examination revealed spasticity, hyperreflexia with up-going plantar reflexes, and muscle strength of 3 in her lower extremities. Anal tone was decreased. A T8 sensory level was detected. Spine MRI revealed a T2/fluid-attenuated inversion recovery (FLAIR) hyperintense signal with associated contrast enhancement and cord swelling from T2 to 7 vertebral segments. What are the next steps in managing this patient?

CLINICAL PRESENTATION

It is important to consider the age and gender of the patient when evaluating myelopathic patients. Older patients (older than 50 years) are more likely to suffer spinal cord infarction. Female patients are at higher risk of having TM. Demographic features are otherwise not particularly useful in distinguishing the etiologic causes of myelopathy.[13]

The temporal profile of the myelopathic features must be elucidated. TM typically has an acute to subacute onset, with neurologic deficits reaching a nadir within a few weeks. An apoplectic onset with deficits reaching the nadir in less than 4 hours indicates a vascular event. An insidious, progressive course in which the deficits continue to worsen beyond 4 weeks is uncharacteristic of TM. Clinically, TM may present as one of several syndromes of the spinal cord. Acute complete TM (ACTM) manifests as paresis/plegia, sensory dysfunction (characterized by numbness, paresthesias, or other manifestations in conjunction with a sensory level), and autonomic impairment below the level of the lesion. Acute partial TM (APTM) results in asymmetric manifestations or deficits specific to particular anatomic tracts; manifestations include the

---

Box 1
Nosology of transverse myelitis

Myelopathy: a broad, generic term referring to a lesion affecting the spinal cord

Myelitis: refers to an inflammatory disease of the spinal cord

Transverse myelitis (TM): classically describes a pathobiologically heterogeneous syndrome characterized by acute or subacute spinal cord dysfunction resulting in paresis, a sensory level, and autonomic impairment below the level of the lesion

Acute Complete TM (ACTM): TM causing paresis of the lower and/or upper extremities, sensory dysfunction (characterized by a sensory level), and autonomic impairment below the level of the lesion. On magnetic resonance imaging (MRI), there is typically a single lesion spanning 1 or 2 vertebral segments; on axial sections, there is either full-thickness involvement, or the central portion of the spinal cord is maximally affected.

Acute Partial TM (APTM): TM causing asymmetric neurologic impairment (localizable to the spinal cord) or deficits attributable to a specific anatomic tract. On MRI, it spans 1 or 2 vertebral segments; there is involvement of a small portion of the spinal cord on axial sections.

Longitudinally-Extensive TM (LETM): a spinal cord lesion that extends over 3 or more vertebral segments on MRI. On axial sections, it typically involves the center of the cord over more than two-thirds of the spinal cord area.

Secondary TM: TM related to a systemic inflammatory autoimmune disorder (eg, lupus, Sjögren syndrome, sarcoidosis). It is typically an ACTM.

Idiopathic TM: TM without any clear etiology despite a thorough investigation. It should meet the criteria listed in **Table 8.**

---

hemi-cord (Brown-Sequard), central cord, or posterior column syndrome, as well as selective tract impairment. **Table 1** describes these syndromes. Distinguishing ACTM and APTM has etiologic and prognostic significance, as discussed later.

Acutely, limb tone and muscle stretch reflexes may be diminished and even absent ("spinal shock syndrome") leading to possible diagnostic confusion with Guillain-Barre syndrome (GBS). Clinically, spinal shock may persist for days to weeks, with a mean duration of 4 to 6 weeks following an insult.[14] Over time, spasticity, hyper-reflexia, and extensor plantar responses (ie, classic features of the upper motor neuron [UMN] syndrome) become evident.

Sensory symptoms (both positive and negative) are common in TM. Some patients report a circumferential band of dysesthesia, attributable to the dermatomes just rostral to the sensory level, around their trunk. In some cases, this may be associated with a constricting sensation (colloquially referred to as the "MS hug") that ranges from mild discomfort to a severe spasmodic or burning pain. In the authors' experience, this symptom may be so distressing that it may be more appropriately called the "anaconda squeeze"! TM-related pain may be a central, deep aching pain or radicular in nature.[3] Exacerbation of spinal pain with recumbency may indicate a neoplastic lesion involving the spinal cord.[15] Phantom limb phenomenon has been observed.[16] Lhermitte phenomenon (paresthesia traveling down the limbs and trunk with neck flexion) suggests an intrinsic cervical spinal cord lesion, typically affecting the dorsal columns. A reverse Lhermitte phenomenon (paresthesia with neck extension) usually indicates a compressive extra-axial cervical lesion.[17] Inverse Lhermitte phenomenon (paresthesia traveling upward) is another reported variation.[18]

Autonomic dysfunction is almost always present in the form of perturbations of bladder, sexual, gastrointestinal, cardiovascular, and thermoregulatory functions. Priapism is a rare acute manifestation.[19,20] These features are discussed later.

Table 1		
Spinal cord syndromes		
Syndrome	**Tracts Involved**	**Clinical Manifestations**
Complete transverse myelitis	All	Paresis, sensory loss, and autonomic impairment below the level of the lesion
Hemicord (Brown-Sequard)	Ipsilateral corticospinal; Ipsilateral dorsal columns; contralateral spinothalamic	Ipsilateral paresis and impaired dorsal column sensation; contralateral pain and temperature loss
Dorsal column	Bilateral dorsal columns	Bilateral loss of vibratory and proprioceptive sensation; Lhermitte phenomenon
Subacute Combined Degeneration	Bilateral dorsal columns and corticospinal tracts	Bilateral dorsal column dysfunction; paresis and upper motor neuron signs below the level of the lesion
Central cord	Crossing spinothalamic fibers, and corticospinal tracts	Dissociated sensory loss (diminished pain and temperature with normal dorsal column function) in a shawl-like pattern. Saddle-sparing sensory loss. Upper motor neuron weakness below the level of the lesion.
Conus medullaris	Sacral autonomic fibers	Early and prominent sphincter and sexual impairment; saddle pattern sensory loss; mild weakness
Tract-specific dysfunction		Depending on involved tract

Certain clinical signs can aid in localizing the level of the lesion and are described in **Table 2**.

The list of differential diagnoses of TM is long; hence, a meticulous history and detailed physical examination are indispensible. A systematic and careful history may help exclude other mimics of TM (these are discussed in **Box 2**). An antecedent infection or prior vaccination may implicate acute disseminated encephalomyelitis (ADEM) or parainfectious TM. Travel abroad may indicate more exotic infectious causes of TM, such as schistosomiasis. Risk factors for or concomitant existence of malignancy may implicate a paraneoplastic etiology.

Women of reproductive age are at higher risk of acquired demyelinating diseases and SAIDs with the exception of Behcet disease (BD) and ankylosing spondylitis (AS). A history of relapsing-remitting attacks of neurologic deficits, eg, acute optic neuritis (AON) or internuclear ophthalmoparesis (INO), would suggest MS. Uhthoff phenomenon (discussed later) may be present in demyelinating diseases. A thorough neurologic examination may reveal evidence of prior neurologic impairments suggestive of MS exacerbations disseminated in time and space. NMO usually causes attacks of severe AON (sometimes bilateral) and brainstem lesions resulting in intractable nausea, vomiting, or hiccups.[21–24] Although the manifestations of NMO may be similar to MS, attacks are typically more devastating.[25] In cases of NMO mistakenly diagnosed as MS, treatment with interferon beta-1a would dramatically increase attacks.[26]

Autoimmune disorders, in particular systemic lupus erythematosus (SLE), BD, AS, Sjögren's syndrome (SS), and antiphospholipid syndrome (APS), are known causes of TM. In some, TM may be the initial clinical manifestation of such a disorder. Fatigue

Table 2
Clinical signs with useful localizing value in myelopathic patients

Clinical Sign	Description	References
Beevor sign	Describes the upward migration of the umbilicus during the act of sitting up from supine position owing to weakness of the lower half of the rectus abdominis (because the upper rectus segments pull in a direction opposite of the lower segments, the movement of the abdomen is upward). In some cases, downward migration of the umbilicus may be observed. This sign indicates a lesion at the level of the T10–12 spinal cord and/or roots.	[22]
Superficial abdominal reflexes	A lesion above T6 segmental cord level will abolish all superficial abdominal reflexes. A lesion at or below T10 spares the upper and middle abdominal reflexes. All the reflexes are present with a lesion below T12.	[23]
Cremasteric reflex	Lost in lesions at or above L2 segmental cord level.	[23]
Bulbocavernous reflex	Mediated by S2–4 nerve roots; hence, is abolished in lesions above S2 segmental cord level.	[24]
Anal wink reflex	Mediated by S2–4 nerve roots; hence, is abolished in lesions above S2 segmental cord level	[24]

Box 2
Red flags arguing against TM in myelopathic patients

1. Apoplectic onset (reaching the nadir less than 4 hours from onset).

2. Insidious progressive course.

3. Older age of onset.

4. Preceding trauma, pain, and/or vertebral tenderness would suggest traumatic myelopathy.

5. Vascular instrumentation (in particular, aortic and cardiac surgery) or maneuvers that increase intra-abdominal pressure (eg, weight-lifting or straining) before the acute/subacute appearance of myelopathic features may implicate spinal cord infarction.

6. Prior bariatric surgical procedures, malabsorption syndromes, dietary restrictions, malnutrition, use of zinc supplements, excessive use of zinc-containing denture cream, alcoholism, and/or drug/toxin exposure may implicate a metabolic or toxic etiology.

7. Prior radiation therapy.

8. Immunocompromised state (HIV/AIDS or immunosuppressive therapy).

9. Features of infection: fever, meningismus, rash, leukocytosis, burning dermatomal pain.

10. Paralysis with dissociated sensory loss (loss of pinprick and temperature but preserved dorsal column function) indicates an anterior spinal artery infarction.

11. The exacerbation of spinal pain with recumbency suggests malignancy.

12. Foix-Alajouanine syndrome (congestive venous myelopathy) is characterized by exacerbation of myelopathic features with exercise and relief with rest.

and constitutional complaints are common in patients with autoimmune disorders. A thorough integumentary examination may offer valuable clinical signs. Systemic (eg, renal, cardiac) and nonmyelopathic neurologic manifestations (eg, mononeuritis multiplex, myositis, cerebellar ataxia) may occur in some SAIDs. The presence of peripheral nervous system deficits rules out MS and NMO, unless there are concomitant disorders in the same patient (eg, diabetic peripheral neuropathy). **Table 3** describes some salient manifestations of selected systemic autoimmune disorders.

EVALUATION AND DIAGNOSIS

Magnetic resonance imaging (MRI) of the complete spinal axis is mandatory in any patient with myelopathic features to exclude structural lesions, particularly those amenable to emergent neurosurgical intervention. The spinal cord cephalad to the suspected level of the lesion should always be imaged owing to possibly misleading signs, eg, paraparesis attributable to cervical lesions. The most sensitive MRI sequence for detecting spinal cord lesions (especially MS plaques) are short-tau inversion recovery (STIR) fast spin-echo and T2-weighted fast spin-echo sequences.[27,28]

The location and length of the cord lesion on MRI may also provide clues about the underlying disease. Based on clinical and radiologic data, TM can first be dichotomized into longitudinally limited and longitudinally extensive TM (LETM). Longitudinally limited TM can be further classified as ACTM or APTM. ACTM and APTM span 1 or 2 vertebral segments. ACTM causes a complete spinal cord syndrome; on axial sections, there is either full-thickness involvement, or the central portion of the spinal cord is maximally affected.[29] APTM results in asymmetric spinal cord involvement or neurologic deficits attributable to a specific anatomic tract; on axial sections, there is involvement of a portion of the spinal cord. Patients with APTM are at increased risk of recurrence and transition to MS.[13,29,30] Conversely, ACTM carries a lower risk of transition to clinically definite multiple sclerosis (CDMS) and is usually related to other

Table 3 Systemic manifestations of autoimmune disorders	
Disorder	**Clinical Sign/Symptom**
Sjögren syndrome	Xerophthalmia, xerostomia, parotid gland enlargement, Raynaud phenomenon, dysphagia, and dry cough (owing to xerotrachea). A positive Schirmer test detects deficient tear production.
Systemic lupus erythematosus	Joint pains, morning stiffness, myalgias, and integumentary manifestations (alopecia, unguium mutilans, perniotic lesions, leuconychia, splinter hemorrhages, nail-fold hyperkeratosis, ragged cuticles, malar rash, Raynaud phenomenon, photosensitivity, and/or discoid lupus).
Antiphospholipid syndrome	History of deep vein thromboses, pulmonary embolism, multiple miscarriages, and/or young-onset stroke.
Behcet disease	Classic triad of recurrent aphthous ulcers, genital ulcers, and uveitis. Other manifestations: ophthalmic (hypopyon and retinal vasculitis) and cutaneous (pseudofolliculitis, erythema nodosumlike lesions, or acneiform lesions). Positive pathergy test.
Ankylosing spondylitis	Back pain, enthesitis, and limited spinal flexion.

causes (eg, SAIDs). LETM refers to lesions that extend over 3 or more vertebral segments; on axial sections, it typically involves more than two-thirds of the spinal cord thickness (maximally affecting the central portion).[3,29] **Box 3** summarizes the differential diagnoses of LETM. The unique radiologic features of different etiologies are explored later.

A brain MRI with and without gadolinium administration should also be obtained on all patients to look for evidence of concomitant or prior lesions that may provide clues about the etiology. The presence of MS-like brain lesions in patients with partial TM portends an 80% risk of transition to clinically definite MS at 3 to 5 years.[13]

Serum vitamin B12 level, thyroid function tests, syphilis, and HIV serologies *always* should be obtained to evaluate for potentially treatable causes of myelopathy. Vitamin E, serum copper, and ceruloplasmin levels are checked in those at risk of deficiency (see later in this article for further details). Serum aquaporin-4–specific autoantibodies (NMO-immunoglobulin [Ig]G) should be checked on all patients with TM because of its high specificity for NMO or NMO spectrum disorders (NMOSD).[31,32] NMO-IgG seropositivity is rarely found in patients with APTM[30] but its presence would have profound implications on treatment. Inflammatory markers (please see **Box 4**) should be checked if SAID is suspected. In suspected parainfectious TM, serologic evidence of recent infection (eg, *Mycoplasma* antibody titers) should be sought. Serum paraneoplastic profiles should be performed in suspected cases of paraneoplastic TM; additionally, in such cases, appropriate investigations should be undertaken to search for the occult malignancy, the identification of which can have profound ramifications for the patient; even a cure if a malignancy can be confirmed and eradicated before pathologic dissemination.

Cerebrospinal fluid (CSF) analysis is essential in the evaluation of TM. CSF cell count, differential, protein, glucose, oligoclonal bands (OCBs) and IgG index should be checked on all patients with TM. Isoelectric focusing is the superior method for the detection of OCBs, providing a much higher yield and specificity.[33] OCBs are useful in predicting conversion to MS, as OCBs are present in 85% to 90% of patients

---

Box 3
Differential diagnosis of LETM

1. Neuromyelitis optica (NMO) or NMO-spectrum disorders

2. Acute disseminated encephalomyelitis (ADEM)

3. Systemic autoimmune disorders: systemic lupus erythematosus (SLE), Sjögren syndrome (SS), neurosarcoidosis, neuro-Behcet disease

4. Parainfectious TM: *Borrelia burgdorferi, Chlamydia psittaci,* mumps virus, cytomegalovirus, coxsackie virus, *Mycobacterium tuberculosis, Mycoplasma pneumoniae,* enterovirus 71, hepatitis C virus, *Brucella melitensis,* Epstein-Barr virus, echovirus type 30, *Ascaris suum, Toxocara canis,* and *Schistosoma* species.

5. Paraneoplastic TM (in particular, anti-collapsin response-mediator protein [CRMP]-5 antibodies)

6. Mimics of TM

   a. Neoplasms: primary intramedullary spinal cord tumors, metastatic intramedullary tumors, lymphoma

   b. Radiation myelitis

   c. Metabolic myelopathies: B12 deficiency, copper deficiency, nitrous oxide toxicity

   d. Vascular myelopathies: anterior spinal artery infarction, spinal dural arteriovenous fistula

---

Box 4
Investigations into suspected TM

Must be obtained on all patients:

1. Magnetic resonance image (MRI) of the spine

2. Brain MRI

3. Cerebrospinal fluid (CSF): cells, differential, protein, glucose, Venereal Disease Research Laboratory (VDRL), immunoglobulin (Ig)G index, oligoclonal bands, cytologic analysis

4. Serum: B12, methylmalonic acid, HIV antibodies, syphilis serologies, thyroid stimulating hormone (TSH), Free T4, 25-hydroxyvitamin D

Must be obtained on all patients with LETM:

1. Serum NMO-IgG

2. Serum erythrocyte sedimentation rate, C-reactive protein, antinuclear antibodies, antibodies to extractable nuclear antigen, rheumatoid factor, antiphospholipid antibodies, and anti-neutrophil cytoplasmic antibodies (ANCA)

3. Visual-evoked potentials

May need to be obtained:

1. Neuro-ophthalmological evaluation

2. Paraneoplastic panel

3. Infectious serologies and CSF studies (cultures and viral polymerase chain reaction)

4. Serum copper and ceruloplasmin

5. Serum vitamin E level

6. Computed tomography of the chest

7. Nerve conduction studies and electromyography

8. Minor salivary gland biopsy

---

with MS, in 20% to 30% of patients with NMO or SAIDs, and rarely in other causes of TM.[13] Bear in mind that their mere presence clearly does not militate against being reflective of a myriad of inflammatory, infectious, and neoplastic or paraneoplastic processes.

A neuro-ophthalmological evaluation is warranted to look for ophthalmic manifestations that may provide valuable diagnostic clues, especially when radiologic and laboratory investigations are unremarkable. For example, different subtypes of uveitis are associated with unique etiologic underpinnings.[34] Demyelinating diseases affecting the brainstem and/or cerebellum commonly cause ocular motor manifestations.[35]

Electrophysiologic tests may be very useful in assessing patients with TM. Nerve conduction studies and electromyography (EMG) may reveal and help characterize any peripheral nervous pathology, the exclusion of which would lend compelling support for a spinal cord process. This latter principle is especially salient in that acute TM can present as a spinal shock variant, one that may mimic a polyneuropathic process like GBS. In early TM, F-waves may be absent,[36] an observation that can serve to misguide even the most experienced neurologic consultant (especially when the MRI is unremarkable) to localize the disease process to the peripheral nervous system. EMG-evidence of anterior horn cell dysfunction may portend a poor prognosis for recovery.[37] Somatosensory evoked potentials may offer evidence of a myelopathy in the presence of a normal spinal cord MRI. In addition, conventional and multifocal visual-evoked potentials (VEP) may provide evidence of subclinical demyelination along the afferent visual pathways not clearly identified on imaging. Evidence of such disruption may support the diagnosis of MS or NMO but are by no means specific for these disease entities (discussed in greater detail later).

A list of investigations into TM is provided in **Box 4**.

CAUSES OF TM

Box 5 summarizes the causes of TM.

Multiple Sclerosis

MS is a disabling progressive neurologic disorder affecting approximately 400,000 people in the United States.[38] First attacks of MS, called clinically isolated syndrome (CIS), usually consist of AON, brainstem syndromes, or APTM. The probability for APTM to transition to CDMS ranges from 10% to 62%.[30,39–43] APTM may be a CIS with a higher risk of conversion to MS.[43]

TM in MS most commonly presents with sensory phenomena. Spine MRI typically reveals an asymmetrically placed lesion (usually occurring in the posterolateral or lateral portion of the spinal cord) less than 2 segments in length (ie, APTM) with a predilection for the cervicothoracic cord.[3,30,39,42,43]

The most important investigation that helps determine the risk of conversion to CDMS is the brain MRI. If it is normal, only 10% of patients with APTM will develop CDMS at 61 months[30]; this increases to 21% risk of progression at 20 years follow-up according to another study of CIS.[44] White matter lesions predict higher risk of conversion to MS (with rates of up to 88% reported).[43,44] If the lesions meet at least 3 of the Barkhof criteria[45] this risk is increased substantially.[43]

Another important factor that helps predict the risk of transition to CDMS is CSF OCBs. In the setting of TM, OCBs have been shown to have a robust predictive value of for predicting conversion to MS.[43,46–48] In patients with TM with normal brain MRIs, the presence of OCBs and/or an elevated IgG index portends a higher risk of developing MS.[49] The risk of developing MS is less than 10% with a normal brain MRI and CSF findings.[43]

Longitudinally extensive lesions in the context of TM is actually quite rare in MS and, when present, is significantly shorter than those seen in NMO. When MS is confirmed, spinal lesions tend to favor a cervical localization, and tend to have less cord swelling and gadolinium-enhancement.[50] In general, patients with LETM have been shown to have a conspicuously low risk of developing MS.[30]

Neuromyelitis Optica

NMO is diagnosed on the basis of the revised Wingerchuk criteria[51] requiring the presence of optic neuritis and TM as well as 2 of 3 of the following: NMO antibodies, LETM, and/or brain MRI lesions inconsistent with MS. NMOSDs include Asian optic-spinal MS, recurrent LETM, recurrent AON, and AON or TM in the context of certain organ-specific and non–organ-specific autoimmune disease. The article on NMO by Sahraian, MA, elsewhere in this issue discusses this disease in detail. Here, we underscore the important features of NMO that give rise to diagnostic confusion.

Diagnostic confusion may arise with SAIDs, as patients with NMO/NMOSD often have accompanying autoimmune diseases and multiple non–organ-specific autoantibodies. Autoimmune diseases observed to coexist with NMO include SS, SLE, autoimmune thyroid disease, type 1 diabetes mellitus, ulcerative colitis, idiopathic

Box 5
Summary of reported causes of TM

1. Acquired demyelinating disorders
   a. Multiple sclerosis
   b. NMO
   c. ADEM
2. Systemic inflammatory autoimmune disorders
   a. SLE
   b. SS
   c. Antiphospholipid syndrome
   d. Behcet disease
   e. Vogt-Koyanagi Harada disease
   f. Ankylosing spondylitis
   g. Mixed connective tissue disease
   h. Others: systemic sclerosis, anti-Jo-1 antibody, urticarial vasculitis, psoriatic arthritis, perinuclear ANCA systemic vasculitis, graft-versus-host disease, common variable immunodeficiency, celiac disease
3. Neurosarcoidosis
4. Parainfectious TM
   a. Viral: hepatitis A, hepatitis B, hepatitis C, hepatitis E, measles, mumps, rubella, varicella zoster, Epstein-Barr, cytomegalovirus, herpes simplex, influenza A/B, lymphocytic choriomeningitis virus, chikungunya, Hanta virus, HIV, human T-cell lymphotropic virus, human herpes virus 6, Japanese encephalitis, Murray Valley encephalitis, St Louis encephalitis, tick-borne encephalitis, vaccinia, Rocky Mountain spotted fever, dengue virus, enterovirus 71, coxsackievirus A and B, West Nile virus, parvovirus B19, human corona virus, and echovirus
   b. Bacterial: *Mycoplasma pneumoniae, Campylobacter jejuni, Borrelia burgdorferi, Acinetobacter baumanii, Coxiella burnetii, Bartonella henselae, Chlamydia psittaci, Leptospira, Chlamydia pneumoniae, Legionella pneumonia, Orientia tsutsugamushi* (scrub typhus), *Salmonella* paratyphi B, *Mycobacterium tuberculosis, Treponema pallidum, Brucellosis melitensis*, and groups A and B streptococci
   c. Fungal: *Actinomyces, Blastomyces, Coccidioides, Aspergillus, Cryptococcus*, and *Cladophialophora bantiana*
   d. Parasitic: *Toxocara* species, *Schistosoma* species, *Gnasthostoma spinigerum, Echinococcus granulosus, Taenia solium, Toxoplasma gondii, Acanthamoeba* species, *Paragonimus westermani*, and *Trypanosoma brucei*
5. Paraneoplastic syndromes
   a. Anti-Ri (ANNA-2) antibody
   b. CRMP-5-IgG antibody
   c. Anti-amphiphysin IgG antibody
   d. Anti-GAD65 antibody
   e. NMDAR antibody
6. Atopic myelitis
7. Drugs and toxins
   a. Tumor necrosis factor-alpha inhibitors

b. Sulfasalazine

c. Epidural anesthesia

d. Chemotherapeutic agents: gemcitabine, cytarabine, cisplatin

e. Heroin

f. Benzene

g. Brown recluse spider toxin

8. Idiopathic TM

thrombocytopenic purpura, myasthenia gravis, rheumatoid arthritis, polymyositis, celiac disease, and Raynaud phenomenon.[52,53]

We propose that all patients with a known SAID (eg, SS or SLE) who present with TM undergo serologic testing for NMO-IgG. The high specificity of NMO-IgG seropositivity[31,54] will establish the additional diagnosis of NMO coexisting with the systemic autoimmune disorder. In patients with NMO or TM, the isolated presence of systemic non–organ-specific antibodies should not be used to make a diagnosis of any particular rheumatic disease; instead, these assays can lend support in corroborating such conditions, when the established clinical criteria for each respective disorder has been fulfilled.

Sjögren Syndrome

SS is a chronic, protean, progressive, systemic autoimmune disorder characterized by mononuclear infiltration and destruction of the salivary and lacrimal glands, leading to keratoconjunctivitis sicca, typically affecting middle-aged to elderly women. SS may appear alone (primary SS) or exist with another autoimmune disease (secondary SS).[55–57]

A wide range of central nervous system (CNS) manifestations may occur, including AON and TM.[56,58,59] The precise prevalence of neurologic manifestations in SS is unclear, and has been reported to range from 8.5% to 70.0%[57]; this large discrepancy may be related to the inclusion or exclusion of psychiatric and cognitive impairment. Neurologic deficits may be the initial presentation in as many as 57% of patients with SS.[57] Spinal cord involvement (either acute TM or progressive myelopathy) may occur in 20% to 35% of patients with SS and may constitute the initial presentation of the disease in up to about 20%.[55,57] The lesions tend to affect the cervical cord and may be longitudinally extensive.[57,60]

CSF typically reveals pleocytosis, mildly increased protein, and a mildly elevated IgG index.[56,60] Cytologic analysis may reveal small round lymphocytes, reactive lymphoid cells, plasma cells, and atypical mononuclear cells.[56] OCBs have been reported in about 30% of patients with SS.[57] SS-A or SS-B antibody seropositivity is not mandatory for the diagnosis of SS, because only 21% of patients with primary SS and neurologic manifestations demonstrate such seropositivity.[57]

Although other CNS manifestations of SS are corticosteroid-responsive,[56] spinal cord involvement is often refractory to steroids.[60] Intravenous (IV) cyclophosphamide is effective[56,57]; there is anecdotal evidence supporting the use of plasmapheresis[61] and IV gammaglobulin.[62] Maintenance immunosuppressive therapy with monthly pulse IV cyclophosphamide may be considered.[56] Rituximab is another promising agent[63] and may be a suitable agent for patients with coexisting NMO or MS, or where there is diagnostic confusion with these diseases.

Careful longitudinal follow-up is important in SS, as recurrent attacks of TM or AON can culminate in substantial disability, and may ultimately lead to a confirmed diagnosis of NMO or MS.

Systemic Lupus Erythematosus

SLE is a chronic, systemic, autoimmune disease. The diagnosis of SLE requires at least 4 of 11 features, as outlined by the American College of Rheumatology.[64] Although neuropsychiatric manifestations of SLE are common, TM accounts for only 1% to 2% of patients,[65] but constitutes the most devastating complication of SLE and one that often portends a poor prognosis.[66] SLE-related TM tends to occur within the first 5 years from diagnosis, is the initial clinical manifestation in almost half of patients, and recurs in 21% to 55% of cases.[67–69] AON and brainstem manifestations may accompany TM in SLE,[70,71] mimicking MS and representing a significant source of diagnostic confusion.

A short period of prodromal symptoms (eg, headache, fever, nausea) typically heralds the onset of thoracic myelopathy with prominent bladder dysfunction.[69,71] In a large series of SLE-related TM, 2 different clinical patterns at presentation were observed: gray and white matter myelitis. Gray matter myelitis demonstrated lower motor neuron (LMN) features, urinary retention, and a more devastating but monophasic course. White matter myelitis demonstrated UMN features and a more indolent but recurrent course.[72] An earlier study suggested that EMG evidence of anterior horn cell dysfunction in patients with TM predicts a poor prognosis for recovery.[37] The features of gray and white matter myelitis are summarized in **Table 4**.

Although low-titer positive antinuclear antibodies (ANA) in idiopathic TM (ITM) cases are similar to that of the general population, much higher serum ANA titers, anti–double-stranded DNA antibodies, and hypocomplementemia are found in SLE-related TM.[68,71] The presence of antiphospholipid antibodies (APLA) in SLE has been suggested to increase the risk of developing TM[73] but this association has been challenged.[67,69] CSF pleocytosis with elevated protein and intrathecal IgG synthesis are typically detected, particularly in LETM[68,69,71,74]; interestingly, OCBs, although unusual, have been observed in APLA-seropositive patients.[69]

The most common MRI finding in SLE-related TM is a longitudinally extensive, T2-hyperintense lesion (accompanied by cord swelling).[68,69,71,74–78] In severe cases, the lesion involves the entire spinal cord and extends into the medulla.[79,80] Radiologic findings may not correlate with the clinical course.[68] Almost a third of patients with SLE-related TM do not have any detectable MRI abnormalities at presentation.[67] On brain MRI, subcortical lesions predominate in APS and SLE, whereas periventricular and callosal lesions are more common in MS.[81]

In a randomized controlled trial, IV cyclophosphamide was found to be more efficacious in treating neuropsychiatric manifestations of SLE compared with IV methylprednisolone.[82] The combination of high-dose IV methylprednisolone and IV cyclophosphamide may be effective in SLE-related TM if instituted promptly, resulting in improvement in a few days to 3 weeks.[67,70,83,84] Relapses are common (50%–60%) during corticosteroid dose taper, emphasizing the need for maintenance immunosuppression.[70] Plasmapheresis has been used in severe cases.[67,71,85,86] There is anecdotal evidence for using intravenous immunoglobulin and rituximab.[71,87,88] Anticoagulation therapy is indicated only in those with a history of thrombotic phenomena.[69,71,73,74] Long-term aspirin use has anecdotal support.[74]

Factors associated with severe neurologic deficits include extensive cord MRI lesions, LMN features and sphincteric dysfunction at onset, APLA, and delayed (>2 weeks) initiation of therapy.[67,72,89]

Table 4
The differences between gray and white matter myelitis in SLE

	Gray Matter Myelitis	White Matter Myelitis
Presentation	Lower motor neuron features with urinary retention (urinary retention always heralds paraplegia)	Upper motor neuron features
Prodrome (fever, nausea, vomiting)	Very frequent	Infrequent
Clinical course	More rapid deterioration; more severe weakness at nadir. Lower motor neuron features persist beyond the time expected for spinal shock. More aggressive immunosuppression needed.	Less severe clinical deterioration; longer time to reach nadir; less severe weakness at nadir.
Long-term Disability	Greater	Less
CSF	Neutrophilic pleocytosis; higher protein; hypoglycorrachia	Mild pleocytosis; mildly elevated protein; normal glucose
MRI	Cord swelling; frequent LETM; less frequent gadolinium-enhancement	Infrequent cord swelling; less frequent LETM; More frequent gadolinium-enhancement
Recurrence	Very rare	More than 70% of patients
Prior optic neuritis	Absent	Frequent
Coexisting NMO and/or NMO-IgG seropositivity	None	Frequent
Higher SLE disease activity	Frequent	Infrequent

Abbreviations: CSF, cerebrospinal fluid; LETM, longitudinally extensive transverse myelitis; NMO, neuromyelitis optica; NMO-IgG, aquaporin-4-antibody; SLE, systemic lupus erythematosus.
Data from Birnbaum J, Petri M, Thompson R, et al. Distinct subtypes of myelitis in systemic lupus erythematosus. Arthritis Rheum 2009;60(11):3378–87.

Antiphospholipid Syndrome

APS is a systemic, autoimmune disorder characterized by recurrent thrombotic events and/or miscarriages, as well as APLA seropositivity (2 or more occasions at least 6 weeks apart) (ie, anticardiolipin, lupus anticoagulant, and anti-beta-2-glycoprotein I antibodies).[90] In secondary APS, the disease coexists with another autoimmune disorder.

TM is an unusual complication of APS, with a prevalence of less than 1%.[91–93] Although typically monophasic, recurrent corticosteroid-responsive LETM has also been observed.[92] Characteristically, acute thoracic cord dysfunction occurs with sphincter involvement.[93] Spine MRI may be normal on presentation in up to 40% of patients, underscoring the importance of repeat imaging in suspected cases.[94] It is hypothesized that interactions between APLA and spinal cord phospholipids are responsible for APS-related TM,[95] explaining the efficacy of and justifying the use of early high-dose corticosteroid therapy.[93] In corticosteroid-refractory patients, cyclophosphamide, plasmapheresis, and rituximab may be needed.[93]

A higher prevalence of APLA seropositivity has been reported in patients with MS and appears to rise with disease duration.[96–100] Although diagnostic confusion may arise in APLA-positive patients with TM, the presence of CSF OCBs and the absence of prior miscarriages or thrombotic phenomena would favor MS rather than APS.

Behcet Disease

BD is a relapsing multisystem inflammatory disorder of unclear etiology resulting in oral aphthous ulcers, genital ulcers, uveitis, cutaneous manifestations, and involvement of other organ systems.[101]

Neurologic involvement in BD (neuro-BD) may follow or precede the onset of systemic manifestations.[102] Neuro-BD typically occurs in the third to fourth decade of life, is more common in men, and is usually associated with ocular involvement.[102–104] The frequency of neuro-BD varies greatly, from 1.3% to 59.0%, with a pooled average of 9.4%.[102,104] Neuro-BD can be classified as parenchymal or nonparenchymal (vascular). Parenchymal neuro-BD commonly manifests as a meningoencephalitic syndrome with headaches and focal neurologic deficits.[102] The manifestations of vascular BD stem from cerebral venous thrombosis (often with subsequent increased intracranial hypertension) and/or rarely, arterial infarctions.[105] Spinal cord involvement ranges between 2.5% and 30.0%, with a predilection for the cervical and thoracic cord segments (in particular the posterolateral cord), and carries a poor prognosis.[102,103,106–109] Isolated TM in neuro-BD is distinctly unusual.[102,105]

Spinal cord lesions are usually longitudinally extensive and involve multiple noncontiguous segments, or even involve the entire cord. Cord swelling and T2-hyperintense, nonenhancing lesions are present in the acute or subacute phase.[106,107,109–114] An unusual report of TM (extending from T9 to the conus) following CT-guided L2 nerve root injection, may be a florid demonstration of the pathergic reaction in the spinal cord.[115]

Brain MRI may reveal T1-hypo/isointense and T2-hyperintense lesions that may or may not show gadolinium enhancement acutely. Characteristically, an upper pontomesencephalic lesion with thalamic, hypothalamic, and basal ganglial extension on one side is seen.[102,105,107,109,116,117] Interestingly, the red nucleus is almost always spared.[107,109] Striking brainstem atrophy, as well as the rarity of periventricular lesions, optic neuropathy, cortical atrophy, and gray matter lesions in neuro-BD,[102,109,117,118] distinguish it from MS.

CSF typically reveals normal glucose, increased protein, and neutrophilic pleocytosis; the IgG index may be elevated, and OCBs are rare.[103–106,108,117]

Acutely, administration of high-dose corticosteroids results in improvement in most patients[103,104,108,110,111,113,119]; corticosteroid therapy also improved pleocytosis.[117] Infliximab, cyclophosphamide, and intravenous immunoglobulin have been used with some success.[104,120]

No randomized controlled trials have been conducted into the treatment of neuro-BD. Azathioprine, mycophenolate mofetil, and methotrexate have been used as initial immunosuppressive therapy. In more aggressive disease, tumor necrosis factor-antagonists or monthly infusions of cyclophosphamide have been used. Colchicine, thalidomide, and pentoxifylline may be used for mucocutaneous lesions.[102–104] Cyclosporin A has been used to treat ophthalmic manifestations but may be neurotoxic and worsen neurologic manifestations.[121–124]

TM in Other Rheumatologic Diseases

TM has been reported in AS, psoriatic arthritis, mixed connective tissue disease, and systemic sclerosis (please refer to **Table 5**).

Table 5
Other dysimmune disorders associated with TM

Disorder	Comment	References
Ankylosing spondylitis	Neurologic involvement is rare and is almost always attributable to compressive myelopathy. Noncompressive myelopathy is exceptionally rare with only 2 clearly documented cases of TM.	368–370
Psoriatic arthritis		371
Mixed connective tissue disease	Female preponderance; predilection for the thoracic cord.	372–377
Systemic sclerosis	Rare and typically compressive in etiology. Progressive myelopathy, subacute TM, and NMO-IgG positive LETM have been reported.	378–381
Anti-Jo-1 antibody	A single report of TM preceding the development of polymyositis and pulmonary fibrosis in a patient with anti-Jo-1 antibody.	382
Urticarial vasculitis	Urticarial vasculitis may be primary disorder or coexist with other autoimmune diseases.	383
pANCA seropositivity	Perinuclear antineutrophil cytoplasmic antibody (pANCA) seropositivity has been reported to cause TM associated with CSF pleocytosis and increased protein with typically absent OCBs.	384,385
Celiac disease	Celiac disease is an immune-mediated disorder characterized by intolerance to dietary gluten.	386
Thymic follicular hyperplasia	Recurrent multifocal TM associated with thymic follicular hyperplasia that resolved following thymectomy.	387
Graft-vs-host disease	TM may be a rare manifestation of graft-vs-host disease following hematopoietic cell transplantation.	388–390
Common variable immunodeficiency	A primary immune deficiency disorder characterized by hypogammaglobulinemia, antibody deficiency, and recurrent infections.	391,392

Abbreviations: CSF, cerebrospinal fluid; LETM, longitudinally extensive transverse myelitis; NMO-IgG, aquaporin-4-antibody; OCB, oligoclonal bands; SLE, systemic lupus erythematosus.

Neurosarcoidosis

Sarcoidosis is a multisystem granulomatous disease with protean manifestations that may affect any organ. Neurologic involvement (neurosarcoidosis) is reported in 5% to 13% of patients with sarcoidosis[125–128] but may be as high as 26%.[129] The usual age of onset is the fourth decade.[127,130] Spinal cord neurosarcoidosis appears to be more common in men.[131,132]

CNS features are the initial manifestation of neurosarcoidosis in up to 70% of patients.[130] Although unusual, spinal cord involvement portends a poor outcome, and may be related to intramedullary, intradural extramedullary, or extradural lesions; cauda equina syndrome; or arachnoiditis.[130,131,133] Although isolated myelopathy has been observed, half of patients with spinal cord neurosarcoidosis demonstrate systemic manifestations.[129,133,134]

Neurosarcoidosis has a predilection for the cervical and thoracic cord[131,132,135–137] and is frequently associated with back pain and radicular symptoms.[131,138–140]

Intramedullary disease typically appears as a longitudinally extensive, T1-hypointense, T2-hyperintense, heterogeneously enhancing lesion with fusiform cord enlargement or myelomalacia.[131,141] Spinal cord lesions may be multifocal; gadolinium enhancement may be nodular or predominate at the periphery of the lesion.[129,131,132] Neurosarcoidosis should be suspected in any infiltrating intramedullary cord lesion with leptomeningeal enhancement. Half of patients with spinal neurosarcoidosis have concomitant intracranial lesions.[131,141]

The diagnosis of spinal cord neurosarcoidosis is challenging, particularly if systemic manifestations are absent. When clinical suspicion is high, even in the absence of systemic symptoms, it is worthwhile performing a high-resolution chest CT, positron emission tomography, ophthalmic examination, or a gallium-67 scan to identify extraneural granulomas that may be amenable to biopsy.[66,140,142]

CSF findings reveal elevated protein, lymphocytic pleocytosis, occasional hypoglycorrachia, and infrequent OCBs. CSF angiotensin-converting enzyme levels are normal in more than half of patients. Hypoglycorrachia is specific and can distinguish neurosarcoidosis from other inflammatory etiologies.[130,131,140,143]

Early corticosteroid therapy results in remarkable recovery but delayed treatment leads to only partial resolution of myelopathic manifestations.[132] A high index of suspicion for the diagnosis is required because early intervention is associated with a favorable outcome.

Vogt-Koyanagi-Harada Syndrome

Vogt-Koyanagi-Harada syndrome (VKH), also known as uveomeningoencephalitis, is a systemic inflammatory disorder affecting the melanin-forming cells in different organs.[144] TM is an infrequent complication of VKH,[145,146] and bilateral AON with papilitis has been reported.[147] These manifestations may mimic MS or NMO. CSF pleocytosis can provide early evidence of disease activity, therefore allowing early treatment with corticosteroids.[148,149]

Acute Disseminated Encephalomyelitis

ADEM is a monophasic disorder that occurs following infections or vaccinations, is associated with multifocal demyelinating lesions, and may include encephalopathy, coma, and/or seizures.[150] TM occurs in about 24% of patients[151] and, in unusual cases, may be the sole manifestation of ADEM.[152] It is possible that some cases of TM represent limited forms of ADEM.[29] Unlike MS and NMO, ADEM may be associated with demyelinating peripheral neuropathies.[153]

ADEM may occur at any age but is most common in the pediatric population (mean age of onset of 5.7 years).[154] Postvaccination ADEM incidence is variable, and the most frequently implicated vaccine is the non-neural measles, mumps, and rubella vaccine.[66,155] An initial attack consistent with a demyelinating event with acute or subacute onset, a stable to stuttering course (evolving over 1 week to 3 months), characteristic MRI features, and concomitant encephalopathy and meningismus, suggests a diagnosis of ADEM.[66]

Radiologically, acute, multiple, symmetric, supratentorial and infratentorial lesions, with one at least 1 cm in diameter are observed; symmetric basal ganglial and thalamic involvement is common.[66,151] The lesions should be of the same age and demonstrate homogeneous gadolinium enhancement, as ADEM is typically monophasic.[156,157] The typical spinal cord lesion is swollen, enhances variably, and predominantly affects the thoracic cord.[151] It may take up to 14 days from the onset of symptoms for the MRI to show abnormalities.[158] CSF in ADEM typically reveals marked pleocytosis, elevated protein, normal IgG index, and no OCBs.[155,159,160]

Treatment with high-dose IV corticosteroid therapy may help diminish inflammation and restore the blood-brain barrier integrity. Early initiation of plasmapheresis (within 15 days of onset) has been shown to result in clinical improvement and should be offered to those who fail steroid therapy.[161–165]

Parainfectious TM

Parainfectious TM (PITM) refers to TM associated with an antecedent infection. It is unclear if it shares the same pathophysiological underpinnings as ADEM (and represents different ends of a spectrum) or if they are separate entities. Both are preceded by typically monophasic, steroid-responsive events preceded by infections. It is difficult to determine if PITM is caused by direct microbial invasion (causing myelitis by either the direct pathogenic destruction, or from the pathogen-triggered immune reaction), or a consequence of immune-mediated, inflammatory mechanisms induced by a remote infection. The antecedent infection has typically resolved before the onset of TM and it is difficult to demonstrate the offending organism in the spinal cord parenchyma.

The hepatitis viruses may cause TM via postinfectious, immune-mediated, inflammatory mechanisms.[166] Hepatitis A virus and Hepatitis B virus infection have been associated with immune-mediated TM.[166] Hepatitis C virus (HCV) is the most commonly implicated hepatitis virus in TM. HCV has been associated with recurrent, corticosteroid-responsive, demyelinating TM (even without hepatic involvement).[166–171] There is a single report of hepatitis E–virus associated TM.[172]

Viruses associated with PITM[155,173–186] are listed in **Box 5**.

CNS manifestations are the most common extrapulmonary complication of *Mycoplasma pneumoniae* infection.[155,187–189] Although encephalitis is the most frequent complication,[189] TM is the most severe and debilitating manifestation.[190] Acute to subacute thoracic myelopathy typically arise 2 to 4 weeks after the antecedent respiratory infection and progress to a nadir in about 3 days; it may be accompanied by meningoencephalitis and/or polyradiculopathy.[190] LETM has been reported.[191–193] A predominantly mononuclear pleocytosis with increased protein and normal glucose levels are frequently found.[190] Serologic detection of anti-*Mycoplasma* antibodies supports the diagnosis. Positive *M pneumoniae* CSF polymerase chain reaction provides reliable diagnostic evidence of preceding infection.

Antecedent *Campylobacter jejuni* infection has been classically associated with GBS, presumably because of molecular mimicry between bacterial lipopolysaccharides and human gangliosides. It has been associated with TM,[194–196] ADEM,[197–199] and 1 case of biopsy-proven CNS vasculitis.[200] In patients with TM with a recent diarrheal illness, stool cultures for *C jejuni* and serologic studies for antiganglioside antibodies should be considered.

Bacteria reported to cause PITM[155,195,201–214] are listed in **Box 5**.

Fungal and parasitic causes of PITM[5,215–223] are rare; these are listed in **Box 5**. These microbes most likely cause myelopathy by direct pathogenic effects. One noteworthy parasite is the pinworm (*Enterobius vermicularis*), which has been reported to cause TM associated with anti-GM1 antibodies (which are also seen in *C jejuni* infection) via molecular mimicry.[224]

Pathogens associated with parainfectious LETM[167–170,186,192,193,201,209,212,213,225–239] are listed in **Box 3**.

It is imperative to remember that the occurrence of TM following an infection does not automatically implicate ADEM or a parainfectious autoimmune response. Longitudinal follow-up is needed and further evaluation may be warranted because infections may trigger TM that heralds the diagnosis MS or NMO. Diagnostic confusion may arise in cases in which concomitant parainfectious AON[240,241] and TM may mimic the appearance of a demyelinating disease. As such, longitudinal follow-up is required to ascertain the nature of the disease.

Paraneoplastic TM

Collapsin response-mediator protein-5 (CRMP-5-IgG) antibodies, observed in small-cell lung cancer, is the paraneoplastic antibody most commonly associated with TM; LETM has also been observed. CRMP-5-IgG–related AON is a recognized manifestation of this paraneoplastic syndrome. A clinical picture resembling MS or NMO may arise.[242,243] Patients demonstrate a subacute, progressive, predominantly motor myelopathy as well as increased CSF protein, elevated IgG index, and mild pleocytosis.[242,244] MRI demonstrates T2-hyperintense lesions with occasional gadolinium enhancement. In more than 40% of patients, LETM may be demonstrated.[242] Other paraneoplastic antibodies associated with TM are listed in **Table 6**.

Atopic Myelitis

Atopic myelitis (AM) demonstrates a chronic persistent or fluctuating course of predominantly cervical myelitis, associated with marked hyper-IgEemia, allergen-specific IgE (most commonly to dust mites), and occasional coexistent atopic diseases (eg, atopic dermatitis, atopic rhinitis, asthma).[245] The vast majority of reported cases occur in Japanese patients, but a there are a few reports of AM in White patients.[246,247] Sensory deficits are the predominant symptom, with infrequent motor and bladder involvement.[248]

On MRI, the lesions are T2-hyperintense with variable gadolinium enhancement, appear to favor the posterior columns of the cervical cord, and are limited to 1 to 2 vertebral bodies.[248,249] Because the clinical and radiologic picture resembles MS, it is imperative to obtain a brain MRI to look for lesions that would be suggestive of MS.[250] CSF cell count and protein are typically normal and OCBs are not seen.[249,250] VEP may be abnormal in more than 20% of patients with AM (and therefore may not help distinguish it from MS), as atopic AON has been reported to occur as well.[250,251]

TM in Other Dysimmune Disorders

Table 5 lists various dysimmune disorders that have been associated with TM.

Table 6
Paraneoplastic antibodies associated with TM aside from collapsin response-mediator protein 5 Ig antibodies

Paraneoplastic Antibody	Comment	References
Anti-Ri (ANNA-2)	Anti-Ri antibodies are usually associated with lung or breast carcinoma	393,394
Anti-amphiphysin IgG	Classically associated with breast cancer and stiff man syndrome	395,396
Anti-glutamic acid decarboxylase (GAD65)	Classically associated with stiff person syndrome, cerebellar ataxia, diabetes mellitus type 1, and limbic encephalitis	244,397
N-methyl-d-aspartate receptor (NMDAR)	Classically associated with limbic encephalitis, and related to ovarian teratomas.	398–400

Drug-induced and Toxin-related TM

Drugs and toxins associated with TM are listed in **Table 7**.

Idiopathic TM

The Transverse Myelitis Consortium Working Group has proposed a set of strict criteria for the diagnosis of ITM,[7] which are summarized in **Table 8**. To make the diagnosis, all inclusion and no exclusion criteria should be present. The application of these criteria has resulted in a fairly homogeneous group of patients in terms of clinical and radiologic data.[252] The reported proportion of patients with TM with ITM varies widely, from 16%[252] to approximately 60%.[253,254]

The overall mean age of disease onset appears to be between 35 and 40 years, with a female preponderance.[252,254] The MRI typically demonstrates a centromedullary lesion, extending over 2 vertebral segments and involving more than two-thirds of the cross-sectional area of the spinal cord, with a predilection for the thoracic cord.[41,252,253,255–259] Cord swelling is seen in half of cases. Gadolinium enhancement (which may be nodular, peripheral, heterogeneous, or moderately diffuse) occurs in approximately one-third to one-half of cases.[41,252,253,255] CSF shows increased protein in most patients; pleocytosis and OCBs are sometimes seen.[41,252,258] Interestingly, unlike other causes of TM, negative OCBs is correlated with recurrence.[252]

ITM is typically monophasic but recurs in about one-quarter to one-third of cases (recurrence of initial insult, expansion of prior lesion, or a new lesion).[8,12,66,252,259] Risk factors for recurrence seem to be the following: (1) male gender; (2) age older than 50 years; (3) severe motor weakness and sphincteric dysfunction; and (4) negative CSF OCBs, normal IgG index, and NMO-IgG seronegativity.[252,258,259] Recurrences are associated with a poor outcome.[259] Interestingly, Kim and colleagues[258] and Alvarenga and colleagues[254] both reported recurrences exceeding 60% in their respective studies despite the low rate of NMO-IgG seropositivity. There are several serologic, CSF, and radiologic differences among the patients with recurrent ITM in these studies and may represent distinct clinical entities that have yet to be characterized. A Korean study of 15 patients with recurrent ITM lends support to the hypothesis that recurrent ITM may represent a unique entity.[260] More longitudinal studies are needed to clearly elucidate the characteristics of recurrent ITM.

Table 7
Drugs and toxins associated with TM

Drug/Toxin	Comment	Reference
TNF-alpha inhibitors	Reported to cause CNS demyelination and TM.	401,402
Sulfasalazine		403
Chemotherapeutic agents	Gemcitabine, cytarabine (cytosine arabinoside), and cisplatin.	404–408
General and epidural anesthesia	The association between TM and general anesthesia is debatable.	409–415
Heroin	Although most of cases of myelopathy in heroin addicts result from anterior spinal artery infarction, there are reports of TM.	416–419
Benzene		420
Brown recluse spider bite	Incomplete TM (anterior spinal syndrome), responsive to corticosteroid therapy.	421

Abbreviations: CNS, central nervous system; TM, transverse myelitis; TNF, tumor necrosis factor.

Table 8
Transverse Myelitis Consortium Working group criteria for the idiopathic transverse myelitis

Inclusion Criteria	Exclusion Criteria
Neurologic impairment attributable to the spinal cord	History of radiation to the spine within 10 y
Bilateral signs or symptoms (may be asymmetric)	Anterior spinal artery distribution of deficits
Clearly defined sensory level	Abnormal flow voids on the spinal cord
Exclusion of extra-axial compressive etiology by neuroimaging	Serologic or clinical evidence of systemic autoimmune disease
Evidence of inflammation in the spinal cord (CSF cells or IgG index, or MRI gadolinium enhancement) seen at onset or within 7 d	CNS manifestations of infectious etiology (eg, syphilis, Lyme, HIV, HTLV-1, *Mycoplasma*)
Progressive worsening to a nadir between 4 h to 21 d after onset	Brain MRI lesions suggestive of MS
	History of optic neuritis

Abbreviations: CNS, central nervous system; CSF, cerebrospinal fluid; HTLV, Human T-Lymphotropic Virus; Ig, immunoglobulin; MRI, magnetic resonance imaging; MS, multiple sclerosis.

Data from Transverse Myelitis Consortium Group. Proposed diagnostic criteria and nosology of acute transverse myelitis. Neurology 2002;59:499–505.

The response of ITM to corticosteroid therapy is usually disappointing.[41,252] In general, one-third of patients with idiopathic acute transverse myelitis recover with little or no sequelae, one-third are left with a moderate degree of permanent disability, and one-third have severe disabilities.[252] Spinal shock at presentation was highly predictive of a poor outcome.[252] Interestingly, a higher CSF glucose level (related to higher serum levels) may portend a poorer outcome.[41]

Pediatric TM

On the whole, the incidence of TM in children is much lower than that of the adult population. There appears to a bimodal distribution: toddlers younger than age 3, and children between 5 and 17 years. Males and females are equally affected. Antecedent infections (typically respiratory) or preceding vaccinations are common.[10,261,262] Because of the association with respiratory infections, there is a clustering of TM cases in the winter months.[262,263]

Compared with adults, pediatric TM is more frequently postinfectious, thoracic, centromedullary, and longitudinally extensive. The risk of conversion to MS is lower and functional recovery is often better than in the adult population.[261–266] Complete recovery appears to be the rule with poor outcome in only a minority of patients.[264,266,267] The course in pediatric TM has been divided into 3 phases: onset, plateau, and recovery. The plateau may last up to 4 weeks; if recovery has not started by the end of this period, the likelihood of recovery diminishes.[262,264,268] Beyond 6 months, any improvement is very improbable.[264]

CSF analysis frequently reveals pleocytosis and elevated protein; OCBs and increased IgG indices are rare.[261,262,264] Although the proportion of pediatric TM cases with LETM is higher than that of adults, the rate of NMO-IgG seropositivity is much lower.[262,269] This low rate of NMO-IgG seropositivity, with the typically monophasic clinical course and benign outcome in pediatric LETM, suggests that the pathobiological underpinnings of LETM in the pediatric population is different from that in adults.

Age younger than 3 years, requirement for respiratory support, severe impairment at onset, flaccid paralysis at onset, a more rapid progression to the nadir of weakness, CSF pleocytosis, and MRI T1-hypointensity at the time of diagnosis were poor prognostic indicators for recovery.[261,264,267,268] Early treatment with IV methylprednisolone had a significant positive effect on outcome.[264] The most common long-term neurologic complication of TM in children is bladder dysfunction.[261,264,266] As in adults, APTM, CSF OCBs, and the brain MRI lesions portend an increased risk for transition to MS; LETM carries a low risk of developing MS.[262]

Table 9 highlights the important CSF and MRI features of the different causes of TM.

PSEUDOEXACERBATION

Pseudoexacerbation is a phenomenon in which patients experience temporary worsening of previously suffered neurologic deficits. In demyelinating disorders, Uhthoff phenomenon is the most common underlying cause of pseudoexacerbation (authors' personal experience). Any condition that increases the patient's body temperature (eg, febrile illness, exercise, hot weather, hot baths, hot showers, stress, menses, dehydration) can cause a pseudoexacerbation. Any infection, particularly urinary tract infections (UTI) may result in pseudoexacerbation. In fact, any metabolic or physiologic derangements (eg, hyperglycemia, hypertension) has the potential to transiently worsen prior neurologic deficits. In conclusion, worsening of prior myelopathic symptoms in a patient with previous TM does not automatically implicate a recurrence or relapse. Pseudoexacerbation should be considered and investigations into the cause of pseudoexacerbation should be undertaken. Treatment of recurrent TM entails immunosuppressive therapy, but treatment of pseudoexacerbation involves addressing the underlying cause (eg, treating the UTI).

MIMICS OF TRANSVERSE MYELITIS

In making the diagnosis of TM, it is essential to remember that many noninflammatory etiologies may mimic the appearance of TM. Recognizing these entities is important, as the treatment and management strategies would be vastly different.

Entities important to recognize include vascular myelopathy, compressive myelopathy, metabolic/toxic myelopathy, neoplasms, and radiation myelitis. Selected etiologies are described in **Table 10**.

MANAGEMENT
Acute Management

Once the diagnosis of TM is made, immunotherapy should be instituted to stop the inflammatory process and therefore allow recovery to commence. In a small open-label trial, high-dose IV methylprednisolone was shown to improve the outcome in pediatric TM.[264] Despite the lack of randomized controlled studies, administration of high-dose IV corticosteroids (IV methylprednisolone 1 g daily for 3–7 days) should be started as early as possible in all patients with TM.[13]

In patients with poor or no response to corticosteroids, plasmapheresis should be offered,[13] with the rationale of removing humoral factors inciting TM. The benefits of plasmapheresis have been proven in acute attacks of CNS demyelinating diseases.[163–165,270] Early initiation of plasmapheresis (within 15 days of onset) is the best predictor of a favorable acute response and of improvement at 6 months.[164,165] The typical regimen is exchanges of 1.5 plasma volumes for 5 treatments over 10 days.[271] Plasmapheresis also has anecdotal support in various systemic autoimmune disorders (described previously).

Table 9
Highlighted CSF and MRI differences for various causes of TM

	CSF	MRI Features of Spinal Cord Lesion	MRI Features of Brain Lesions	Comments
Multiple sclerosis	OCB Increased IgG index	APTM Cigar-shaped Posterior cord	Periventricular plaques (Dawson fingers) Juxtacortical lesions T1 black holes Cortical atrophy	
Neuromyelitis optica	OCB rare	LETM	Periventricular lesions (not perpendicularly oriented), hypothalamic, lesions around 3rd and 4th ventricles, or brainstem lesions. Clinically silent lesions rare. "Cloudlike" gadolinium enhancement	NMO-IgG seropositivity
Neurosarcoidosis	Lymphocytic pleocytosis OCB rare Low glucose	LETM Favors cervical and thoracic cord Patchy enhancement Leptomeningeal enhancement	Leptomeningeal enhancement	Cranial neuropathies Pulmonary manifestations
Systemic lupus erythematosus	Pleocytosis OCBs infrequent	LETM Cord swelling	Subcortical lesions	Gray and white matter myelitis
Sjögren syndrome	Pleocytosis OCBs in a third of patients	Favors cervical cord LETM	Basal ganglial lesions Corpus callosal lesions rare	Cochlear neuropathy
Behcet disease	Mixed pleocytosis OCBs rare	LETM Posterolateral cord	Unilateral upper brainstem-diencephalic-basal ganglial Brainstem atrophy	
ADEM	Marked pleocytosis Increased protein No OCB IgG index negative	LETM	Acute, multiple, symmetric, supratentorial and infratentorial lesions, with one at least 1 cm in diameter Symmetric basal ganglial and thalamic lesions	Typically monophasic Antecedent infection or vaccination

(continued on next page)

Table 9 (continued)				
	CSF	MRI Features of Spinal Cord Lesion	MRI Features of Brain Lesions	Comments
Atopic Myelitis	Bland CSF No OCB	APTM Cervical cord Posterior columns	No brain lesions	Marked hyperIgEemia
Idiopathic transverse myelitis	Increased protein OCBs may be seen	LETM Involves two-thirds of cross-sectional cord area Predilection for thoracic cord	No brain lesions	Typically monophasic Negative OCBs correlate with recurrence

Abbreviations: ADEM, acute disseminated encephalomyelitis; APTM, acute partial transverse myelitis; CSF, cerebrospinal fluid; LETM, longitudinally extensive transverse myelitis; MRI, magnetic resonance imaging; NMO-IgG, aquaporin-4-antibody; OCB, oligoclonal bands.

Although plasmapheresis may provide benefit beyond that obtained with steroids, patients with American Spinal Injury Association (ASIA) A level of disability may need IV cyclophosphamide as well.[272] IV cyclophosphamide appears to be efficacious in active inflammatory MS[273,274] and other autoimmune conditions. The major concern with cyclophosphamide is the adverse effect profile, which includes nausea, hemorrhagic cystitis, and malignancies.

In high cervical cord lesions extending into the medulla, respiratory failure may be fatal[275]; therefore, in such patients, vital signs and respiratory function should be vigilantly monitored. Other acute issues that may arise include immobility (and the complications thereof), urinary retention, constipation, and gastroparesis. These are discussed later in this article.

In cases of TM attributable to systemic autoimmune disease or acquired demyelinating disease, commencement of long-term immunomodulatory therapies would help prevent future attacks.[3] A discussion of these therapies is beyond the scope of this article.

The Importance of a Multidisciplinary Approach to Neurorehabilitation

A very important aspect of managing TM focuses on the multiple complications arising from the disease. The main thrust of long-term management is neurorehabilitation, the active process by which those disabled by injury or disease achieve a full recovery or, if full recovery is not possible, realize their optimal physical, mental, and social potential and are integrated into their most appropriate environment.[276] Successful neurorehabilitation is dependent on a multidisciplinary assessment that can develop goal-oriented programs tailored for the patient's specific needs; therefore, early consultation with the physical medicine and rehabilitation physician, physical therapist, occupational therapist, and psychologist/psychiatrist is vital. In fact, there is evidence that a multidisciplinary comprehensive care center is a highly efficient and cost-effective care delivery system that minimizes adverse events, lowers rehospitalization rate, and improves patients' perception.[277]

Mobility and Gait Impairment

Acute immobility

In the acute phase of TM, weakness may be severe and care should be taken to avoid the complications of prolonged immobility. Low molecular weight heparin or

Table 10
Mimics of TM

Etiology	Description	References
Vitamin B12 deficiency	May present as an isolated myelopathy or in combination with neuropathy, encephalopathy, and/or behavioral changes. Dorsal column impairment is the most common manifestation, followed by pyramidal dysfunction (the classic subacute combined degeneration of the cord). Hematologic manifestations may be absent up to 30% of patients with neurologic manifestations. MRI reveals T2-hyperintense signal in the posterior columns (the "inverted V" or "inverted rabbit ear" sign on axial views). In severe cases, MRI shows the "anchor" sign (because of involvement of the posterior, anterior, and pyramidal tracts).	422–425
Vitamin E deficiency	May cause a predominantly dorsal column syndrome associated with a peripheral neuropathy because of axonal degeneration. Preferentially affects the cervical cord. Clinically and radiologically similar to B12 deficiency.	426–428
Copper deficiency	May cause both myelopathy and optic neuropathy. Causes of acquired copper deficiency include malnutrition, zinc toxicity, Menke disease, bariatric surgery, gastrectomy, malabsorption syndromes, and use of copper chelating agents. Clinically and radiologically indistinguishable from B12 deficiency.	429–433
Nitrous oxide (N2O) toxicity	Analgesic gas commonly abused because of euphoric effects. N2O inactivates vitamin B12 by irreversible oxidation of the cobalt center of methylcobalamine, thereby inhibiting the methionine synthesis pathway. In healthy subjects, this does not cause clinical manifestations. In subclinically B12-deficient individuals, N2O exhausts residual stocks of vitamin B12, leading to neurologic manifestations.	434–436
Neurolathyrism and neurocassivism	Neurolathyrism is caused by consumption of grass pea. Neurocassavism (konzo) is caused by bitter cassava root consumption. Both are found in malnourished populations, and are characterized by subacute paraparesis with prominent UMN features.	437

Intramedullary primary spinal cord tumors	May be ependymomas, astrocytomas, or hemangioblastomas. Typically cause an insidious, progressive myelopathy. Hemorrhage or infarction of the tumor may result in an acute presentation and radiologic appearance mimicking TM. [5]
Primary CNS lymphoma	May give rise to a clinical and radiologic picture mimicking TM compounded by its corticosteroid-responsiveness. [438–440] Congenital or acquired immunodeficiency is the only established risk factor. More common in middle-aged and older men. Insidious onset of myelopathy with back pain and constitutional symptoms. Serum lactate dehydrogenase may be elevated. CSF: lymphocytic pleocytosis, markedly elevated protein, and hypoglycorrachia. OCBs and IgG index are absent. Cytologic analysis may demonstrate malignant cells (large-volume CSF examination can increase the diagnostic yield). MRI: T2-hyperintensity, gadolinium enhancement, cord swelling, conus medullaris involvement, and concomittant brain lesions.
Intravascular lymphoma	Predominantly affects vessels in the skin and neurologic system. [441–446] May mimic TM and even LETM. CSF: lymphocytic pleocytosis and increased protein, but no malignant cells. MRI: affects the conus medullaris (unlike TM).
Radiation myelitis	Early radiation myelopathy: begins 10–16 weeks after starting radiotherapy with predominantly sensory phenomena (including Lhermitte) and typically resolves spontaneously. [447–450] Delayed radiation myelopathy: begins months or years following radiation exposure and manifests as a subacute or insidious myelopathy. Concurrent use of chemotherapeutic agents may cause widespread white matter necrosis owing to synergistic toxicity. Preexisting myelopathy from any cause may be risk factors for radiation myelitis. MRI: cord swelling on T1-weighted images, intramedullary T2-hyperintensity, ring-like gadolinium enhancement.

Abbreviations: CNS, central nervous system; CSF, cerebrospinal fluid; Ig, immunoglobulin; LETM, longitudinally extensive transverse myelitis; MRI, magnetic resonance imaging; OCB, oligoclonal bands; TM, transverse myelitis; UMN, upper motor neuron.

fondaparinux can be used to prevent venous thromboembolism.[278] Respiratory therapy may prevent atelectasis. In severely weak patients, pressure sores are a serious complication. Addressing risk factors (eg, malnutrition, impaired circulation), conscientious use of pressure-reducing measures (eg, frequent and regular turning, pressure-distributing positioning aids, sheepskins), and early mobilization are critical.[279]

Long-term mobility

Decreased mobility is a factor associated with diminished quality of life (QOL) following spinal cord injury (SC)I.[280] Improving mobility in an energy-efficient manner may thus improve health-related QOL following TM and should be a priority of rehabilitation.[281]

Bipedal locomotion is a complex phenomenon that requires intricate interactions between central pattern generators and peripheral reflexes that involve multiple neural networks, including the visual, vestibular, proprioceptive, and corticospinal systems.[282] Walking parameters can be affected by age, weight, spasticity, lower limb strength, balance, pain, duration of rehabilitation, cord lesion level, and the presence of other comorbidities. Functional walking has several requisites, including safety (which dictates the need for walking aids), speed, comfort, and distance.[283]

Velocity is one of the most important parameters in determining functional ambulation, particularly community ambulation[283]; SCI patients have tremendous difficulty achieving the speed needed to cross an intersection safely.[284] Following nontraumatic SCI, although inpatient rehabilitation may improve walking abilities, gait speed often remains impaired and insufficient to safely negotiate community environments.[285] **Table 11** describes concepts and strategies in managing mobility following TM.

The benefits of physical exercise extend beyond improvements in strength and functional capacity; mood, fatigue, balance, and QOL can also improve.[286] Exercise also carries anti-inflammatory benefits.[287]

Spasticity

Spasticity is the velocity-dependent increase in muscle tone owing to disruption of the descending corticospinal, vestibulospinal, and reticulospinal pathways. It often affects the patient by causing muscle stiffness, spasms, pain, and clonus. Paroxysmal tonic spasms are sudden, episodic, brief, painful, stereotypic, dystonic contractions that may occur following TM.[3,288] Spasticity may result in pain, interrupted sleep, and impaired ambulation.[288]

Although some degree of spasticity may protect against osteoporosis,[289] and is needed for weight bearing to allow ambulation, excessive spasticity can disrupt activities of daily living (eg, transferring, hygiene, sexual activity). Successful treatment of spasticity can be attained with an integrated multidisciplinary approach. **Table 12** summarizes management options for spasticity.

Movement Disorders

Movement disorders that may be complicate TM include propriospinal myoclonus (PSM), periodic limb movement disorder (PLMS) and restless leg syndrome (RLS). PSM is an unusual movement disorder, sometimes seen after spinal cord lesions, characterized by myoclonic jerks arising in muscles corresponding to a myelomere (myoclonic generator) and spreading rostrally and caudally to the other myotomes.[290] Drug therapy of PSM is disappointing but there are reports of treatment with benzodiazepines, zonisamide, and valproate.

Table 11
Management options for addressing long term mobility issues following transverse myelitis

Therapy/Device/ Concept	Description	References
Conventional therapy	Focuses on compensatory strategies for nonremediable neurologic deficits. Focuses on strengthening muscles above the level of the lesion, and unaffected muscles below the level of the lesion.	
Activity-based therapy	Interventions that provide activation of the neuromuscular system below the level of lesion with the goal of retraining the nervous system to recover a specific motor task.	451
Ankle-foot orthoses (AFOs)	AFOs can support the weakened musculature around the ankle. AFOs address excess plantar flexion during initial contact, stabilize the ankle for effective push-off during late stance, and prevent toe-drag during swing.	452
Functional electrical stimulator devices	Can reduce toe drag, circumduction, pelvic obliquity, and genu recurvatum, improving energy efficiency and facilitating safety and walking duration. Long-term use results in stable improvements of walking performance that persist even when the device is turned off. Adherent use of a dorsiflexion assist device may enhance the fidelity of activation of motor cortical regions and the descending corticospinal connections that control the swing phase of ambulation.	286,453,454
Robot-assisted gait training	Different systems are commercially available, including the "Lokomat," the "LokoHelp," and the "Gait trainer."	455
Neuromuscular electrical stimulation (NMES)	Helpful in improving interlimb coordination during locomotion	456
Dalframpridine	Dalframpridine is the extended-release, oral form of 4-aminopyridine approved by the Food and Drug Administration that has been shown to improve the walking ability in patients with multiple sclerosis by improving conduction along demyelinated axons.	457

PLMS and RLS have been reported as a consequence of spinal cord pathologies, including TM, and may be related to the emergence of spasticity.[291] These disorders may impair sleep quality and, as such, should be treated. Serum ferritin levels should be ascertained, as iron-deficiency anemia is a common and treatable cause of RLS.[291] Caffeine, alcohol, nicotine, and medications that may aggravate RLS should be avoided. The first-line choice for pharmacologic therapy is a dopaminergic agonist (eg, ropinorole, pramipexole). Other options include levodopa, opiates, gabapentin, lamotrigine, or clonazepam.[292]

Bladder Dysfunction

Bladder dysfunction remains one of the most common and disabling consequences of TM[293]; UTI is the most common medical complication in myelopathic patients.[294]

Table 12
Management options for spasticity in patients with transverse myelitis

Management Strategy	Comment
Nonpharmacologic measures	Physical therapy, stretching exercises, orthotics, and aquatic therapy Useful for mild cases.
Pharmacologic therapy	Baclofen Tizanadine Dantrolene (must monitor liver function tests) Anticonvulsants Benzodiazepines Anticonvulsants and benzodiazepines are useful for paroxysmal tonic spasms. Sedation may limit the use of the above-mentioned drugs.
Botolinum neurotoxin	Particularly useful for nonambulatory patients with severe adductor spasms that complicate adequate perineal hygiene.
Intrathecal baclofen (ITB)	May be used when oral medications cause too much sedation. Patients must be carefully evaluated before ITB use because of serious risks associated with baclofen withdrawal.

Despite complete motor recovery following TM, bladder dysfunction often persists.[295] In general, 3 forms of bladder dysfunction may be present: detrusor overactivity (failure to store), detrusor-sphincter dyssynergia (DSD), and detrusor hypocontractility (failure to empty).

In acute TM, urinary retention from a hypocontractile "shocked" bladder (detrusor areflexia or hyporeflexia) often necessitates placement of a urinary catheter.[293,295] Similar to how UMN signs appear following spinal shock, detrusor hyperreflexia typically develops, characterized by frequency, urgency, urge incontinence, and the sensation of bladder spasms[295,296]; in fact, the resolution of spinal shock and subsequent emergence of UMN signs may parallel similar changes in the bladder.[293] Some patients experience DSD, where insufficient external urinary sphincter relaxation during detrusor contraction results in urinary retention, increasing the risk for vesicoureteral reflux, infection, and nephrolithiasis.[296] Patients with DSD can also report urgency, frequency, incontinence, urinary hesitancy, and a sensation of incomplete bladder emptying after voiding.[297] More infrequently, a hypotonic, overly compliant bladder (failure to empty) may present with frequency, overflow incontinence, and signs of incomplete emptying.[297,298] Urinary symptoms are unreliable in differentiating poor bladder compliance from urinary retention.[3]

Although ultrasonographic assessment of postvoid residual urine volume is useful, urodynamic studies (and hence, urologic consultation) and renal ultrasound are often required to properly characterize the nature of bladder dysfunction, plan management, and identify those at risk for future complications.[295,298] **Table 13** summarizes the various problems of bladder dysfunction and management options.

Gastrointestinal Dysfunction

TM may result in gastrointestinal dysfunction following perturbation of the autonomic pathways of the spinal cord. In the setting of spinal shock, there is an increased risk for gastroduodenal ulceration and hemorrhage, paralytic ileus, acute gastric dilatation, and atypical presentations of acute abdominal pathology.[299]

Table 13
Managing the urinary dysfunction following transverse myelitis

	Treatment Options	Comments
Detrusor hyperreflexia (failure to store)	• Anticholinergic agents (eg, trospium, fesoterodine, oxybutynin, tolterodine) • Selective M2- and M3-antimuscarinics (darifenacin and solifenacin) • Intravesical atropine, oxybutinin, capsaicin, or resiniferatoxin • Detrusor muscle botulinum toxin A injection • Suprapubic vibration ("Queen Square bladder stimulator")	Common side effects include dry mouth and constipation. Contraindicated in patients with angle-closure glaucoma and mechanical bladder outlet obstruction. Nonselective agents should be used cautiously, if at all, in patients with cognitive dysfunction.
Detrusor-sphincter dyssynergia	• Alpha-1 adrenergic antagonists (eg, tamsulosin) • Clean intermittent catheterization (CIC) • Suprapubic vibration ("Queen Square bladder stimulator") • Neuromodulation (InterStim) • Intrasphincteric botulinum toxin • Indwelling Foley catheter • Suprapubic catheter	Alpha antagonists may cause hypotension, tachycardia, and bladder incontinence, particularly in those patients with coincident bladder spasms. CIC should be considered if postvoid residual volume exceeds 100 mL. Patients with sacral nerve stimulators cannot undergo MRIs. Indwelling Foley catheters are contraindicated in females.
Frequent urinary tract infections	Appropriate antibiotics Prophylactic antibiotic therapy Cranberry preparations Vitamin C supplementation	Cystoscopic evaluation may be needed to look for bladder trabeculations that serve as a nidus for infections.
Painful bladder spasms	Pharmacotherapy Timed voiding Neuromodulation	Pharmacotherapy: baclofen, benzodiazepines, hyoscine butylbromide, gabapentin and cannabinoids.
Nocturia	Behavioral measures Pelvic floor exercises Imipramine Desmopressin (DDAVP) Bladder rehabilitation	Avoid alcoholic and caffeinated beverages after 5 PM, to limit fluid intake in the evening, to avoid any fluids 2 h before bedtime and to void before going to bed.

Data from Refs.[3,297,298,458–465]

Gastroparesis

Gastroparesis (presenting with nausea, vomiting, pain, bloating, and/or early satiety) increases the risk of reflux and aspiration of gastric contents. It has been reported following cervical cord, thoracic cord, and cervico-medullary junction lesions.[300–303]

Gastroparesis may occur in the acute and chronic phases of TM. **Table 14** summarizes the management of gastroparesis.

Neurogenic bowel dysfunction

Bowel dysfunction is a source of considerable psychosocial disability, limiting the ability to work and affecting patients' QOL.[304] It may manifest as either constipation or fecal incontinence. The exact pathophysiology of bowel dysfunction in TM is unclear, but may because of disruption of the extrinsic neurologic control of gut and sphincter function, pelvic floor musculature, autonomic dysfunction, and/or impaired anorectal sensation.[304] Psychiatric disorders and medications also contribute to bowel dysfunction. For example, although opioid narcotics and anticholinergic drugs cause constipation, baclofen can theoretically alter the response to rectal distension and the threshold of conscious rectal sensation and cause fecal incontinence.[304] Management strategies for neurogenic bowel dysfunction are summarized in **Table 14**. Transanal irrigation (TAI) can be carried out using either a rectal balloon catheter or a cone-shaped colostomy tip. In a retrospective study of 348 patients (either constipation or fecal incontinence) during a 10-year period, TAI showed benefit in treating neurogenic bowel dysfunction.[305]

Miscellaneous gastrointestinal disorders

Hemorrhoids (and hemorrhage) are more frequent in patients with bowel dysfunction and is likely a consequence of straining and the use of suppositories and enemas.[299]

Gallbladder disease is also more prevalent following SCI.[299]

Superior mesenteric artery syndrome (where the third part of the duodenum is intermittently compressed by the vessel) causes vomiting when supine. Rapid weight loss, prolonged supine positioning, and the use of spinal orthosis are predisposing factors.[299]

Sexual Dysfunction

Sexuality is a fundamental aspect of health at the core of individual identity and influences a person's well-being.[306] Sexual dysfunction is a frequent complication of spinal cord lesions and has been shown to increase the risk of suicide.[307] As the incidence of TM is higher in the second and fourth decades of life, it affects adolescents or young adults who are sexually active.

Sexual dysfunction may be a direct consequence of damage to the autonomic and sensory pathways in the spinal cord following TM. Indirectly, complications of TM, including the psychological response to disability, spasticity, immobility, pressure ulcers, pain, and sphincter dysfunction, affect sexual function. Psychological dysfunction contributes more to sexual dysfunction than the actual physical disabilities.[308] Comorbidities (eg, mood disorders, diabetes) and medications are other important contributors to sexual dysfunction.

An open, frank, and nonjudgmental discussion about sexual function, expectations, beliefs, preferences, and the potential complications from TM should be undertaken with the patient. Including the patient's partner in such discussions is often helpful. A medical assessment of the reproductive system should be conducted as part of the multidisciplinary approach to TM.[306] Skin, bladder, and bowel care before sexual activity is important.[306] Autonomic dysreflexia (see later in this article) is a potentially dangerous consequence of sexual activity. Because of diminished or absent sensation, skin breakdown may occur from excessive friction, and in men, there is an increased risk of penile trauma.

Following spinal cord damage, most men can have some form of erection (psychogenic or reflexogenic) but these are often insufficiently predictable, rigid, or long

Table 14
Management of gastrointestinal dysfunction in patients with transverse myelitis

Problem	Management Strategies
Gastroparesis	Stop drugs that inhibit gastrointestinal motility (eg, narcotics, calcium channel blockers, anticholinergics).
	Consultation with a gastroenterologist for endoscopy, gastric emptying studies, and investigations to characterize the nature of dysmotility.
	Gastric decompression with a nasogastric tube, bowel rest, intravenous fluids, and proton-pump inhibitors or gastric H2-receptor blockers should be considered.
	Prokinetic agents (eg, metoclopramide, macrolide antibiotics, bethanecol or pyridostigmine) may be used. Tardive dyskinesia is a risk of metoclopramide use.
	Gastric electrical stimulation (Enterra therapy) and endoscopic injection of botulinum neurotoxin may be of potential benefit.
	In refractory cases, surgical interventions like pyloroplasty may be needed.
Constipation	*General measures*: high-fiber diet, bulking agents, increased fluid intake (at least 2 L daily), physical exercise, and establishing a regular toileting routine (best accomplished after breakfast to take advantage of the gastrocolic response, which peaks about 30 minutes after eating).
	Stimulant or osmotic laxatives (senna and bisacodyl) can be titrated to produce a satisfactory response (without producing liquid stool).
	Osmotic laxatives, although effective, can produce liquid stool with subsequent incontinence.
	Rectal stimulants have a predictable time of response. Begin with a glycerine suppository, progressing to bisacodyl, sodium citrate micro-enema, and ultimately a phosphate enema.
	Biofeedback may help, particularly in pelvic floor incoordination.
	Neostigmine in combination with glycopyrrolate has been shown to be effective.
	4-aminopyridine may improve constipation.
	Digital stimulation of the anal canal serves to manually disimpact the rectum.
	Abdominal massage may be helpful.
	For refractory cases: colostomy, neuromodulation, Malone Antegrade Continence Enema.
	Transanal irrigation (TAI).
Fecal incontinence	Mild and infrequent: loperamide, codeine phosphate.
	Antidiarrheal drugs should be used with caution if incontinence and constipation coexist, and periodic checks for impaction may be required. Fecal impaction is a common complication and patients experience anorexia, nausea, and spurious diarrhea (liquid stool passing around the blockage).
	Biofeedback is another useful tool.
	Anal plugs or pads may be needed.
	Severe cases: surgical intervention (eg, dynamic graciloplasty, artificial bowel sphincter, and sacral nerve stimulation).
	TAI

Data from Refs.[299,304,305,466,467]

lasting to allow sexual intercourse.[309–311] Only 25% of men with SCI have erections adequate for sexual intercourse[312]; erectile dysfunction is a great source of distress in men with SCI, even more so than the loss of functional independence or sphincter dysfunction.[313] A precise coordination of sympathetic, parasympathetic, and somatic divisions of the nervous system is essential for normal antegrade ejaculation. This intricate neural network is easily disrupted following spinal cord damage, leading to ejaculatory dysfunction and, hence, infertility. Intact genital sensation is the most important positive predictive factor of male sexual function, whereas an important negative predictor of sexuality is the presence of spasticity.[314]

The effects of spinal cord lesions on female sexuality is much less studied than in males, mainly because of the preponderance of male patients with traumatic SCI and partly because female fertility is not affected.[308,315] Manifestations include decreased libido, lack of arousal, vaginal dryness, dyspareunia, and decreased genital sensation.[316]

An important point to emphasize to all patients is that although genital sensation is diminished, individuals are more likely to develop new erotogenous areas above the level of the lesion, or with time, learn to interpret altered autonomic input from genitoperineal stimulation[317,318]; it is, therefore, important to explore new methods of sexual expression. Also, access to programs for sexual rehabilitation that include a multidisciplinary spinal cord team, as well as support groups, may be a pivotal part of treatment. **Table 15** summarizes some management strategies for sexual dysfunction.

Autonomic Dysregulation

Autonomic dysfunction may occur in the acute or chronic phases of TM and appears to be present in lesions above the upper thoracic segments.

Acute spinal cord lesions may cause neurogenic shock. In addition, cardiac dysrhythmias (eg, bradycardia and arrest) may occur.[319] Initial management may require hemodynamic monitoring and management in an intensive care setting.

Orthostatic hypotension

Orthostatic hypotension (OH) may occur in both the acute and chronic phases of TM. OH is defined as a decrease in systolic blood pressure of 20 mm Hg or more or a decrease in diastolic blood pressure of 10 mm Hg or more when the subject moves from an upright to supine posture, regardless of whether symptoms occur.[320] Clinical manifestations include pallor, diaphoresis, light-headed dizziness, syncope, anxiety, and nausea.

It is more common with lesions above the upper thoracic spinal segments.[321] Loss of sympathetic nervous activity and reflex vasoconstriction lead to pooling of venous blood in the abdominal organs and lower limbs; ultimately, cardiac output (and arterial pressure) drops. The reflex tachycardia that occurs often cannot adequately compensate for this. Cerebral hypoperfusion from reduced cardiac output is responsible for its manifestations.

Thermodysregulation

Although classically reported following traumatic SCI, thermodysregulation is another potential complication of TM with lesions at T6 and above; it can be classified as poikilothermia, "quad fever," and exercise-induced hyperthermia.[319]

Disruption of the interomediolateral columns of the spinal cord and hypothalamic lesions likely contribute to thermodysregulation following TM.[322] Perturbed heat dissipation mechanisms, in particular defective sweating (possibly owing to disruption of the descending sudomotor pathways), is believed to be a major contributor to thermodysregulation. Urinary dysfunction following TM often leads to voluntary restriction of fluid intake; further exacerbating thermodysregulation.[323]

"Quad fever" can occur in the acute phase and patients often present with fever.[319] Needless to say, a thorough workup should be undertaken to rule out infection, thromboembolism, inflammation, and atelectasis before attributing pyrexia to "quad fever."

Table 15
Management strategies for sexual dysfunction in patients with transverse myelitis

Problem	Management Strategies
Reduced libido	Stop any offending medication (particularly selective serotonin reuptake inhibitors). Consider using bupropion. Check free testosterone levels (in both men and women) - testosterone replacement therapy for deficient states.
Erectile dysfunction	Phosphodiesterase 5 inhibitors (sildenafil, tadalafil, and vardenafil). If unresponsive to oral agents, intracavernosal alprostadil injection, intraurethral alprostadil pellet, penile tension rings, vacuum devices, implantable penile prostheses, and sacral neuromodulation (Sacral Anterior Root Stimulator Implants) may be considered.
Ejaculatory dysfunction (affecting fertility)	Strong afferent stimulation and intense activation of the autonomic nervous system is needed to trigger the ejaculatory reflex. Penile vibratory stimulation (PVS) is the first line of treatment. Midodrine may be used as an adjunct to PVS in men who failed PVS alone. Rectal probe electro-ejaculation may be used but frequently results in retrograde ejaculation and may cause significant discomfort. Surgical techniques for sperm retrieval (eg, Brindley reservoir, microsurgical aspiration of spermatozoa from the vas deferens, or testicular biopsy) may also be considered if other measures fail.
Female orgasmic dysfunction	Manual and vibratory clitoral stimulation (eg, Eroscillator). Clitoral vacuum suction device (Eros) is approved by the Food and Drug Administration for female orgasmic dysfunction.
Lubrication dysfunction	Lubricants Topical estrogen Clitoral vacuum suction device (Eros) Estrogen replacement therapy

A description of the various considerations and measures to improve sexual activity and function in patients with spinal cord lesions is beyond the scope of this article. An excellent resource is the clinical practice guideline published by the Consortium for Spinal Cord Medicine.[306]
    Data from Refs.[306,317,465,468–472]

Exercise-induced hyperthermia as a result of Uhthoff phenomenon and heat-induced fatigue is important to recognize.[323] Approximately 60% to 80% of patients with MS experience transient worsening of neurologic symptoms as a result of elevated body temperature (ie, Uhthoff phenomenon).[323]

In addition to defective sweating (hypohidrosis), profuse sweating (hyperhidrosis) can occur above the level of the lesion with little or no sweating below it. Episodic hyperhidrosis may be associated with episodes of autonomic dysreflexia.[319]

Autonomic dysreflexia
Autonomic dysreflexia (AD) is a well-recognized chronic complication of SCI and may occur following TM. It usually occurs in subjects with lesions above the outflow to the splanchnic and renal vascular beds (T5-6). AD is characterized by paroxysms of excessive, uninhibited sympathetic output leading to hypertension, bradycardia

(although tachycardia may occur), pounding headache, piloerection, nasal congestion, anxiety, nausea, chills and shivering, flushing, and profuse sweating above the level of the lesion[319,324–326]; severe cases may result in myocardial ischemia, seizures, retinal detachment, intracranial hemorrhage, hypertensive emergency, reversible posterior leukoencephalopathy, and even death.[325,327–329]

The higher the level of the lesion, the more severe the cardiovascular dysfunction; complete SCI is associated with a higher incidence of AD compared with incomplete lesions.[325] Any stimuli below the affected spinal level may precipitate AD, including bladder catheterization, manipulation of an indwelling catheter, DSD, UTI, bladder percussion, sexual activity, fecal impaction, pressure sores, ingrown toenails, sacral stress fracture, and use of devices for ejaculation.[319,325,330–332] In most cases, AD is related to bladder distention or bowel impaction.[325,333]

Table 16 summarizes the management strategies for AD.

Pain and Sensory Complaints

Sensory phenomena are a common complication of TM. Early recognition and intervention may prevent chronic pain syndromes.[261] TM-related pain may be classified as nociceptive or neuropathic. Nociceptive pain is related to musculoskeletal and visceral (eg, biliary colic) sources. Neuropathic pain may be related to complex regional pain syndromes, segmental deafferentation, radiculopathy, or cord damage. Two unique types of neuropathic pain are recognized: (1) a segmentally distributed radicular pain at the level of the lesion; and (2) a late-onset central dysesthesia syndrome below the level of the lesion, characterized by a stimulus-independent, continuous pain.[334]

Treatments include oral tricyclic antidepressants, anticonvulsants, serotonin-norepinephrine reuptake inhibitors, nonsteroidal anti-inflammatory drugs, or narcotics. Lidocaine patches, topical capsaicin, and botulinum neurotoxin are other options.[3,297] Anticonvulsants may be useful for Lhermitte phenomenon.[335] Biofeedback, physical therapy, acupuncture, and transcutaneous electrical nerve stimulation are nonpharmacologic measures that can be considered. Dorsal root entry zone ablation is useful for radicular pain at the level of the lesion. Consultation with a pain management team may be needed.

A rare complication of TM is neurogenic pruritus, characterized by a dermatomal distribution of pruritus that is often associated with hypoesthesia or hyperesthesia; it responds poorly to medical therapy.[336]

Osteoporosis

Osteoporosis is a known complication of SCI[337,338] and may be a consequence of both the cord lesion, subsequent immobilization, and neuroendocrinological dysfunction.[339,340] The duration of paralysis correlates with the degree of bone loss.[340] The pathobiological underpinnings of bone demineralization are unclear and, interestingly, its pattern differs from that seen in endocrine-related osteoporosis.[339]

Bone loss begins immediately after SCI and is greater below the level of the lesion. In the first months, demineralization occurs exclusively in the sublesional areas and predominantly in weight-bearing skeletal sites.[339,340] The largest decrease in bone mass occurs during the first 6 months after injury and stabilizes after 12 to 16 months, at which point approximately two-thirds of the original bone mass is close to the threshold for pathologic fractures.[341] Hypercalcemia and hypercalciuria resulting from increased bony resorption may increase the risk of nephrolithiasis.[339,340] Women are at greater risk of osteoporosis following SCI.[340]

Supplementation with calcium and vitamin D is a cost-effective and easily implemented method of addressing bone loss. Physical exercise (weight-bearing activities,

Table 16
Management strategies for autonomic dysregulation following transverse myelitis

Problem	Management Strategy
Orthostatic hypotension	*Nonpharmacologic*: increasing fluid intake; a high salt diet (>8 g/d); avoiding a hot environment; avoiding large carbohydrate-rich meals; avoiding prolonged recumbency; application of external counterpressure (eg, abdominal binding, compression stockings); functional electrical stimulator devices (induces intermittent muscle contractions and therefore increasing venous return); exercise training may also induce positive changes in autonomic cardiovascular regulation. *Pharmacologic*: midodrine; L-threo-3,4-dihydroxyphenylserine (L-DOPS); fludrocortisone.
Thermodysregulation	Adequate hydration. Exercising or working during cooler hours of the day. Cold showers. Regional cooling devices. Precooling by immersing the lower extremities in cold water before thermal stress, allows the lower limbs to serve as "heat sinks." Dalfampridine.
Autonomic dysreflexia	*Acute Management* Identify the possible trigger and decrease afferent stimulation. Sit the patient up to cause an orthostatic decrease in the blood pressure. Loosen the clothing and other constrictive devices. Check the blood pressure every 2–5 minutes until the patient is stable. The best antihypertensive medications have a rapid onset and short duration of action (eg, nitrates, hydralazine and immediate-release nifedipine); 10 mg nifedipine may be given using the "bite and swallow" method. Alternatively, 1 inch of 2% nitropaste can be applied above the level of the lesion and wiped off when the hypertensive episode subsides. *Preventive Measures* Preventative measures are the most effective approach. Prevention of pressure sores and addressing urinary and bowel dysfunction are imperative. Individuals should carry a medical emergency card for AD. Pharmacologic prevention: Alpha-1 antagonists (terazosin and prazosin); gabapentin; prostaglandin E2; phenozybenzamine.

Data from Refs.[323,325,473–480]

verticalization, and aided-walking systems) has been shown to have an osteogenic influence in healthy subjects and in those with SCI. Functional electrical stimulator–induced mechanical loading has also been shown to conserve bone density, but this benefit is seen only if it is started as early as possible following spinal cord damage (less than 6 months postinjury). Bisphosphonates and salmon calcitonin are potentially beneficial therapies.[339]

Vitamin D Deficiency

Vitamin D deficiency is commonly found in patients with both acute and chronic SCI.[342] It may lead to elevated parathyroid hormone levels that subsequently increase bone loss.[343] Aside from its role in osteoporosis, Vitamin D is important in the immunopathogenesis of TM.

Low vitamin D levels have been linked to TM[344] as well as various autoimmune disorders, including MS,[345,346] SLE,[347] and AS.[348] In MS, suboptimal vitamin D levels increase the relapse rate as well as the risk of developing the disease. Interestingly, low vitamin D levels have been shown to correlate with an increased risk for recurrent TM.[349,350] The immunologic role of vitamin D is fascinating but remains unclear. Reductions in proinflammatory agents, such as interleukin (IL)-6, IL-1-beta, gamma-interferon, and IL-17 have been observed with vitamin D supplementation.[351,352] Optimal vitamin D levels have been shown to suppress Th17-mediated autoimmunity[353] and augment T-cell regulatory cell populations, providing a putative mechanism for preventing autoimmunity.[354]

Factors contributing to vitamin D deficiency include inadequate dietary intake and sun exposure. The primary source of vitamin D in humans is sunlight.[355] TM-related complications, including immobility and thermodysregulation, as well as photosensitivity in some autoimmune disorders, limit sunlight exposure. Many patients also harbor the misconception that consuming foods with calcium and vitamin D causes nephrolithiasis.[342] The use of hepatically metabolized anticonvulsants to treat various complications of TM further exacerbates vitamin D deficiency.[356]

The "normal" value of 25-hydroxyvitamin D levels remains 10 to 20 ng/mL in many institutions and commercial laboratories.[342] Unfortunately, recommendations about vitamin D intake from health agencies lags behind developments in the field.[357] An amount of 5000 IU per day has been shown to reduce the number of MS relapses[358] and intakes up to 10,000 IU per day appear safe.[359] Vitamin D3 appears superior to vitamin D2[360] and is available at all retail pharmacies in the United States for a low price. Patients seen at the neuroimmunologic disease clinic at our institution are encouraged to take between 5000 and 10,000 IU of vitamin D3 daily to achieve serum levels of between 60 and 80 ng/mL.

Adequate vitamin D levels have several other notable benefits, including a decreased risk of breast and colon cancer,[361,362] improved muscle strength,[363] decreased frequency of falls,[364] and diminished musculoskeletal pain.[365]

Psychological Considerations

In patients presenting for the first time with TM, consultation with a clinical psychologist or psychiatrist is valuable in addressing its understandably devastating impact on the patient's QOL. Indeed, a recent study found that almost 90% of parents of children with TM perceive a need for psychiatric care but only a quarter receive it.[277]

The loss of functional independence, along with sphincter and sexual dysfunction, would be expected to negatively affect the patient's psychological constitution and adversely affect future expectations. Mood disorders and emotional changes following TM may also be a consequence of the pathobiological changes engendered by the underlying disease process. Mood disorders, fatigue, and cognitive impairment are well-recognized sequelae of MS and autoimmune disorders like BD, SS, and SLE.[56,102,103,105,366] Additionally, certain immunomodulatory drugs (eg, interferon-beta) may cause depression.[367]

Recognition of the neuropsychiatric symptoms associated with TM is important because it affects the patient's QOL. Formal neuropsychological testing may help identify the mood disorder or cognitive domain(s) affected. Consultation with a clinical psychologist and/or psychiatrist is useful is deciding if the patient can be managed with counseling, psychotherapy, group therapy, and/or pharmacotherapy. Cognitive dysfunction may be treated with memantine or anticholinesterase inhibitors like donepezil.[297]

SUMMARY

TM constitutes a pathobiologically heterogeneous syndrome, with immune-mediated, inflammatory damage of the spinal cord at its core. A detailed history and thorough physical examination are indispensible. The most important investigation to undertake is an MRI of the entire spinal axis and the brain. The location and length of the lesion are important discriminators with etiologic and prognostic significance.

APTM is commonly attributable to MS. Although LETM is characteristic of NMO, longitudinally extensive lesions may occur in other diseases as well. The brain MRI and CSF OCBs are powerful predictors of conversion to MS. NMO-IgG seropositivity has a high specificity for NMO.

The epidemiologic, clinical, radiologic, and longitudinal data seen in pediatric TM suggests that the pathobiological underpinnings are distinct from TM in the adult population. As such, caution should be exercised when applying findings from studies in the adult population to children and vice versa.

Although the application of set criteria for diagnosing ITM has resulted in a fairly homogeneous group of patients (clinically and radiologically), it remains possible that recurrent ITM represents a unique disease entity. More longitudinal studies are needed to elucidate the nature of recurrent ITM.

REFERENCES

1. Oppenheim H. Zum Capitel der Myelitis. Berl Klin Wchnschr 1891;28:761.
2. Cree BA, Wingerchuk DM. Acute transverse myelitis: is the "idiopathic" form vanishing? Neurology 2005;65:1857–8.
3. Frohman EM, Wingerchuk DM. Clinical practice. Transverse myelitis. N Engl J Med 2010;363(6):564–72.
4. de Seze J, Stojkovic T, Breteau G, et al. Acute myelopathies: clinical, laboratory, and outcome profiles in 79 cases. Brain 2001;124:1509–21.
5. Jacob A, Weinshenker BG. An approach to the diagnosis of acute transverse myelitis. Semin Neurol 2008;28:105–20.
6. Wingerchuk DM. Postinfectious encephalomyelitis. Curr Neurol Neurosci Rep 2003;3:256–64.
7. Transverse Myelitis Consortium Group. Proposed diagnostic criteria and nosology of acute transverse myelitis. Neurology 2002;59:499–505.
8. Berman M, Feldman S, Alter M, et al. Acute transverse myelitis: incidence and etiologic considerations. Neurology 1981;31:966–71.
9. Jeffrey DR, Mandler RN, Davis LE. Transverse myelitis. Retrospective analysis of 33 cases, with differentiation of cases associated with multiple sclerosis and parainfectious events. Arch Neurol 1993;50:532–5.
10. Bhat A, Naguwa S, Cheema G, et al. The epidemiology of transverse myelitis. Autoimmun Rev 2010;9:A395–9.
11. Debette S, de Seze J, Pruvo JP, et al. Long-term outcome of acute and subacute myelopathies. J Neurol 2009;256:980–8.
12. Christensen PB, Wermuth L, Mulder DW, et al. Clinical course and long-term prognosis of acute transverse myelopathy. Acta Neurol Scand 1990;81:431–5.
13. Scott TF, Frohman EM, de Seze J, et al. Evidence-based guideline: clinical evaluation and treatment of transverse myelitis: report of the Therapeutics and

Technology Assessment Subcommittee of the American Academy of Neurology. Neurology 2011;77(24):2128–34.

14. Ditunno JF, Little JW, Tessler A, et al. Spinal shock revisited: a four-phase model. Spinal Cord 2004;42(7):383–95.

15. Fogelson J, Williams K. Compressive and traumatic myelopathies. Continuum (Minneap Minn) 2008;14(3):110–33.

16. Bakheit AM. Phantom limb sensations after complete thoracic transverse myelitis. J Neurol Neurosurg Psychiatry 2000;69(2):275–6.

17. Kempster PA, Rollinson RD. The Lhermitte phenomenon: variant forms and their significance. J Clin Neurosci 2008;15(4):379–81.

18. Layzer RB. Myeloneuropathy after prolonged exposure to nitrous oxide. Lancet 1978;312(8102):1227–30.

19. Todd NV. Priapism in acute spinal cord injury. Spinal Cord 2011;49(10):1033–5.

20. Hammond ER, Kerr DA. Priapism in infantile transverse myelitis. Arch Neurol 2009;66(7):894–7.

21. Kim SM, Go MJ, Sung JJ, et al. Painful tonic spasm in neuromyelitis optica: incidence, diagnostic utility and clinical characteristics. Arch Neurol 2012;69(8): 1026–31.

22. Tashiro K. Charles Edward Beevor. J Neurol 2001;248:635–6.

23. Brazis PW, Masdeu JC, Biller J. Spinal cord. In: Localization in clinical neurology. 5th edition. Philadelphia: Lippincott Williams & Wilkins; 2007. p. 99–123.

24. Blumenfeld H. The neurologic exam as a lesson in neuroanatomy. In: Neuroanatomy through clinical cases. Sunderland (MA): Sinauer Associates, Inc; 2002. p. 49–82.

25. Wingerchuk DM, Hogancamp WF, O'Brien PC, et al. The clinical course of neuromyelitis optica (Devic's syndrome). Neurology 1999;53(5):1107–14.

26. Palace J, Leite MI, Nairne A, et al. Interferon beta treatment in neuromyelitis optica: increase in relapses and aquaporin 4 antibody titers. Arch Neurol 2010;67(8):1016–7.

27. Bot JC, Barkhof F, Lycklama à Nijeholt GJ, et al. Comparison of a conventional cardiac-triggered dual spin-echo and a fast STIR sequence in detection of spinal cord lesions in multiple sclerosis. Eur Radiol 2000;10(5):753–8.

28. Campi A, Pontesilli S, Gerevini S, et al. Comparison of MRI pulse sequences for investigation of lesions of the cervical spinal cord. Neuroradiology 2000;42(9): 669–75.

29. Scott TF. Nosology of idiopathic transverse myelitis syndromes. Acta Neurol Scand 2007;115:371–6.

30. Scott TF, Kassab SL, Singh S. Acute partial transverse myelitis with normal cerebral magnetic resonance imaging: transition rate to clinically definite multiple sclerosis. Mult Scler 2005;11(4):373–7.

31. Lennon VA, Wingerchuk DM, Kryzer TJ, et al. A serum autoantibody marker of neuromyelitis optica: distinction from multiple sclerosis. Lancet 2004;364: 2106–12.

32. Weinshenker BG, Wingerchuk DM, Vukusic S, et al. Neuromyelitis optica IgG predicts relapse after longitudinally extensive transverse myelitis. Ann Neurol 2006;59:566–9.

33. McLean BN, Luxton RW, Thompson EJ. A study of immunoglobulin G in the cerebrospinal fluid of 1007 patients with suspected neurological disease using isoelectric focusing and the log IgG-index. A comparison and diagnostic applications. Brain 1990;113(Pt 5):1269–89.

34. Rodriguez A, Calogne M, Pedroza-Seres M, et al. Referral patterns of uveitis in a tertiary eye care center. Arch Ophthalmol 1996;114(5):593–9.
35. Frohman EM, Frohman TC, Zee DS, et al. The neuro-ophthalmology of multiple sclerosis. Lancet Neurol 2005;4(2):111–21.
36. Syme JA, Kelly JJ. Absent F-waves early in a case of transverse myelitis. Muscle Nerve 1994;17:462–5.
37. Misra UK, Kalita J. Can electromyography predict the prognosis of transverse myelitis? J Neurol 1998;245:741–4.
38. Frohman EM, Racke MK, Raine CS. Multiple sclerosis—the plaque and its pathogenesis. N Engl J Med 2006;354:942–55.
39. Cordonnier C, de Seze J, Breteau G, et al. Prospective study of patients presenting with acute partial transverse myelopathy. J Neurol 2003;250(12):1447–52.
40. Harzheim M, Schlegel U, Urbach H, et al. Discriminatory features of acute transverse myelitis: a retrospective analysis of 45 patients. J Neurol Sci 2004;217: 217–23.
41. Bruna J, Martinez-Yelamos S, Martinez-Yelamos A, et al. Idiopathic acute transverse myelitis: a clinical study and prognostic markers in 45 cases. Mult Scler 2006;12(2):169–73.
42. Sellner J, Luthi N, Buhler R, et al. Acute partial transverse myelitis: risk factors for conversion to multiple sclerosis. Eur J Neurol 2008;15(4):398–405.
43. Bourre B, Zephir H, Ongagna JC, et al. Long-term follow-up of acute partial transverse myelitis. Arch Neurol 2012;69(3):357–62.
44. Fisniku LK, Brex PA, Altmann DR, et al. Disability and T2 MRI lesions: a 20-year follow-up of patients with relapse onset of multiple sclerosis. Brain 2008;131: 808–17.
45. Barkhof F, Filippi M, Miller DH, et al. Comparison of MRI criteria at first presentation to predict conversion to clinically definite multiple sclerosis. Brain 1997; 120(pt 11):2059–69.
46. Bashir K, Whitaker JN. Importance of paraclinical and CSF studies in the diagnosis of MS in patients presenting with partial cervical transverse myelopathy and negative cranial MRI. Mult Scler 2000;6:312–6.
47. O'Riordan JI, Thompson AJ, Kingsley DP, et al. The prognostic value of brain MRI in clinically isolated syndromes of the CNSA 10-year follow up. Brain 1998;121:495–503.
48. Martinelli V, Comi G, Rovaris M, et al. Acute myelopathy of unknown etiology: a clinical, neurophysiological and MRI study of short and long-term prognostic factors. J Neurol 1995;242:497–503.
49. Perumal J, Zabad R, Caon C, et al. Acute transverse myelitis with normal brain MRI: long-term risk of MS. J Neurol 2008;255(1):89–93.
50. Qiu W, Wu JS, Zhang MN, et al. Longitudinally extensive myelopathy in Caucasians: a West Australian study of 26 cases from the Perth Demyelinating Diseases Database. J Neurol Neurosurg Psychiatry 2010;81:209–12.
51. Wingerchuk DM, Lennon VA, Pittock SJ, et al. Revised diagnostic criteria for neuromyelitis optica. Neurology 2006;66:1485–9.
52. Pittock SJ, Lennon VA, de Seze J, et al. Neuromyelitis optica and non organ-specific autoimmunity. Arch Neurol 2008;65:78–83.
53. Wingerchuk DM, Lennon VA, Lucchinetti CF, et al. The spectrum of neuromyelitis optica. Lancet Neurol 2007;6:805–15.
54. Jarius S, Jacobi C, de Seze J, et al. Frequency and specificity of antibodies to aquaporin-4 in neurological patients with rheumatic disorders. Mult Scler 2011; 17(9):1067–73.

55. Vitali C, Bombardieri S, Jonsson R, et al. Classification criteria for Sjögren's syndrome: a revised version of the European criteria proposed by the American-European Consensus Group. Ann Rheum Dis 2002;61:554–8.
56. Govoni M, Padovan M, Rizzo N, et al. CNS involvement in primary Sjogren's syndrome: prevalence, clinical aspects, diagnostic assessment and therapeutic approach. CNS Drugs 2001;15:597–607.
57. Delalande S, de Seze J, Fauchais AL, et al. Neurologic manifestations in primary Sjögren syndrome: a study of 82 patients. Medicine (Baltimore) 2004;83: 280–91.
58. Alexander EL, Provost TT, Stevens MD, et al. Neurologic complications of primary Sjögren's syndrome. Medicine (Baltimore) 1982;61:247–57.
59. Escudero D, Latorre P, Codina M, et al. Central nervous system disease in Sjögren's syndrome. Ann Med Interne (Paris) 1995;146:239–42.
60. Kim SM, Water P, Vincent A, et al. Sjögren's syndrome myelopathy: spinal cord involvement in Sjogren's syndrome might be a manifestation of NMO. Mult Scler 2009;15:1062–8.
61. Konttinen YT, Kinnunen E, Von Bonsdorff M, et al. Acute transverse myelopathy successfully treated with plasmapheresis and prednisone in a patient with primary Sjogren's syndrome. Arthritis Rheum 1987;30:339–44.
62. Canhao H, Fonseca JE, Rosa A. Intravenous gammaglobulin in the treatment of central nervous system vasculitis associated with Sjögren's syndrome. J Rheumatol 2000;27:1102–3.
63. Alcântara C, Gomes MJ, Ferreira C. Rituximab therapy in primary Sjögren's syndrome. Ann N Y Acad Sci 2009;1173:701–5 (Contemporary Challenges in Autoimmunity).
64. Hochberg MC. Updating the American College of Rheumatology revised criteria for the classification of systemic lupus erythematosus. Arthritis Rheum 1997; 40(9):1725.
65. West SG. Neuropsychiatric lupus. Rheum Dis Clin North Am 1994;20(1):129–58.
66. Eckstein C, Saidha S, Levy M. A differential diagnosis of central nervous system demyelination: beyond multiple sclerosis. J Neurol 2012;259(5):801–16.
67. Kovacs B, LaVerty T, Brent L, et al. Transverse myelopathy in systemic lupus erythematosus: an analysis of 14 cases and review of the literature. Ann Rheum Dis 2000;59:120–4.
68. Schulz SW, Shenin M, Mehta A, et al. Initial presentation of acute transverse myelitis in systemic lupus erythematosus: demographics, diagnosis, management and comparison to idiopathic cases. Rheumatol Int 2012;32(9): 2623–7.
69. Katsiari CG, Giavri I, Mitsikostas DD, et al. Acute transverse myelitis and anti-phospholipid antibodies in lupus. No evidence for anticoagulation. Eur J Neurol 2011;18(4):556–63.
70. Bertsias GK, Ioannidis JP, Aringer M, et al. EULAR recommendations for the management of systemic lupus erythematosus with neuropsychiatric manifestations: report of a task force of the EULAR standing committee for clinical affairs. Ann Rheum Dis 2010;69(12):2074–82.
71. Espinosa G, Mendizabal A, Minguez S, et al. Transverse myelitis affecting more than 4 spinal segments associated with systemic lupus erythematosus: clinical, immunological, and radiological characteristics of 22 patients. Semin Arthritis Rheum 2010;39(4):246–56.
72. Birnbaum J, Petri M, Thompson R, et al. Distinct subtypes of myelitis in systemic lupus erythematosus. Arthritis Rheum 2009;60(11):3378–87.

73. D'Cruz DP, Mellor-Pita S, Joven B, et al. Transverse myelitis as the first manifestation of systemic lupus erythematosus or lupus-like disease: good functional outcome and relevance of antiphospholipid antibodies. J Rheumatol 2004;31:280–5.
74. Tellez-Zenteno JF, Remes-Troche JM, Negrete-Pulido RO, et al. Longitudinal myelitis associated with systemic lupus erythematosus: clinical features and magnetic resonance imaging of six cases. Lupus 2001;10:851–6.
75. Provenzale JM, Barboriak DP, Gaensler RL, et al. Lupus-related myelitis: serial MR findings. Am J Neuroradiol 1994;15:1911–7.
76. Salmaggi A, Lamperti E, Eoli M, et al. Spinal cord involvement and systemic lupus erythematosus: clinical and magnetic resonance findings in 5 patients. Clin Exp Rheumatol 1994;12:389–94.
77. Mok CC, Lau CS, Chan EYT, et al. Acute transverse myelopathy in systemic lupus erythematosus: clinical presentation, treatment and outcome. J Rheumatol 1998;25:467–73.
78. Deodhar AA, Hochenedl T, Bennett RM. Longitudinal involvement of the spinal cord in a patient with lupus related transverse myelitis. J Rheumatol 1999;26:446–9.
79. Neumann-Andersen G, Lindgren S. Involvement of the entire spinal cord and medulla oblongata in acute catastrophic-onset transverse myelitis in SLE. Clin Rheumatol 2000;19:156–60.
80. Katramados AM, Rabah R, Adams MD, et al. Longitudinal myelitis, aseptic meningitis, and conus medullaris infarction as presenting manifestations of pediatric systemic lupus erythematosus. Lupus 2008;17:332–6.
81. Theodoridou A, Settas L. Demyelination in rheumatic diseases. Postgrad Med J 2008;84:127–32.
82. Barile-Fabris L, Ariza-Andraca R, Olguin-Ortega L, et al. Controlled clinical trial of IV cyclophosphamide versus IV methylprenisolone in severe neurological manifestations in systemic lupus erythematous. Ann Rheum Dis 2005;64:620–5.
83. Sherer Y, Hassin S, Shoenfeld Y, et al. Transverse myelitis in patients with antiphospholipid antibodies—the importance of early diagnosis and treatment. Clin Rheumatol 2002;21:207–10.
84. Harisdangkul V, Doorenbos D, Subramony SH. Lupus transverse myelopathy: better outcome with early recognition and aggressive high-dose intravenous corticosteroid pulse treatment. J Neurol 1995;242:326–31.
85. Neuwelt CM. The role of plasmapheresis in the treatment of severe central nervous system neuropsychiatric systemic lupus erythematosus. Ther Apher Dial 2003;7:173–82.
86. Bartolucci P, Bréchignac S, Cohen P, et al. Adjunctive plasma exchanges to treat neuropsychiatric lupus: a retrospective study on 10 patients. Lupus 2007;16:817–22.
87. Armstrong DJ, McCarron MT, Wright GD. SLE-associated transverse myelitis successfully treated with rituximab (anti-CD20 monoclonal antibody). Rheumatol Int 2006;26:771–2.
88. Ye Y, Qian J, Gu Y, et al. Rituximab in the treatment of severe lupus myelopathy. Clin Rheumatol 2011;30(7):981–6.
89. Lu X, Gu Y, Wang Y, et al. Prognostic factors of lupus myelopathy. Lupus 2008;17:323–8.
90. Wilson WA, Gharavi AE, Koike T, et al. International consensus statement on preliminary classification criteria for definite antiphospholipid syndrome: report of an international workshop. Arthritis Rheum 1999;42(7):1309–11.

91. Cervera R, Piette JC, Font J, et al. Antiphospholipid syndrome: clinical and immunologic manifestations and patterns of disease expression in a cohort of 1000 patients. Arthritis Rheum 2002;46:1019–27.

92. Kim JH, Lee SI, Park SI, et al. Recurrent transverse myelitis in primary antiphospholipid syndrome: case report and literature review. Rheumatol Int 2004;24: 244–6.

93. Rodrigues CE, de Carvalho JF. Clinical, radiologic, and therapeutic analysis of 14 patients with transverse myelitis associated with antiphospholipid syndrome: report of 4 cases and review of the literature. Semin Arthritis Rheum 2011;40(4): 349–57.

94. Tristano AG. Acute transverse myelitis as part of the catastrophic antiphospholipid syndrome in a systemic lupus erythematosus patient. Neurologia 2004;19: 774–5.

95. Rodrigues CE, Carvalho JF, Shoenfeld Y. Neurological manifestations of antiphospholipid syndrome. Eur J Clin Invest 2010;40(4):350–9.

96. Tourbah A, Clapin A, Gout O, et al. Systemic autoimmune features and multiple sclerosis. A 5-year follow up. Arch Neurol 1998;55:517–21.

97. Roussel V, Yi F, Jauberteau O, et al. Prevalence and clinical significance of antiphospholipid antibodies in multiple sclerosis: a study of 89 patients. J Autoimmun 2000;14:259–65.

98. Gaarg N, Zivadinov R, Ramanathan M, et al. Clinical and MRI correlates of autoreactive antibodies in multiple sclerosis patients. J Neuroimmunol 2007;187: 159–65.

99. Stosic M, Ambrus J, Garg N, et al. MRI characteristics of patients with antiphospholipid syndrome and multiple sclerosis. J Neurol 2010;257(1):63–71.

100. Szmyrka-Kaczmarek M, Pokryszko-Dragan A, Pawlik B, et al. Antinuclear and antiphospholipid antibodies in patients with multiple sclerosis. Lupus 2012;21: 412–20.

101. The International Study Group for Behcet's disease. Criteria for diagnosis of Behcet's disease. Lancet 1990;335:1078–80.

102. Al-Araji A, Kidd D. Neuro-Behcet's disease: epidemiology, clinical characteristics, and management. Lancet Neurol 2009;8:192–204.

103. Yesilot N, Mutlu M, Gungoer O, et al. Clinical characteristics and course of spinal cord involvement in Behcet's disease. Eur J Neurol 2007;14:729–37.

104. Ideguchi H, Suda A, Takeno M, et al. Neurological manifestations of Behcet's disease in Japan: a study of 54 patients. J Neurol 2010;257(6):1012–20.

105. Akman-Demir G, Serdaroglu P, Tasci B, et al. Clinical patterns of neurological involvement in Behçet's disease: evaluation of 200 patients. Brain 1999;122: 2171–81.

106. Moskau S, Urbach H, Hartmann A, et al. Multifocal myelitis in Behcet's disease. Neurology 2003;60(3):517.

107. Kocer N, Islak C, Siva A, et al. CNS involvement in neuro-Behcet syndrome: an MR study. AJNR Am J Neuroradiol 1999;20:1015–24.

108. Monaco AL, Corte RL, Caniatti L, et al. Neurological involvement in North Italian patients with Behcet's disease. Rheumatol Int 2006;26:1113–9.

109. Lee SH, Yoon PH, Park SJ, et al. MRI findings in neuro-Behcet's disease. Clinical Radiol 2001;56:485–94.

110. Fukae J, Noda K, Fujishima K, et al. Subacute longitudinal myelitis associated with Behcet's disease. Intern Med 2010;49:343–7.

111. Morrissey SP, Miller DH, Hermaszewski R, et al. Magnetic resonance imaging of the central nervous system in Behcet's disease. Eur Neurol 1993;33:287–93.

112. Yoshioka H, Matsubara T, Miyanomae Y, et al. Spinal cord MRI in neuro-Behcet's disease. Neuroradiology 1996;38:661-2.
113. Mascalchi M, Cosottini M, Cellerini M, et al. MRI of spinal cord involvement in Behcet's disease: case report. Neuroradiology 1998;40(4):255-7.
114. Green AL, Mitchell PJ. Spinal cord neuro-Behcet's disease detected on magnetic resonance imaging. Australas Radiol 2000;44(2):201-3.
115. Desphande DM, Krishnan C, Kerr DA. Transverse myelitis after lumbar steroid injection in a patient with Behcet's disease. Spinal Cord 2005;43:735-7.
116. Vuolo L, Bonzano L, Roccatagliata C, et al. Reversibility of brain lesions in a case of neuro-Behcet's disease studied by MR diffusion. Neurol Sci 2010; 31(2):213-5.
117. Kidd D, Steuer A, Denman AM, et al. Neurological complications in Behçet's syndrome. Brain 1999;122:2183-94.
118. Coban O, Bahar S, Akman-Demir G, et al. Masked assessment of MRI findings: is it possible to differentiate neuro-Behcet's disease from other central nervous system. Neuroradiology 1999;41:255-60.
119. Zhao B, He L, Lai XH. A case of neuro-Behcet's disease presenting with lumbar spinal cord involvement. Spinal Cord 2010;48:172-3.
120. Piptone N, Olivieri I, Padula A, et al. Infliximab for the treatment of neuro-Behcet's disease: a case series and review of the literature. Arthritis Rheum 2008; 59:285-90.
121. Serkova NJ, Christians U, Benet LZ. Biochemical mechanisms of cyclosporine neurotoxicity. Mol Interv 2004;4:97-107.
122. Kotake S, Higashi K, Yoshikawa K, et al. Central nervous system symptoms in patients with Behçet disease receiving cyclosporine therapy. Ophthalmology 1999;106:586-9.
123. Kato Y, Numaga J, Kato S, et al. Central nervous system symptoms in a population of Behçet's disease patients with refractory uveitis treated with cyclosporine A. Clin Experiment Ophthalmol 2001;29:335-6.
124. Kötter I, Günaydin I, Batra M, et al. CNS involvement occurs more frequently in patients with Behçet's disease under cyclosporin A (CSA) than under other medications: results of a retrospective analysis of 117 cases. Clin Rheumatol 2006;25:482-6.
125. Lower EE, Broderick JP, Brott TG, et al. Diagnosis and management of neurological sarcoidosis. Arch Intern Med 1997;157(16):1864-8.
126. Chapelon C, Ziza JM, Piette JC, et al. Neurosarcoidosis: signs, course and treatment in 35 confirmed cases. Medicine (Baltimore) 1990;69(5):261-76.
127. Stern BJ, Krumholz A, Johns C, et al. Sarcoidosis and its neurological manifestations. Arch Neurol 1985;42(9):909-17.
128. Delaney P. Neurologic manifestations in sarcoidosis: review of the literature, with a report of 23 cases. Ann Intern Med 1977;87(3):336-45.
129. Saleh S, Saw C, Marzouk K, et al. Sarcoidosis of the spinal cord: literature review and report of eight cases. J Natl Med Assoc 2006;98:965-76.
130. Joseph FG, Scolding NJ. Neurosarcoidosis: a study of 30 new cases. J Neurol Neurosurg Psychiatry 2009;80(3):297-304.
131. Cohen-Aubart F, Galanaud D, Grabli D, et al. Spinal cord sarcoidosis: clinical and laboratory profile and outcome of 31 patients in a case-control study. Medicine (Baltimore) 2010;89(2):133-40.
132. Christoforidis GA, Spickler EM, Recio MV, et al. MR of CNS sarcoidosis: correlation of imaging features to clinical symptoms and response to treatment. AJNR Am J Neuroradiol 1999;20(4):655-69.

133. Bhagavati S, Choi J. Intramedullary cervical spinal cord sarcoidosis. Spinal Cord 2009;47:179–81.
134. Terada T, Shigeno K, Hori M, et al. Isolated spinal neurosarcoidosis: an autopsy case. Spinal Cord 2010;48:776–8.
135. Lidar M, Dori A, Levy Y, et al. Sarcoidosis presenting as "corset-like" myelopathy: a description of six cases and literature review. Clin Rev Allergy Immunol 2010;38(2–3):270–5.
136. Marangoni S, Argentiero V, Tavolato B, Neurosarcoidosis. Clinical description of 7 cases with a proposal for a new diagnostic strategy. J Neurol 2006;253(4): 488–95.
137. Spencer TS, Campellone JV, Maldonado I, et al. Clinical and magnetic resonance imaging manifestations of neurosarcoidosis. Semin Arthritis Rheum 2005;34:649–61.
138. Kumar N, Frohman EM. Spinal neurosarcoidosis mimicking an idiopathic inflammatory demyelinating syndrome. Arch Neurol 2004;61(4):586–9.
139. Sakushima K, Yabe I, Nakano F, et al. Clinical features of spinal cord sarcoidosis: analysis of 17 neurosarcoidosis patients. J Neurol 2011;258(12):2163–7.
140. Zajicek JP, Scolding NJ, Foster O, et al. Central nervous system sarcoidosis—diagnosis and management. QJM 1999;92(2):103–7.
141. Shah R, Roberson GH, Cure JK. Correlation of MR imaging findings and clinical manifestations in neurosarcoidosis. AJNR Am J Neuroradiol 2009;30:953–61.
142. Sulavik SB, Spencer RP, Weed DA, et al. Recognition of distinctive patterns of gallium-67 distribution in sarcoidosis. J Nucl Med 1990;31:1909–14.
143. Dale JC, O'Brien JF. Determination of angiotensin-converting enzyme levels in cerebrospinal fluid is not a useful test for the diagnosis of neurosarcoidosis. Mayo Clin Proc 1999;74(5):535.
144. Read RW, Holland GN, Rao NA, et al. Revised diagnostic criteria for Vogt-Koyanagi-Harada disease: report of the international committee on nomenclature. Am J Ophthalmol 2001;131(5):647–52.
145. Lubin JR, Lowenstein JI, Fredrick AR. VKH syndrome with focal neurological signs. Am J Ophthalmol 1981;91(3):332–41.
146. Dahbour SS. MRI documented acute myelitis in a patient with Vogt-Koyanagi-Harada syndrome: first report. Clin Neurol Neurosurg 2009;111(2):200–2.
147. Rajendram R, Evans M, Khurana RN, et al. Vogt-Koyanagi-Harada disease presenting as optic neuritis. Int Ophthalmol 2007;27(2–3):217–20.
148. Tahara T, Sekitani T. Neurotological evaluation of Harada's disease. Acta Otolaryngol Suppl 1995;519:110–3.
149. Miyanaga M, Kawaguchi T, Shimuzu K, et al. Influence of early cerebrospinal fluid-guided diagnosis and early high-dose corticosteroid therapy on ocular outcomes of Vogt-Koyanagi-Harada disease. Int Ophthalmol 2007;27(2–3): 183–8.
150. Miller DH, Weinshenker BG, Filippi M, et al. Differential diagnosis of suspected multiple sclerosis: a consensus approach. Mult Scler 2008;14(9):1157–74.
151. Tenenbaum S, Chitnis T, Ness J, et al. Acute disseminated encephalomyelitis. Neurology 2007;68(16 Suppl 2):S32–6.
152. Straussberg R, Schonfeld T, Weitz R, et al. Improvement of atypical acute disseminated encephalomyelitis with steroids and intravenous immunoglobulins. Pediatr Neurol 2001;24:139–43.
153. Aimoto Y, Moriwaka F, Matsumoto K, et al. A case of acute disseminated encephalomyelitis (ADEM) associated with demyelinating peripheral neuropathy. No To Shinkei 1996;48:857–60.

154. Torisu H, Kira R, Ishizaki Y, et al. Clinical study of childhood acute disseminated encephalomyelitis, multiple sclerosis, and acute transverse myelitis in Fukuoka Prefecture, Japan. Brain Dev 2010;32(6):454–62.
155. Huynh W, Cordato DJ, Kehdi E, et al. Post-vaccination encephalomyelitis: literature review and illustrative case. J Clin Neurosci 2008;15(12):1315–22.
156. Callen DJ, Shroff MM, Branson HM, et al. Role of MRI in the differentiation of ADEM from MS in children. Neurology 2009;72(11):968–73.
157. Kesselring J, Miller DH, Robb SA, et al. Acute disseminated encephalomyelitis. MRI findings and the distinction from multiple sclerosis. Brain 1990;113: 291–302.
158. Kimura S, Nezu A, Ohtsuki N, et al. Serial magnetic resonance imaging in children with postinfectious encephalitis. Brain Dev 1996;18:461–5.
159. Franciotta D, Columba-Cabezas S, Andreoni L, et al. Oligoclonal IgG band patterns in inflammatory demyelinating human and mouse diseases. J Neuroimmunol 2008;200(1–2):125–8.
160. Stuve O, Nessler S, Hartung HP, et al. Acute disseminated encephalomyelitis: pathogenesis, diagnosis, treatment, and prognosis. Nervenarzt 2005;76(6): 701–7.
161. Straub J, Chofflon M, Delavelle J. Early high-dose intravenous methylprednisolone in acute disseminated encephalomyelitis: a successful recovery. Neurology 1997;49(4):1145–7.
162. Stricker RB, Miller RG, Kiprov DD. Role of plasmapheresis in acute disseminated (post-infectious) encephalomyelitis. J Clin Apher 1992;7(4):173–9.
163. Weinshenker BG, O'Brien PC, Petterson TM, et al. A randomized trial of plasma exchange in acute CNS inflammatory demyelinating disease. Ann Neurol 1999; 46:878–86.
164. Llufriu S, Castillo J, Blanco Y, et al. Plasma exchange for acute attacks of CNS demyelination: predictors of improvement at 6 months. Neurology 2009;73(12): 949–53.
165. Keegan M, Pineda AA, McClelland RL, et al. Plasma exchange for severe attacks of CNS demyelination: predictors of response. Neurology 2002;58: 143–6.
166. Stübgen JP. Immune-mediated myelitis associated with hepatitis virus infections. J Neuroimmunol 2011;239(1–2):21–7.
167. Takahashi-Fujigasaki J, Takagi S, Sakamoto T, et al. Spinal cord biopsy findings of anti-aquaporin-4 antibody-negative recurrent longitudinal myelitis in a patient with sicca symptoms and hepatitis C viral infection. Neuropathology 2009;29(4): 472–9.
168. Aktipi KM, Ravaglia S, Ceroni M, et al. Severe recurrent myelitis in patients with hepatitis C virus infection. Neurology 2007;68:468–9.
169. Pacheco VH, Acharya JN. Recurrent myelopathy and hepatitis C infection. Ann Neurol 2006;60(Suppl 3):S45.
170. Grewal AK, Lopes MB, Berg CL, et al. Recurrent demyelinating myelitis associated with hepatitis C viral infection. J Neurol Sci 2004;224:101–6.
171. Sobukawa E, Sakimura K, Hoshino S, et al. Hepatic myelopathy: an unusual neurological complication of advanced hepatic disease. Intern Med 1994;33: 718–22.
172. Mandal K, Chopra N. Acute transverse myelitis following hepatitis E virus infection. Indian Pediatr 2006;43:365–6.
173. Seet RC, Lim EC, Wilder-Smith EP. Acute transverse myelitis following dengue virus infection. J Clin Virol 2006;35(3):310–2.

174. Kusuhara T, Nakajima M, Inoue H, et al. Parainfectious encephalomyeloradiculitis associated with herpes simplex virus 1 DNA in cerebrospinal fluid. Clin Infect Dis 2002;34(9):1199–205.
175. Larik A, Chiong Y, Lee LC, et al. Longitudinally extensive transverse myelitis associated with dengue fever. BMJ Case Rep 2012. http://dx.doi.org/10.1136/bcr.12.2011.5378. pii: bcr1220115378.
176. Chanthamat N, Sathirapanya P. Acute transverse myelitis associated with dengue viral infection. J Spinal Cord Med 2010;33(4):425–7.
177. Kincaid O, Lipton HL. Viral myelitis: an update. Curr Neurol Neurosci Rep 2006; 6(6):469–74.
178. Roos KL. West Nile encephalitis and myelitis. Curr Opin Neurol 2004;17:343–6.
179. Solomon T, Dung NM, Kneen R, et al. Japanese encephalitis. J Neurol Neurosurg Psychiatry 2000;68:405–15.
180. Einsiedel L, Kat E, Ravindran J, et al. MR findings in Murray Valley encephalitis. AJNR Am J Neuroradiol 2003;24:1379–82.
181. Bender A. Severe tick borne encephalitis with simultaneous brain stem, bithalamic, and spinal cord involvement documented by MRI. J Neurol Neurosurg Psychiatry 2005;76:135–7.
182. Scheibe F, Hofmann J, Ruprecht K. Parainfectious myelitis associated with parvovirus B19 infection. J Neurol 2010;257:1557–8.
183. Barton LL, Hyndman NJ. Lymphocytic choriomeningitis virus: reemerging central nervous system pathogen. Pediatrics 2000;105:e35.
184. Arpino C, Curatolo P, Rezza G. Chikungunya and the nervous system: what we do and do not know. Rev Med Virol 2009;19(3):121–9.
185. Huisa BN, Chapin JE, Adair JC. Central nervous system complications following Hanta virus cardiopulmonary syndrome. J Neurovirol 2009;15(2):202–5.
186. Unay B, Kendirli T, Meral C, et al. Transverse myelitis due to echovirus type 30. Acta Paediatr 2005;94(12):1863–4.
187. Ponka A. Central nervous system manifestations associated with serologically verified Mycoplasma pneumoniae infection. Scand J Infect Dis 1980;12:175–84.
188. Cassell GH, Cole BC. Mycoplasmas as agents of human disease. N Engl J Med 1981;304:80–9.
189. Koskiniemi M. CNS manifestations associated with Mycoplasma pneumoniae infections: summary of cases at the University of Helsinki and review. Clin Infect Dis 1993;17(Suppl 1):S52–7.
190. Tsiodras S, Kelesidis TH, Kelesidis I, et al. Mycoplasma pneumoniae-associated myelitis: a comprehensive review. Eur J Neurol 2006;13:112–24.
191. Isoda H, Ramsey R. MR imaging of acute transverse myelitis (myelopathy). Radiat Med 1998;16:179–86.
192. Goebels N, Helmchen C, Abele-Horn M, et al. Extensive myelitis associated with Mycoplasma pneumoniae infection: magnetic resonance imaging and clinical long-term follow-up. J Neurol 2001;248:204–8.
193. Csabi G, Komaromy H, Hollody K. Transverse myelitis as a rare, serious complication of Mycoplasma pneumoniae infection. Pediatr Neurol 2009;41(4):312–3.
194. Gozzard P, Orr D, Sanderson F, et al. Acute transverse myelitis as a rare manifestation of Campylobacter diarrhoea with concomitant disruption of the blood brain barrier. J Clin Neurosci 2012;19:316–8.
195. Baar I, Jacobs BC, Govers N, et al. Campylobacter jejuni-induced acute transverse myelitis. Spinal Cord 2007;45:690–4.
196. Aberle J, Kluwe J, Pawlas F, et al. Severe myelitis following infection with Campylobacter enteritis. Eur J Clin Microbiol Infect Dis 2004;23:134–5.

197. Huber S, Kappos L, Fuhr P, et al. Combined acute disseminated encephalomy-elitis and acute motor axonal neuropathy after vaccination for hepatitis A and infection with *Campylobacter jejuni*. J Neurol 1999;246:1204–6.
198. Orr D, McKendrick MW, Sharrack B. Acute disseminated encephalomyelitis temporally associated with *Campylobacter* gastroenteritis. J Neurol Neurosurg Psychiatry 2004;75:792–3.
199. Gaig C, Valldeoriola F, Saiz A. Acute disseminated encephalomyelitis associ-ated with *Campylobacter jejuni* infection and antiganglioside GM1 IgG anti-bodies. J Neurol 2005;252:613–4.
200. Nasralla CA, Pay N, Goodpasture HC, et al. Postinfectious encephalopathy in a child following *Campylobacter jejuni* enteritis. AJNR Am J Neuroradiol 1993; 14:444–8.
201. Bigi S, Aebi C, Nauer C, et al. Acute transverse myelitis in Lyme neuroborrelio-sis. Infection 2010;38(5):413–6.
202. Pourhassan A, Shoja MM, Tubbs RS, et al. Acute transverse myelitis secondary to *Salmonella paratyphi* B infection. Infection 2008;36(2):170–3.
203. Ubogu EE, Lindenberg JR, Werz MA. Transverse myelitis associated with *Acine-tobacter baumanii* intrathecal pump catheter-related infection. Reg Anesth Pain Med 2003;28(5):470–4.
204. Waltereit R, Küker W, Jürgens S, et al. Acute transverse myelitis associated with *Coxiella burnetii* infection. J Neurol 2001;249(10):1459–61.
205. Schimmel MS, Schlesinger Y, Berger I, et al. Transverse myelitis: unusual sequelae of neonatal group B streptococcus disease. J Perinatol 2002;22(7): 580–1.
206. Pickerill RG, Milder JE. Transverse myelitis associated with cat-scratch disease in an adult. JAMA 1981;246:2840–1.
207. Salgado CD, Weisse ME. Transverse myelitis associated with probable cat-scratch disease in a previously healthy pediatric patient. Clin Infect Dis 2000; 31(2):609–11.
208. Williams W, Sunderland R. As sick as a pigeon; psittacosis myelitis. Arch Dis Child 1989;64:1626–8.
209. Crook T, Bannister B. Acute transverse myelitis associated with *Chlamydia psit-taci* infection. J Infect 1996;32(2):151–2.
210. de Lau LM, Siepman DA, Remmers MJ, et al. Acute disseminating encephalo-myelitis following Legionnaires disease. Arch Neurol 2010;67(5):623–6.
211. Lee KL, Lee JK, Yim YM, et al. Acute transverse myelitis associated with scrub typhus: case report and a review of literature. Diagn Microbiol Infect Dis 2008; 60(2):237–9.
212. Feng Y, Guo N, Liu J, et al. Mycobacteria infection in incomplete transverse myelitis is refractory steroids: a pilot study. Clin Dev Immunol 2011;2011: 501369.
213. Krishnan C, Kaplin AI, Graber JS, et al. Recurrent transverse myelitis following neurobrucellosis: immunologic features and beneficial response to immunosup-pression. J Neurovirol 2005;11:225–31.
214. Baylor P, Garoufi A, Karpathios T, et al. Transverse myelitis in 2 patients with *Bartonella henselae* infection (cat scratch disease). Clin Infect Dis 2007;45: e42–5.
215. Gumbo T, Hakim JG, Mielke J, et al. Cryptococcus myelitis: atypical presenta-tion of a common infection. Clin Infect Dis 2001;32:1235–6.
216. Shields GS, Castillo M. Myelitis caused by *Cladophialophora bantiana*. AJR Am J Roentgenol 2002;179:278–9.

217. Jabbour RA, Kanj SS, Sawaya RA, et al. *Toxocara canis* myelitis: clinical features, magnetic resonance imaging (MRI) findings, and treatment outcome in 17 patients. Medicine (Baltimore) 2011;90(5):337–43.
218. Dauriac-Le Masson V, Chochon F, Demeret S, et al. *Toxocara canis* meningo-myelitis. J Neurol 2005;252(10):1267–8.
219. Marx C, Lin J, Masruha MR, et al. Toxocariasis of the CNS simulating acute disseminated encephalomyelitis. Neurology 2007;69(8):806–7.
220. Helsen G, Vandecasteele SJ, Vanopdenbosch LJ. Toxocariasis presenting as encephalomyelitis. Case Report Med 2011;2011:503913. http://dx.doi.org/10.1155/2011/503913.
221. Ross AG, McManus DP, Farrar J, et al. Neuroschistosomiasis. J Neurol 2012;259:22–32.
222. Bunyaratavej K, Pongpunlert W, Jongwutiwes S, et al. Spinal gnathostomiasis resembling an intrinsic cord tumor/myelitis in a 4-year-old boy. Southeast Asian J Trop Med Public Health 2008;39:800–3.
223. Kibiki GS, Murphy DK. Transverse myelitis due to trypanosomiasis in a middle aged Tanzanian man. J Neurol Neurosurg Psychiatry 2006;77:684–5.
224. Drulovic J, Dujmovic I, Stojsavljevic N. Transverse myelopathy in the antiphos-pholipid antibody syndrome: pinworm infestation as a trigger? J Neurol Neuro-surg Psychiatry 2000;68:246–56.
225. Lesca G, Deschamps R, Lubetzki C, et al. Acute myelitis in early *Borrelia burg-dorferi* infection. J Neurol 2002;249:1472–4.
226. Baumann M, Birnbacher R, Koch J, et al. Uncommon manifestations of neuro-borreliosis in children. Eur J Paediatr Neurol 2010;14:274–7.
227. Bajaj NPS, Rose P, Clifford-Jones R, et al. Acute transverse myelitis and Guillain-Barre overlap syndrome with serological evidence for mumps viraemia. Acta Neurol Scand 2001;104:239–42.
228. Venketasubramanian N. Transverse myelitis following mumps in an adult—a case report with MRI correlation. Acta Neurol Scand 1997;96:328–31.
229. Rigamonti A, Usai S, Ciusani E, et al. Atypical transverse myelitis due to cyto-megalovirus in an immunocompetent patient. Neurol Sci 2005;26:351–4.
230. Ku B, Lee K. Acute transverse myelitis caused by Coxsackie virus B4 infection: a case report. J Korean Med Sci 1998;13:449–53.
231. Minami K, Tsuda Y, Maeda H, et al. Acute transverse myelitis caused by Coxsackie virus B5 infection. J Paediatr Child Health 2004;40:66–8.
232. Chortis P. Study in the therapy of transverse myelitis occurring during tubercu-lous meningitis. Dis Chest 1958;33:506–12.
233. McMinn P, Stratov I, Nagarajan L, et al. Neurological manifestations of Entero-virus 71 infection in children during an outbreak of hand, foot, and mouth disease in Western Australia. Clin Infect Dis 2001;32(2):236–42.
234. Gruhn B, Meerbach A, Egerer R, et al. Successful treatment of Epstein-Barr virus-induced transverse myelitis with ganciclovir and cytomegalovirus hyperim-mune globulin following unrelated bone marrow transplantation. Bone Marrow Transplant 1999;24:1355–8.
235. Caldas C, Bernicker E, Dal Nogare A, et al. Case report: transverse myelitis associated with Epstein-Barr virus infection. Am J Med Sci 1994;307:45–8.
236. Corssmit EP, Leverstein-van Hall M, Portegies P, et al. Severe neurological complications in association with Epstein-Barr virus infection. J Neurovirol 1997;3:460–4.
237. Umehara F, Ookatsu H, Hayashi D, et al. MRI studies of spinal visceral larva migrans syndrome. J Neurol Sci 2006;249:7–12.

238. Lee IH, Kim ST, Oh DK, et al. MRI findings of spinal visceral larva migrans of *Toxocara canis*. Eur J Radiol 2010;75:236–40.
239. Joshi TN, Yamazaki MK, Zhao H, et al. Spinal schistosomiasis: differential diagnosis for acute paraparesis in a U.S. resident. J Spinal Cord Med 2010;33(3): 256–60.
240. Hull TP, Bates JH. Optic neuritis after influenza vaccination. Am J Ophthalmol 1997;124:703–4.
241. Ray CL, Dreizin IJ. Bilateral optic neuropathy associated with influenza vaccination. J Neuroophthalmol 1996;16:182–4.
242. Keegan BM, Pittock SJ, Lennon VA. Autoimmune myelopathy associated with collapsin response-mediator protein-5 immunoglobulin G. Ann Neurol 2008; 63(4):531–4.
243. Cross SA, Salomao DR, Parisi JE, et al. Paraneoplastic autoimmune optic neuritis with retinitis defined by CRMP-5 IgG. Ann Neurol 2003;54:38–50.
244. Pittock SJ, Yoshikawa H, Ahlskog JE, et al. Glutamic acid decarboxylase autoimmunity with brainstem, extrapyramidal, and spinal cord dysfunction. Mayo Clin Proc 2006;81:1207–14.
245. Tanaka M, Matsushita T, Tateishi T, et al. Distinct CSF cytokine/chemokine profiles in atopic myelitis and other causes of myelitis. Neurology 2008;71(13): 974–81.
246. Zoli A, Mariano M, Fusari A, et al. Atopic myelitis: first case report outside Japan? Allergy 2005;60:410–1.
247. Gregoire SM, Mormont E, Laloux P, et al. Atopic myelitis: a clinical, biological, radiological and histopathological diagnosis. J Neurol Sci 2006;247:231–5.
248. Kira J, Kawano Y, Horiuchi I, et al. Clinical, immunological and MRI features of myelitis with atopic dermatitis (atopic myelitis). J Neurol Sci 1999;162(1):56–61.
249. Kira J, Yamasaki K, Kawano Y, et al. Acute myelitis associated with hyperIgEemia and atopic dermatitis. J Neurol Sci 1997;148(2):199–203.
250. Isobe N, Kanamori Y, Yonekawa T, et al. First diagnostic criteria for atopic myelitis with special reference to discrimination from myelitis-onset multiple sclerosis. J Neurol Sci 2012;316:30–5.
251. Constantinescu CS, Thomas M, Zaman AG. Atopic optic neuritis. Ocul Immunol Inflamm 2006;14:125–7.
252. de Seze J, Lanctin C, Lebrun C, et al. Idiopathic acute transverse myelitis: application of the recent diagnostic criteria. Neurology 2005;65(12):1950–3.
253. Krishnan C, Kaplin A, Deshpande D, et al. Transverse myelitis: pathogenesis, diagnosis and treatment. Front Biosci 2004;9:1483–99.
254. Alvarenga MP, Thuler LC, Neto SP, et al. The clinical course of idiopathic acute transverse myelitis in patients from Rio de Janeiro. J Neurol 2010;257(6):992–8.
255. Choi KH, Lee KS, Chung SO, et al. Idiopathic transverse myelitis: MR characteristics. AJNR Am J Neuroradiol 1996;17:1151–60.
256. Alper G, Petropoulou KA, Fitz CR, et al. Idiopathic acute transverse myelitis in children: an analysis and discussion of MRI findings. Mult Scler 2011;17:74–80.
257. Young J, Quinn S, Hurrell M, et al. Clinically isolated acute transverse myelitis: prognostic features and incidence. Mult Scler 2009;15(11):1295–302.
258. Kim SH, Kim SM, Vincent A, et al. Clinical characteristics, prognosis, and seropositivity to the anti-aquaporin-4 antibody in Korean patients with longitudinally extensive transverse myelitis. J Neurol 2010;257(6):920–5.
259. Ravaglia S, Bastianello S, Franciotta D, et al. NMO-IgG-negative relapsing myelitis. Spinal Cord 2009;47:531–7.
260. Kim KK. Idiopathic recurrent transverse myelitis. Arch Neurol 2003;60:1290–4.

261. Pidcock FS, Krishnan C, Crawford TO, et al. Acute transverse myelitis in childhood: center-based analysis of 47 cases. Neurology 2007;68:1474–80.
262. Thomas T, Branson HM, Leonard H, et al. The demographic, clinical and magnetic resonance imaging (MRI) features of transverse myelitis in children. J Child Neurol 2012;27:11–21.
263. Andronikou S, Albuquerque-Jonathan G, Wilmshurst J, et al. MRI findings in acute idiopathic transverse myelopathy in children. Pediatr Radiol 2003;33: 624–9.
264. Defresne P, Hollenberg H, Husson B, et al. Acute transverse myelitis in children: clinical course and prognostic factors. J Child Neurol 2003;18:401–6.
265. Knebusch M, Strassburg HM, Reiners K. Acute transverse myelitis in childhood: nine cases and review of the literature. Dev Med Child Neurol 1998;40:631–9.
266. Dunne K, Hopkins IJ, Shield LK. Acute transverse myelopathy in childhood. Dev Med Child Neurol 1986;28:198–204.
267. Yiu EM, Kornberg AJ, Ryan MM, et al. Acute transverse myelitis and acute disseminated encephalomyelitis in childhood: spectrum or separate entities? J Child Neurol 2009;24:287–96.
268. De Goede CG, Holmes EM, Pike MG. Acquired transverse myelopathy in children in the United Kingdom—a 2 year prospective study. Eur J Paediatr Neurol 2010;14:479–87.
269. Banwell B, Tenembaum S, Lennon VA, et al. Neuromyelitis optica-IgG in childhood inflammatory demyelinating CNS disorders. Neurology 2008;70:344–52.
270. Wang KC, Wang SJ, Lee CL, et al. The rescue effect of plasma exchange for neuromyelitis optica. J Clin Neurosci 2011;18:43–6.
271. Gwathmey K, Balogun RA, Burns T. Neurologic indications for therapeutic plasma exchange: an update. J Clin Apher 2011;26(5):261–8.
272. Greenberg BM, Thomas KP, Krishnan C, et al. Idiopathic transverse myelitis: corticosteroids, plasma exchange, or cyclophosphamide. Neurology 2007; 68(19):1614–7.
273. Khan OA, Zvartau-Hind M, Caon C, et al. Effect of monthly intravenous cyclophosphamide in rapidly deteriorating multiple sclerosis patients resistant to conventional therapy. Mult Scler 2001;7:185–8.
274. Smith D. Preliminary analysis of a trial of pulse cyclophosphamide in IFN-beta-resistant active MS. J Neurol Sci 2004;223:73–9.
275. Borchers AT, Gershwin ME. Transverse myelitis. Autoimmun Rev 2012;11: 231–48.
276. Thompson AJ. Neurorehabilitation in multiple sclerosis: foundations, facts and fiction. Curr Opin Neurol 2005;18:267–71.
277. Trecker CC, Kozubal DE, Quigg M, et al. Quality care in transverse myelitis: a responsive protocol. J Child Neurol 2009;24:577–83.
278. Yavin Y, Cohan AT. Venous thromboembolism prophylaxis for the medical patient: where do we stand? Semin Respir Crit Care Med 2008;29(1):75–82.
279. Anders J, Heinemann A, Carsten L, et al. Decubitus ulcers: pathophysiology and primary prevention. Dtsch Arztebl Int 2010;107(21):371–82.
280. Putzke J, Richards J, Hicken B, et al. Predictors of life satisfaction: a spinal cord injury cohort study. Arch Phys Med Rehabil 2002;83:555–61.
281. Ditunno PL, Patrick M, Stineman M, et al. Who wants to walk? Preferences for recovery after SCI: a longitudinal and cross-sectional study. Spinal Cord 2008;46:500–6.
282. Dietz V. Neurophysiology of gait disorders: present and future applications. Electroencephalogr Clin Neurophysiol 1997;103(3):333–55.

283. Scivoletto G, Romanelli A, Mariotti A, et al. Clinical factors that affect walking level and performance in chronic spinal cord lesion patients. Spine (Phila Pa 1976) 2008;33(3):259–64.
284. Lapointe R, Lajoie Y, Serresse O, et al. Functional community ambulation requirements in incomplete spinal cord injured subjects. Spinal Cord 2001;39: 327–35.
285. Sturt RN, Holland AE, New PW. Walking ability at discharge from inpatient rehabilitation in a cohort of non-traumatic spinal cord injury patients. Spinal Cord 2009;47(10):763–8.
286. Courtney AM, Castro-Borrero W, Davis SL, et al. Functional treatments in multiple sclerosis. Curr Opin Neurol 2011;24(3):250–4.
287. Golzari Z, Shabkhiz F, Soudi S, et al. Combined exercise training reduces IFN-g and IL-17 levels in the plasma and the supernatant of peripheral blood mononuclear cells in women with multiple sclerosis. Int Immunopharmacol 2010;10: 1415–9.
288. Hawker K, Frohman E, Racke M. Levetiracetam for phasic spasticity in multiple sclerosis. Arch Neurol 2003;60:1772–4.
289. Rittweger J, Gerrits K, Altenburg T, et al. Bone adaptation to altered loading after spinal cord injury: a study of bone and muscle strength. J Musculoskelet Neuronal Interact 2006;6:269–76.
290. Roze E, Bounolleau P, Ducreux D, et al. Propriospinal myoclonus revisited: clinical, neurophysiologic, and neuroradiologic findings. Neurology 2009;72(15): 1301–9.
291. Brown LK, Heffner JE, Obbens EA. Tranverse myelitis associated with restless legs syndrome and periodic movements of sleep responsive to an oral dopaminergic agent but not to intrathecal baclofen. Sleep 2000;23(5):1–4.
292. Natarajan R. Review of periodic limb movement and restless leg syndrome. J Postgrad Med 2010;56(2):157–62.
293. Kalita J, Shah S, Kapoor R, et al. Bladder dysfunction in acute transverse myelitis: magnetic resonance imaging and neurophysiological and urodynamic correlations. J Neurol Neurosurg Psychiatry 2002;73(2):154–9.
294. Gupta A, Taly AB, Srivastava A, et al. Non-traumatic spinal cord lesions: epidemiology, complications, neurological and functional outcome of rehabilitation. Spinal Cord 2009;47:307–11.
295. Tanaka ST, Stone AT, Kurzrock EA. Transverse myelitis in children: long-term urological outcomes. J Urol 2006;175(5):1864–8.
296. Lemack GE, Frohman EM, Zimmern PE, et al. Urodynamic distinctions between idiopathic detrusor overactivity and detrusor overactivity secondary to multiple sclerosis. Urology 2006;67:960–4.
297. Samkoff LM, Goodman AD. Symptomatic management in multiple sclerosis. Neurol Clin 2011;29(2):449–63.
298. Fowler CJ, Panicker JN, Drake M, et al. A UK consensus on the management of the bladder in multiple sclerosis. Postgrad Med J 2009;85(1008):552–9.
299. Ebert E. Gastrointestinal involvement in spinal cord injury: a clinical perspective. J Gastrointestin Liver Dis 2012;21(1):75–82.
300. Raghav S, Kipp D, Watson J, et al. Gastroparesis in multiple sclerosis. Mult Scler 2006;12(2):243–4.
301. Reddymasu SC, Bonino J, McCallum RW. Gastroparesis secondary to a demyelinating disease: a case series. BMC Gastroenterol 2007;7:3.
302. Atkinson K, Romano W, Prokopiw I. An unusual cause of gastroparesis: demyelinating disease of the medulla. Dig Dis Sci 1998;43:1430–3.

303. Read SJ, Leggett BA, Pender MP. Gastroparesis with multiple sclerosis. Lancet 1995;346(8984):1228.
304. Wiesel PH, Norton C, Glickman S, et al. Pathophysiology and management of bowel dysfunction in multiple sclerosis. Eur J Gastroenterol Hepatol 2001; 13(4):441–8.
305. Christensen P, Krogh K, Buntzen S, et al. Long-term outcome and safety of transanal irrigation for constipation and fecal incontinence. Dis Colon Rectum 2009;52:286–92.
306. Consortium for Spinal Cord Medicine. Sexuality and reproductive health in adults with spinal cord injury: a clinical practice guideline for health-care professionals. J Spinal Cord Med 2010;33(3):281–336.
307. Lombardi G, Mondaini N, Iazzetta P, et al. Sexuality in patients with spinal cord injuries due to attempted suicide. Spinal Cord 2008;46(1):53–7.
308. Forsythe E, Horsewell JE. Sexual rehabilitation of women with a spinal cord injury. Spinal Cord 2006;44:234–41.
309. Courtois FJ, Charvier KF, Leriche A, et al. Sexual function in spinal cord injury men. Assessing sexual capability. Paraplegia 1993;31:771–84.
310. Courtois FJ, Goulet MC, Charvier KF, et al. Posttraumatic erectile potential of spinal cord injured men: How physiologic recordings supplement subjective reports. Arch Phys Med Rehabil 1999;80:1268–72.
311. Alexander MS, Biering-Sorensen F, Bodner D, et al. International standards to document remaining autonomic function after spinal cord injury. Spinal Cord 2009;47:36–43.
312. Stone AR. The sexual needs of the injured spinal cord patient. Probl Urol 1987;1: 529–36.
313. Barbonetti A, Cavallo F, Felzani G, et al. Erectile dysfunction is the main determinant of psychological distress in men with spinal cord injury. J Sex Med 2012;9(3):830–6.
314. Anderson KD, Borisoff JF, Johnson RD, et al. Long-term effects of spinal cord injury on sexual function in men: implications for neuroplasticity. Spinal Cord 2007;45:338–48.
315. Lombardi G, Del Popolo G, Macchiarella A, et al. Sexual rehabilitation in women with spinal cord injury: a critical review of the literature. Spinal Cord 2010;48(12): 842–9.
316. Lombardi G, Mondaini N, Macchiarella A, et al. Female sexual dysfunction and hormonal status in spinal cord injured (SCI) patients. J Androl 2007;28(5):722–6.
317. Soler JM, Previnaire JG. Ejaculatory dysfunction in spinal cord injury is suggestive of dyssynergic ejaculation. Eur J Phys Rehabil Med 2011;47:677–81.
318. Kreuter M, Taft C, Siösteen A, et al. Women's sexual functioning and sex life after spinal cord injury. Spinal Cord 2011;49(1):154–60.
319. Krassioukov AV, Karlsson AK, Wecht AK, et al. Assessment of autonomic dysfunction following spinal cord injury: rationale for additions to International Standards for Neurological Assessment. J Rehabil Res Dev 2007;44(1):103–12.
320. Consensus statement on the definition of orthostatic hypotension, pure autonomic failure, and multiple system atrophy. The Consensus Committee of the American Autonomic Society and the American Academy of Neurology. Neurology 1996;46(5):1470.
321. Sidorov EV, Townson AF, Dvorak MF, et al. Orthostatic hypotension in the first month following acute spinal cord injury. Spinal Cord 2008;46(1):65–9.
322. Andersen EB, Nordenbo AM. Sympathetic vasoconstrictor responses in multiple sclerosis with thermo-regulatory dysfunction. Clin Auton Res 1997;7:13–6.

323. Davis SL, Wilson TE, White AT, et al. Thermoregulation in multiple sclerosis. J Appl Physiol 2010;109(5):1531–7.
324. Krassioukov AV, Furlan JC, Fehlings MG. Autonomic dysreflexia in acute spinal cord injury: an under-recognized clinical entity. J Neurotrauma 2003;20(8):707–18.
325. Krassioukov A, Warburton DE, Teasell R, et al. A systematic review of the management of autonomic dysreflexia after spinal cord injury. Arch Phys Med Rehabil 2009;90(4):682–95.
326. Braddom RL, Rocco JF. Autonomic dysreflexia. Am J Phys Med Rehabil 1991; 70:234–41.
327. Ho CP, Krassioukov AV. Autonomic dysreflexia and myocardial ischemia. Spinal Cord 2010;48(9):714–5.
328. Chaves CJ, Lee G. Reversible posterior leukoencephalopathy in a patient with autonomic dysreflexia: a case report. Spinal Cord 2008;46(11):760–1.
329. Dolinak D, Balraj E. Autonomic dysreflexia and sudden death in people with traumatic spinal cord injury. Am J Forensic Med Pathol 2007;28(2):95–8.
330. Beard JP, Wade WH, Barber DB. Sacral insufficiency stress fracture as etiology of positional autonomic dysreflexia: case report. Paraplegia 1996;34(3):173–5.
331. Claydon VE, Elliott SL, Sheel AW, et al. Cardiovascular responses to vibrostimulation for sperm retrieval in men with spinal cord injury. J Spinal Cord Med 2006; 29(3):207–16.
332. Szasz G, Carpenter C. Clinical observations in vibratory stimulation of the penis of men with spinal cord injury. Arch Sex Behav 1989;18(6):461–74.
333. Blackmer J. Rehabilitation medicine: 1. Autonomic dysreflexia. CMAJ 2003; 169(9):931–5.
334. Sjölund BH. Pain and rehabilitation after spinal cord injury: the case of sensory spasticity? Brain Res Brain Res Rev 2002;40:250–6.
335. Pollmann W, Feneberg W. Current management of pain associated with multiple sclerosis. CNS Drugs 2008;22(4):291–324.
336. Bond LD Jr, Keough GC. Neurogenic pruritus: a case of pruritus induced by transverse myelitis. Br J Dermatol 2003;149(1):204–5.
337. Biering-Sorensen F, Bohr H, Schaadt O. Bone mineral content of the lumbar spine and lower extremities years after spinal cord lesion. Paraplegia 1988; 26:293–301.
338. Roberts D, Lee W, Cuneo RC, et al. Longitudinal study of bone turnover after acute spinal cord injury. J Clin Endocrinol Metab 1998;83:415–22.
339. Maïmoun L, Fattal C, Micallef JP, et al. Bone loss in spinal cord-injured patients: from physiopathology to therapy. Spinal Cord 2006;44(4):203–10.
340. Dionyssiotis Y. Spinal cord injury-related bone impairment and fractures: an update on epidemiology and physiopathological mechanisms. J Musculoskelet Neuronal Interact 2011;11(3):257–65.
341. Naftchi NE, Viau AT, Sell GH, et al. Mineral metabolism in spinal cord injury. Arch Phys Med Rehabil 1980;61:139–42.
342. Oleson CV, Patel PH, Wuermser LA. Influence of season, ethnicity, and chronicity on vitamin D deficiency in traumatic spinal cord injury. J Spinal Cord Med 2010;33(3):202–13.
343. Pepe J, Romagnoli E, Nofroni I, et al. Vitamin D status as the major factor determining the circulating levels of parathyroid hormone: a study in normal subjects. Osteoporos Int 2005;16(7):805–12.
344. Hiremath GS, Cettomai D, Baynes M, et al. Vitamin D status and effect of low-dose cholecalciferol and high-dose ergocalciferol supplementation in multiple sclerosis. Mult Scler 2009;15(6):735–40.

345. Asherio A, Munger KL, Simon KC. Vitamin D and multiple sclerosis. Lancet Neurol 2010;9(6):599–612.
346. Munger KL, Levin LI, Hollis BW, et al. Serum 25-hydroxyvitamin D levels and risk of multiple sclerosis. JAMA 2006;296(23):2832–8.
347. Birmingham DJ, Hebert LA, Song H, et al. Evidence that abnormally large seasonally declines in vitamin D status may trigger SLE flare in non-African Americans. Lupus 2012;21(8):855–64.
348. Braun-Moscovici Y, Toledano K, Markovits D, et al. Vitamin D level: is it related to disease activity in inflammatory joint disease? Rheumatol Int 2011;31(4):493–9.
349. Mealy MA, Newsome S, Greenberg BM, et al. Low vitamin D levels and recurrent inflammatory spinal cord disease. Arch Neurol 2012;69(3):352–6.
350. Gannage-Yared MH, Azoury M, Mansour I, et al. Effects of a short-term calcium and vitamin D treatment on serum cytokines, bone markers, insulin and lipid concentrations in healthy post-menopausal women. J Endocrinol Invest 2003; 26(8):748–53.
351. Dickie LJ, Church LD, Coulthard LR, et al. Vitamin D3 down-regulates intracellular Toll-like receptor 9 expression and Toll-like receptor 9-induced IL-6 production in human monocytes. Rheumatology (Oxford) 2010;49(8):1466–71.
352. Correale J, Ysrraelit MC, Gaitán MI. Immunomodulatory effects of vitamin D in multiple sclerosis. Brain 2009;132(5):1146–60.
353. Tang J, Zhou R, Luger D, et al. Calcitriol suppresses antiretinal autoimmunity through inhibitory effects on the Th17 effector response. J Immunol 2009; 182(8):4624–32.
354. Prietl B, Pilz S, Wolf M, et al. Vitamin D supplementation and regulatory T cells in apparently healthy subjects: vitamin D treatment for autoimmune diseases? Isr Med Assoc J 2010;12(3):136–9.
355. Holick MF. Vitamin D: the underappreciated D-lightful hormone that is important for skeletal and cellular health. Current Opin Endocrinol Diabetes 2002;9(1): 87–98.
356. Hahn TJ, Hendin BA, Scharp CR, et al. Effect of chronic anticonvulsant therapy on serum 25-hydroxycholecalciferol levels in adults. N Engl J Med 1972; 287(18):900–4.
357. Vieth R. Critique of the considerations for establishing the tolerable upper intake for vitamin D: critical need for revision upwards. J Nutr 2006;136:1117–22.
358. Goldberg P, Flemin MC, Picard EH. Multiple sclerosis: decreased relapse rate through dietary supplementation with calcium, magnesium and vitamin D. Med Hypotheses 1986;21:193–200.
359. Heaney RP, Davies KM, Chen TC, et al. Human serum 25-hydroxycholecalciferol response to extended oral dosing with cholecalciferol. Am J Clin Nutr 2003;77: 204–10.
360. Trang HM, Cole DE, Rubin LA, et al. Evidence that vitamin D3 increases serum 25-hydroxyvitamin D more efficiently than does vitamin D2. Am J Clin Nutr 1998; 68(4):854–8.
361. Giovannucci E, Liu Y, Rimm EB, et al. Prospective study of predictors of vitamin D status and cancer incidence and mortality in men. J Natl Cancer Inst 2006; 98(7):451–9.
362. Robsahm TE, Tretli S, Dahlback A, et al. Vitamin D3 from sunlight may improve the prognosis of breast, colon, and prostate cancer (Norway). Cancer Causes Control 2004;15(2):149–58.
363. Mowe M, Haug E, Bohmer T. Low serum calcidiol concentration in older adults with reduced muscular function. J Am Geriatr Soc 1999;47(2):220–6.

364. Pfeifer M, Begerow B, Minne HW, et al. Vitamin D status, trunk muscle strength, body sway, falls, and fractures among 237 postmenopausal women with osteoporosis. Exp Clin Endocrinol Diabetes 2001;109(2):87–92.
365. Plotkinoff GA, Quigley BA. Prevalence of severe hypovitaminosis D in patients with persistent, nonspecific musculoskeletal pain. Mayo Clin Proc 2003; 78(12):1463–70.
366. Patten SB, Beck CA, Williams JV, et al. Major depression in multiple sclerosis: a population-based perspective. Neurology 2003;61:1524–7.
367. Mohr DC, Goodkin DE, Likosky W, et al. Treatment of depression improves adherence to interferon B-1b therapy for multiple sclerosis. Arch Neurol 1997;54:531–3.
368. Edgar MA. Nervous system involvement in ankylosing spondylitis. BMJ 1974;1: 394.
369. Oh DH, Jun JB, Kim HT, et al. Transverse myelitis in a patient with longstanding ankylosing spondylitis. Clin Exp Rheumatol 2001;19:195–6.
370. Lan HH, Chen DY, Chen CC, et al. Combination of transverse myelitis and arachnoiditis in cauda equina syndrome of long-standing ankylosing spondylitis: MRI features and its role in clinical management. Clin Rheumatol 2007;26:1963–7.
371. Rath JJG, Ronday HK, Wirtz PW. Acute transverse myelitis in psoriatic arthritis. J Neurol 2010;257:457–8.
372. Weiss TD, Nelson JS, Woolsey RM, et al. Transverse myelitis in mixed connective tissue disease. Arthritis Rheum 1978;21(8):982–6.
373. Pedersen C, Bonen H, Boesen F. Transverse myelitis in mixed connective tissue disease. Case report. Clin Rheumatol 1987;6:290–2.
374. Flechtner KM, Baum K. Mixed connective tissue disease: recurrent episodes of optic neuropathy and transverse myelopathy. Successful treatment with plasmapheresis. J Neurol Sci 1994;126:146–8.
375. Mok CC, Lau CS. Transverse myelopathy complicating mixed connective tissue disease. Case report. Clin Neurol Neurosurg 1995;97:259–60.
376. Weatherby SJM, Davies MB, Hawkins CP. Transverse myelopathy, a rare complication of mixed connective tissue disease: comparison with SLE related transverse myelopathy. J Neurol Neurosurg Psychiatry 2000;68:532–41.
377. Bhinder S, Harbour K, Majithia V. Transverse myelitis, a rare neurological manifestation of mixed connective tissue disease—a case report and a review of literature. Clin Rheumatol 2007;26:445–7.
378. Torabi AM, Patel RK, Wolfe GI, et al. Transverse myelitis in systemic sclerosis. Arch Neurol 2004;61:126–8.
379. Franciotta D, Zardini E, Caporali R, et al. Systemic sclerosis in aquaporin-4 antibody-positive longitudinally extensive transverse myelitis. J Neurol Sci 2011; 303:139–41.
380. Brown JJ, Murphy MJ. Transverse myelopathy in progressive systemic sclerosis. Ann Neurol 1985;17:615–7.
381. Averbuch-Heller L, Steiner I, Abramski O. Neurologic manifestations of progressive systemic sclerosis. Arch Neurol 1992;49:1292–5.
382. Ray DW, Bridger J, Hawnaur J, et al. Transverse myelitis as the presentation of Jo-1 antibody syndrome (myositis and fibrosing alveolitis) in long-standing ulcerative colitis. Br J Rheumatol 1993;32:1105–8.
383. Bolla G, Disdier P, Verrot D, et al. Acute transverse myelitis and primary urticarial vasculitis. Clin Rheumatol 1998;17:250–2.
384. Nakashima I, Fujihara K, Endo M, et al. Clinical and laboratory features of myelitis patients with anti-neutrophil cytoplasmic antibodies. J Neurol Sci 1998;157(1):60–6.

385. Hamilton AJ, Whitehead DJ, Bull MD, et al. Systemic pANCA-associated vasculitis with central nervous involvement causing recurrent myelitis: case report. BMC Neurol 2010;10:118.

386. Bürk K, Farecki ML, Lamprecht G, et al. Neurological symptoms in patients with biopsy proven celiac disease. Mov Disord 2009;24:2358–62.

387. Hammond ER, Pardo CA, Kerr DA. Thymic hyperplasia in a patient with recurrent transverse myelitis with clinical resolution after thymectomy. J Neurol Neurosurg Psychiatry 2008;79:334–5.

388. Drobyski WR, Potluri J, Sauer D, et al. Autoimmune hemolytic anemia following T-cell-depleted allogeneic bone marrow transplantation. Bone Marrow Transplant 1996;17:1093–9.

389. Richard S, Fruchtman S, Scigliano E, et al. An immunological syndrome featuring transverse myelitis, Evans syndrome and pulmonary infiltrates after unrelated bone marrow transplant in a patient with severe aplastic anemia. Bone Marrow Transplant 2000;26:1225–8.

390. Perez-Montes R, Richard C, Baro J, et al. Acute transverse myelitis and autoimmune pancytopenia after unrelated hematopoietic cell transplantation. Haematologica 2001;86(5):556–7.

391. Kumar N, Hagan JB, Abraham RS, et al. Common variable immunodeficiency-associated myelitis: report of treatment with infliximab. J Neurol 2008;255(11):1821–4.

392. Hermaszewski RA, Webster AD. Primary hypogammaglobulinemia: a survey of clinical manifestations and complications. Q J Med 1993;86:31–42.

393. Leypoldt F, Eichhorn P, Saager C, et al. Successful immunosuppressive treatment and long-term follow-up of anti-Ri-associated paraneoplastic myelitis. J Neurol Neurosurg Psychiatry 2006;77(10):1199–200.

394. Pittock SJ, Lucchinetti CF, Lennon VA. Anti-neuronal nuclear autoantibody type 2: paraneoplastic accompaniments. Ann Neurol 2003;53(5):580–7.

395. Pittock SJ, Lucchinetti CF, Parisi JE, et al. Amphiphysin autoimmunity: paraneoplastic accompaniments. Ann Neurol 2005;58:96–107.

396. Chamard L, Magnin E, Berger E, et al. Stiff leg syndrome and myelitis with anti-amphiphysin antibodies: a common physiopathology? Eur Neurol 2011;66:253–5.

397. Saiz A, Blanco Y, Sabater L, et al. Spectrum of neurological syndromes associated with glutamic acid decarboxylase antibodies: diagnostic clues for this association. Brain 2008;131:2553–63.

398. Vitaliani R, Mason W, Ances B, et al. Paraneoplastic encephalitis, psychiatric symptoms and hypoventilation in ovarian teratoma. Ann Neurol 2005;58:594–604.

399. Kruer MC, Koch TK, Bourdette DN, et al. NMDA receptor encephalitis mimicking seronegative neuromyelitis optica. Neurology 2010;74:1473–5.

400. Pennington C, Livingstone S, Santosh C, et al. N-Methyl-D-aspartate receptor antibody encephalitis associated with myelitis. J Neurol Sci 2012;317:151–3.

401. Cay HF, Gungor HA, Sezer I, et al. Adverse effect of TNF-alpha blocker? Demyelination in an ankylosing spondylitis patient: a case report. J Clin Pharm Ther 2006;31(6):645–8.

402. Saieg NA, Luzar MJ. Etanercept induced multiple sclerosis and transverse myelitis. J Rheumatol 2006;33:1202–4.

403. Oleginski TP, Harrington TM, Carlson JP. Transverse myelitis secondary to sulfasalazine. J Rheumatol 1991;18(2):304.

404. Zhang M, Li B, Li J. Acute transverse myelopathy probably related to intravenous gemcitabine plus cisplatin. Ann Pharmacother 2011;45(4):544–5.

405. Wang MY, Arnold AC, Vinters HV, et al. Bilateral blindness and lumbosacral myelopathy associated with high-dose carmustine and cisplatin therapy. Am J Ophthalmol 2000;130:367–8.
406. Baker WJ, Royer GL Jr, Weiss RB. Cytarabine and neurologic toxicity. J Clin Oncol 1991;9:679–93.
407. Resar L, Phillips P, Kastan M, et al. Acute neurotoxicity after intrathecal cytosine arabinoside in two adolescents with acute lymphoblastic leukemia of B-cell type. Cancer 1993;71:117–23.
408. Crawford S, Rustin G, Bagshawe K. Acute neurological toxicity of intrathecal cytosine arabinoside: a case report. Cancer Chemother Pharmacol 1986;16: 306–7.
409. Dinsdale T. Spinal analgesia and cauda equina lesions. Anaesthesia 1947;2: 17–27.
410. Dawkins CJ. An analysis of the complications of extradural and caudal block. Anaesthesia 1969;24:554–63.
411. Newberry JM. Paraplegia following general anaesthesia. Anaesthesia 1977;32: 78–9.
412. Schreiner EJ, Lipson SF, Bromage PR, et al. Neurological complications following general anaesthesia. Three cases of major paralysis. Anaesthesia 1983;38:226–9.
413. Kitching A, Taylor S. A postoperative neurological problem. Anaesthesia 1989; 44:695–6.
414. Gutowsky NJ, Davies AO. Transverse myelitis following general anaesthesia. Anaesthesia 1993;48:44–5.
415. Martinez-Garcia E, Pelaez E, Roman JC, et al. Transverse myelitis following general and epidural anaesthesia in a paediatric patient. Anaesthesia 2005; 60:921–3.
416. Richter RW, Rosenberg RN. Transverse myelitis associated with heroin addiction. JAMA 1968;206(6):1255–7.
417. Ell JJ, Uttley D, Silver JR. Acute myelopathy in association with heroin addiction. J Neurol Neurosurg Psychiatry 1981;44:448–50.
418. McCreary M, Emerman C, Hanna J, et al. Acute myelopathy following intranasal insufflation of heroin: a case report. Neurology 2000;55:316–7.
419. Sahni V, Garg D, Garg S, et al. Unusual complications of heroin abuse: transverse myelitis, rhabdomyolysis, compartment syndrome, and ARF. Clin Toxicol (Phila) 2008;46(2):153–5.
420. Herregods P, Chappel R, Mortier G. Benzene poisoning as a possible cause of transverse myelitis. Paraplegia 1984;22:305–10.
421. Sauer GC. Transverse myelitis and paralysis from a brown recluse spider bite. Mo Med 1975;72(10):603–4.
422. Misra UK, Kalita K. Comparison of clinical and electrodiagnostic features in B12 deficiency neurological syndromes with and without antiparietal cell antibodies. Postgrad Med J 2007;83(976):124–7.
423. Lindenbaum J, Healton EB, Savage DG, et al. Neuropsychiatric disorders caused by cobalamin deficiency in the absence of anemia or macrocytosis. N Engl J Med 1988;318(26):1720–8.
424. Naidich MJ, Ho SU. Case 87: subacute combined degeneration. Radiology 2005;237:101–5.
425. Paliwal VK, Malhotra HS, Chaurasia RN, et al. "Anchor"-shaped bright posterior column in a patient with vitamin B12 deficiency myelopathy. Postgrad Med J 2009;85:186.

426. Vorgerd M, Tegenthoff M, Kuhne D, et al. Spinal MRI in progressive myeloneuropathy associated with vitamin E deficiency. Neuroradiology 1996;38:S111–3.

427. Gutmann L, Shockor W, Gutmann L, et al. Vitamin E-deficient spinocerebellar syndrome due to intestinal lymphangiectasia. Neurology 1986;36(4):554–6.

428. Nelson JS, Fitch CD, Fischer VW, et al. Progressive neuropathologic lesions in vitamin E deficient rhesus monkeys. J Neuropathol Exp Neurol 1981;40:166–86.

429. Pineles SL, Wilson CA, Balcer LJ, et al. Combined optic neuropathy and myelopathy secondary to copper deficiency. Surv Ophthalmol 2010;55(4):386–92.

430. Naismith RT, Shepherd JB, Weihl CC, et al. Acute and bilateral blindness due to optic neuropathy associated with copper deficiency. Arch Neurol 2009;66(8):1025–7.

431. Nations SP, Boyer PJ, love LA, et al. Denture cream: an unusual source of excess zinc leading to hypocupremia and neurologic disease. Neurology 2008;71(9):639–43.

432. Kumar N. Copper deficiency myelopathy (human swayback). Mayo Clin Proc 2006;81(10):1371–84.

433. Jaiser SR, Winston GP. Copper deficiency myelopathy. J Neurol 2010;257: 869–81.

434. Tatum WO, Bui DD, Grant EG, et al. Pseudo-Guillain-Barre syndrome due to "whippet"-induced myeloneuropathy. J Neuroimaging 2010;20(4):400–1.

435. Renard D, Dutray A, Remy A, et al. Subacute combined degeneration of the spinal cord caused by nitrous oxide anaesthesia. Neurol Sci 2009;30(1):75–6.

436. Ng J, O'Grady G, Pettit T, et al. Nitrous oxide use in first-year students at Auckland University. Lancet 2009;361:1349–50.

437. Spencer PS, Ludoph AC, Kisby GE. Neurologic diseases associated with use of plant components with toxic potential. Environ Res 1993;62:106–13.

438. Gerstner ER, Batchelor TT. Primary central nervous system lymphoma. Arch Neurol 2010;67(3):291–7.

439. Herrlinger U, Weller M, Kuker W. Primary CNS lymphoma in the spinal cord: clinical manifestations may precede MRI detectability. Neuroradiology 2002;44(3): 239–44.

440. Flanagan EP, O'Neill BP, Porter AB, et al. Primary intramedullary spinal cord lymphoma. Neurology 2011;77(8):784–91.

441. Beristain X, Azzarelli B. The neurological masquerade of intravascular lymphomatosis. Arch Neurol 2002;59:439–43.

442. Grove CS, Robbins PD, Kermode AG. Intravascular lymphoma presenting as progressive paraparesis. J Clin Neurosci 2008;15:1056–8.

443. Yang T, Tian L, Li Q, et al. A case of intravascular B-cell lymphoma presenting as myelopathy and diagnosed postmortem. J Neurol Sci 2008;272:196–8.

444. Kumar N, Keegan AM, Rodriguez FJ, et al. Intravascular lymphoma presenting as a longitudinally-extensive myelitis: diagnostic challenges and etiologic clues. J Neurol Sci 2011;303:146–9.

445. Podnar S. Epidemiology of cauda equina and conus medullaris lesions. Muscle Nerve 2007;35:529–31.

446. Schwarz S, Zoubaa S, Knauth M, et al. Intravascular lymphomatosis presenting with a conus medullaris syndrome mimicking disseminated encephalomyelitis. Neuro Oncol 2002;4(3):187–91.

447. Zeng M, Knisely J. Post-radiotherapy myelitis observed in an AIDS patient with a meningioma: case report and review of the literature. J Neurooncol 1999; 45(2):167–74.

448. Rampling R, Symonds P. Radiation myelopathy. Curr Opin Neurol 1998;11(6): 627–32.

449. Bleyer A, Choi M, Wang SJ, et al. Increased vulnerability of the spinal cord to radiation or intrathecal chemotherapy during adolescence: a report from the Children's Oncology Group. Pediatr Blood Cancer 2009;53:1205–10.

450. Alfonso ER, De Gregorio MA, Mateo P, et al. Radiation myelopathy in over-irradiated patients: MR imaging findings. Eur Radiol 1997;7(3):400–4.

451. Behrman AL, Harkema SJ. Physical rehabilitation as an agent for recovery after spinal cord injury. Phys Med Rehabil Clin N Am 2007;18(2):183–202.

452. Atrice MB. Lower extremity orthotic management for the spinal-cord-injured client. Spinal Cord Inj Rehabil 2000;5(4):1–10.

453. Bailey SN, Hardin EC, Kobetic R, et al. Neurotherapeutic and neuroprosthetic effects of implanted functional electrical stimulation for ambulation after incomplete spinal cord injury. J Rehabil Res Dev 2010;47(1):7–16.

454. Everaert DG, Thompson AK, Chong SL, et al. Does functional electrical stimulation for foot drop strengthen corticospinal connections? Neurorehabil Neural Repair 2010;24:168–77.

455. Swinnen E, Duerinck S, Baeyens JP, et al. Effectiveness of robot-assisted gait training in persons with spinal cord injury: a systematic review. J Rehabil Med 2010;42:520–6.

456. Jung R, Belanger A, Kanchiku T, et al. Neuromuscular stimulation therapy after incomplete spinal cord injury promotes recovery of interlimb coordination during locomotion. J Neural Eng 2009;6(5):055010. http://dx.doi.org/10.1088/1741-2560/6/5/055010.

457. Goodman AD, Brown TR, Edwards KR, et al. A phase 3 trial of extended release oral dalfampridine in multiple sclerosis. Ann Neurol 2010;68(4):494–502.

458. Kalsi V, Gonzales G, Popat R, et al. Botulinum injections for the treatment of bladder symptoms of multiple sclerosis. Ann Neurol 2007;62(5):452–7.

459. Morton SC, Shekelle PG, Adams JL, et al. Antimicrobial prophylaxis for urinary tract infection in persons with spinal cord dysfunction. Arch Phys Med Rehabil 2002;83:129–38.

460. Hess MJ, Hess PE, Sullivan MR, et al. Evaluation of cranberry tablets for the prevention of urinary tract infections in spinal cord injured patients with neurogenic bladder. Spinal Cord 2008;46:622–6.

461. Bosma R, Wynia K, Havlikova E, et al. Efficacy of desmopressin in patients with multiple sclerosis suffering from bladder dysfunction: a meta-analysis. Acta Neurol Scand 2005;112(1):1–5.

462. Khan F, Pallant JF, Pallant JI, et al. A randomised controlled trial: outcomes of bladder rehabilitation in persons with multiple sclerosis. J Neurol Neurosurg Psychiatry 2010;81:1033–8.

463. Dasgupta P, Haslam C, Goodwin R, et al. The 'Queen Square bladder stimulator': a device for assisting emptying of the neurogenic bladder. Br J Urol 1997;80(2):234–7.

464. Prasad RS, Smith SJ, Wright H. Lower abdominal pressure versus external bladder stimulation to aid bladder emptying in multiple sclerosis: a randomized controlled study. Clin Rehabil 2003;17(1):42–7.

465. Schwendimann RN. Treatment of symptoms in multiple sclerosis. Neurol Res 2006;28:306–15.

466. Bywater A, While A. Management of bowel dysfunction in people with multiple sclerosis. Br J Community Nurs 2006;11(8):333–41.

467. Wiesel PH, Norton C, Roy AJ, et al. Gut focused behavioural treatment (biofeedback) for constipation and faecal incontinence in multiple sclerosis. J Neurol Neurosurg Psychiatry 2000;69(2):240–3.

468. Lombardi G, Macchiarella A, Cecconi F, et al. Ten-year follow-up of sildenafil use in spinal cord-injured patients with erectile dysfunction. J Sex Med 2009;6(12): 3449–57.

469. Lombardi G, Nelli F, Celso M, et al. Treating erectile dysfunction and central neurological diseases with oral phosphodiesterase type 5 inhibitors. Review of the literature. J Sex Med 2012;9(4):970–85.

470. Dimitriadis T, Karakitsios K, Tsounapi P, et al. Erectile function and male reproduction in men with spinal cord injury: a review. Andrologia 2010;42(3):139–65.

471. Sipski ML, Alexander CJ, Gomez-Marin O, et al. Effects of vibratory stimulation on sexual response in women with spinal cord injury. J Rehabil Res Dev 2005; 42(5):609–16.

472. Billups KL, Berman L, Berman J, et al. A new non-pharmacological vacuum therapy for female sexual dysfunction. J Sex Marital Ther 2001;27:435–41.

473. Lahrmann H, Cortelli P, Hilz M, et al. EFNS guidelines on the diagnosis and management of orthostatic hypotension. Eur J Neurol 2006;13(9):930–6.

474. Faghri PD, Yount J. Electrically induced and voluntary activation of physiologic muscle pump: a comparison between spinal cord-injured and able-bodied individuals. Clin Rehabil 2002;16(8):878–85.

475. Raymond J, Davis GM, Bryant G, et al. Cardiovascular responses to an orthostatic challenge and electrical-stimulation-induced leg muscle contractions in individuals with paraplegia. Eur J Appl Physiol Occup Physiol 1999;80(3): 205–12.

476. Low PA, Gilden JL, Freeman R, et al. Efficacy of midodrine vs placebo in neurogenic orthostatic hypotension. A randomized, double-blind multicenter study. Midodrine study group. JAMA 1997;277(13):1046–51.

477. Singer W, Sandroni P, Opfer-Gehrking TL, et al. Pyridostigmine treatment trial in neurogenic orthostatic hypotension. Arch Neurol 2006;63(4):513–8.

478. Mathias CJ, Senard JM, Braune S, et al. L-threo-dihydroxyphenylserine (L-threo-DOPS; droxidopa) in the management of neurogenic orthostatic hypotension: a multi-national, multi-center, dose-ranging study in multiple system atrophy and pure autonomic failure. Clin Auton Res 2001;11:235–42.

479. Rabchevsky AG, Patel SP, Duale H, et al. Gabapentin for spasticity and autonomic dysreflexia after severe spinal cord injury. Spinal Cord 2011;49(1): 99–105.

480. Frankel HL, Mathias CJ. Severe hypertension in patients with high spinal cord lesions undergoing electro-ejaculation—management with prostaglandin E2. Paraplegia 1980;18(5):293–9.

Neuromyelitis Optica
Clinical Manifestations and Neuroimaging Features

Mohammad Ali Sahraian, MD[a],*, Ernst-Wilhelm Radue, MD[b],
Alireza Minagar, MD[c]

KEYWORDS

- Neuromyelitis optica • Central nervous system • Autoimmune • Channelopathy

KEY POINTS

- Neuromyelitis optica (NMO) was initially described as a severe monophasic necrotizing demyelinating disease with pure involvement of optic nerves and spinal cord.
- During the last century, and especially the last 2 decades, understanding of the diagnosis, clinical presentation, and pathophysiology of NMO has changed.
- The discovery in 2004 of NMO immunoglobulin G was an important step in accurate and early recognition of NMO and its related disorders.
- With such improvements in diagnosis and early description of cases over the past decade, NMO is still considered a disabling disease of the central nervous system and future studies should be planned for better management of relapses and prevention of disability.

INTRODUCTION

Neuromyelitis optica (NMO or Devic disease) is a chronic inflammatory, demyelinating disease of the central nervous system (CNS) that is characterized by severe attacks of optic neuritis and myelitis that spares the brain in the early stages.[1] The disease was first described in 1870 by Allbutt who reported a patient with "sympathetic disorder of the eye" after an acute myelitis.[2] Twenty-four years later, in 1894, Devic and his student Gault described the clinical characteristics of NMO, optic neuritis and acute transverse myelitis, based on 16 cases from the literature in addition to 1 of their own, and the syndrome was eponymously coined Devic disease.[3]

Controversy about whether NMO is a subtype of multiple sclerosis (MS) or a different disease has persisted for years. However, a series of clinical, radiological, histopathologic, and immunologic studies provide evidence that NMO and NMO spectrum

Disclosure statement: The authors have nothing to disclose.
[a] Sina MS Research Center, Iranian Center for Neurological Research, Sina Hospital, Hassan abad Square, Tehran, Iran; [b] Medical Image Analysis Center, University Hospital, Basel, Switzerland; [c] Louisiana State University Health Sciences Center, Department of Neurology, 1501 Kings Highway, Shreveport, LA 71130, USA
* Corresponding author.
E-mail address: msahrai@sina.tums.ac.ir

Neurol Clin 31 (2013) 139–152
http://dx.doi.org/10.1016/j.ncl.2012.09.010
0733-8619/13/$ – see front matter © 2013 Published by Elsevier Inc.

neurologic.theclinics.com

disorders are distinct from MS in spite of common pathologic characteristics, like demyelination of CNS.[4]

After its first description, NMO was considered to be a severe monophasic syndrome characterized by bilateral optic neuritis (ON) and myelitis occurring in rapid succession. Subsequent reports included patients with less severe clinical attacks, unilateral ON, and myelitis with intervals of several months or years.

The discovery of highly specific NMO immunoglobulin G (NMO-IgG) in 2004 opened a new era in the classification and understanding the pathogenesis of NMO.[4] NMO-IgG binds to aquaporin-4, which is the main channel that regulates water homoeostasis in the CNS.[5] NMO-IgG has also been detected in NMO spectrum disorders, which at present consist of limited forms of the disease such as recurrent ON or longitudinally extensive transverse myelitis (LETM). This article discusses the epidemiology, clinical manifestation, immunopathogenesis, and imaging of NMO. In addition, it reviews the preferred therapeutic options for this condition, which differ from those for MS.

EPIDEMIOLOGY

The incidence and prevalence of NMO and its spectrum are poorly characterized. Cases of NMO have been reported from different parts of the world and different races, although the disease is more prevalent in areas with black, Asian, and Indian populations, in which NMO constitutes from 15% to 57% of demyelinating diseases. Most studies on the epidemiology of NMO have been carried out in small populations mostly based on cases from tertiary hospitals, with the inherent risk of bias.[6] Studies from Japan, Cuba, Denmark, Mexico, and the French West Indies suggest incidence rates of 0.053 to 0.4 per 100,000 patient-years and prevalence rates of 0.52 to 4.4 per 100,000 people.[6–10] Men and women are affected equally in the monophasic course but, in the more frequent relapsing course, women (ratio 5:1–10:1) are overrepresented.[11] The disease is 3 to 9 times more prevalent in women than in men, and the age of onset ranges from childhood to late adulthood, with a median of 35 to 45 years among adults and 4.4 years among children.[1,12–15] The disease is mainly sporadic, although a few familial cases have been reported.[16]

NMO prevalence is estimated to be approximately 1% to 2% that of MS in the United States.[17] The average age of onset was 41.1 (range 3–81) years among 187 patients with NMO and Neuromyelitis optica spectrum disorders (NMOSD). The female/male ratio was 6.5:1 in their patients and 68.3% were NMO-IgG positive.[17]

CLINICAL MANIFESTATIONS

Sequential or simultaneous optic neuritis (ON) and transverse myelitis are typical features of NMO. ON usually presents with unilateral or, less often, bilateral ocular pain and visual loss. It tends to be more severe and leaves a greater impairment compared with MS-associated ON. Bilateral simultaneous or sequential ON in rapid succession is suggests NMO rather than MS. Other clinical features including ocular pain and visual field deficits do not differ from MS. Spinal cord lesions usually involve the cervical part and typically present as LETM with a length of 3 or more vertebral segments.[18] Myelitis caused by NMO, unlike those of MS, often present with complete transverse myelitis with tetraplegia or paraplegia and a well-defined sensory level and sphincter dysfunction, and may be accompanied by pain and paroxysmal tonic spasms of the trunk and the extremities. Prominent dysesthetic, radicular pain, possibly associated with Lhermitte symptoms, is common and may occur in up to 35% of acute severe myelitis attacks in relapsing NMO.[1,19] The lesion may extend toward the brain stem and cause hiccups, intractable nausea, or respiratory failure.[1,19,20] Although NMO was considered to be confined to the optic nerves and spinal cord, recent evidence shows that patients commonly present with brain symptoms at their first manifestation. Involvement of the CNS beyond the optic nerves and spinal cord has been reported 59% of patients with NMO.[21] The patient may present with characteristic brainstem symptoms such as intractable hiccup and vomiting. In review of 144 cases of NMO spectrum disorders, 30 patients (21%) had hiccups and nausea, in 21% and 17% respectively.[22] Medullary involvement in the area postrema and the nucleus tractus solitaries, which are sites of high AQP4 expression, may cause severe vomiting or intractable hiccup.[20,23] Other brainstem symptoms, including vertigo, hearing loss, facial weakness, trigeminal neuralgia, diplopia, ptosis, and nystagmus, have been reported.[18,24] Encephalopathy mimicking acute disseminated encephalomyelitis or posterior reversible encephalopathy syndrome (PRES) are other extraopticospinal manifestations of NMO.[25,26] Amenorrhea, galactorrhea, diabetes insipidus, hypothyroidism, or hyperphagia have been reported as endocrinopathies associated with NMO.[27] Patients with NMO can have a monophasic or relapsing course. In monophasic NMO, simultaneous or closely related ON and LETM (<30 days) occur without any further relapse, but 80% to 90% of the patients follow a relapsing course.[11] ON and myelitis may be separated by several months or years but 55% of patients experience their first optic nerve or spinal cord relapse within 1 year after the initial clinical event; this reaches 78% after 3 years, and 90% within 5 years.[26] The median interval from disease onset to the development of both ON and myelitis, and to fulfillment of the 2006 criteria, were 17 and 28 months, respectively.[28] Predictors of a relapsing course are associated with female sex, older age at onset, longer time interval between the first 2 attacks, and presence of other autoimmune diseases.[29] An antecedent viral illness was reported in 30% of patients with monophasic and 23% of patients with recurrent NMO.[1]

DIAGNOSIS

Severe attacks of myelitis or ON should raise awareness for NMO. The first diagnostic criteria were proposed by Wingerchuk and colleagues[1] in 1999 and were helpful in distinguishing NMO from MS. Based on these criteria, the patient must have all absolute criteria including myelitis, ON, and no clinical disease outside the optic nerves and spinal cord, with 1 major or 2 minor supporting criteria. The major supporting criteria are:

1. Brain magnetic resonance imaging (MRI) not meeting diagnostic criteria for MS
2. LETM on spinal cord MRI
3. Cerebrospinal fluid (CSF) pleocytosis (>50 white blood cells [WBC]/mm^3) or more than 5 neutrophils/mm^3

Bilateral ON, severe ON with fixed visual acuity worse than 20/200 in at least 1 eye and severe, fixed, attack-related weakness (Medical Research Council grade <2) in 1 or more limbs were defined as minor supporting criteria.[1] Because of its limitation in imaging patients with brain abnormalities on MRI, extraopticospinal manifestations and discovery of NMO-IgG, Wingerchuk and colleagues[18] proposed revised diagnostic criteria based on radiologic and clinical evidence in 96 patients. The 2006 revised criteria need both optic neuritis and myelitis as absolute criteria and at least 2 of the following 3 supporting criteria for diagnosis of NMO:

1. Presence of a contiguous spinal cord MRI lesion extending over 3 or more vertebral segments
2. MRI criteria not satisfying the revised McDonald diagnostic criteria for MS
3. NMO-IgG in serum

The revised diagnostic criteria have been also validated in an independent study of Spanish and Italian patients that showed acceptable power in differentiating NMO from MS in most instances, when the clinical findings were inconclusive.[30] This diagnostic combination was 99% sensitive and 90% specific for NMO.[31] An international task force affiliated to proposed diagnostic criteria for NMO in 2008 similar to the revised criteria by Wingerchuk and colleagues[18] (**Table 1**).[32] Spinal MRI at the initial clinical event should be considered for diagnosis because LETM may break up and appear in multiple shorter plaques of less than 3 vertebral segments during a remission phase.[33]

NEUROIMAGING
Spinal Cord

Spinal cord lesions extending over 3 or more vertebral segments are the most reliable MRI finding for the diagnosis of NMO. However, MRI lesions are subject to timing issues; normal-appearing or shorter lesions can be found early during the relapse phase or they might have contracted or resolved over time in the residual atrophic stage.[18] Lesions are predominantly located in the cervical and thoracic cord with a central gray matter pattern, reflected by hyperintensities on T2-weighted axial scans and corresponding T1 hypointensities.[11] Acute spinal cord lesions tend to occupy most of the cross-sectional area of an affected segment and are associated with swelling and gadolinium enhancement (detectable days to months following relapse).[34] In a study on LETM relapses in NMO (N = 11), gadolinium enhancement vanished in all patients following treatment with high-dose methylprednisolone, and lesions may almost entirely disappear during remission. Snake-eye or owl-eye signs are common features of spinal artery ischemia that have been reported to be transiently observed at an early stage of NMO.[35] Recent studies including histopathological analysis and advanced imaging have shown that the cord damage is more extensive than the macroscopic lesions seen on conventional MRI which introduces the concept of normal-appearing spinal cord (NASC).[36] The area of microscopic damage that has normal signal intensity on conventional MRI sequences is called NASC. Such areas are better evaluated with advanced MRI techniques, such as diffusion tensor imaging.[37] Pessôa and colleagues[38] showed that there is extensive NASC damage in patients with NMO, including peripheral areas of the cervical spinal cord, affecting the white matter, mainly caused by demyelination in comparison with patients with MS.

Spinal cord lesions expanding for more than 2 vertebral segments are rarely found in MS.[39] MS lesions in spinal cord usually appear as short segments, are asymmetric, and are often in the posterior column.[40,41]

Brain

Brain MRI is initially normal in most patients with NMO. Between 55% and 84% of patients with NMO have normal brain MRI at presentation but serial scans may depict lesions in up to 85%.[32,42,43] Brain lesions usually corresponded with structures with high AQP4 expression such, as ependymal cells, hypothalamus, and brainstem.[24] Brain involvement has been reported more frequently in children than in adults. Brain MRI lesions are usually nonspecific in 60% of patients but may fulfill the Barkhof criteria for dissemination in space.[24] The lesions may be different in size, shape, and location and may range from nonspecific punctate or small round dots, located in juxtacortical, subcortical, and deep white matter, to large, edematous lesions in different areas. Involvement of corpus callosum is commonly seen in MS and has been reported as a sensitive and specific indicator of MS.[40,44,45] Acute, large, edematous callosal lesions with a heterogeneous intensity occasionally develop in patients with NMO (marbled

Table 1
2008 International Consensus Diagnostic Criteria for NMO

Major Criteria (All Required)	Minor Criteria (At Least One Required)	
Optic neuritis in 1 or more eyes	—	Brain MRI not fulfilling McDonald diagnostic criteria	Unspecific brain MRI abnormalities Lesions in dorsal medulla, with or without contiguous spinal cord signal abnormalities Hypothalamic or brainstem lesions Linear callosal lesions not in configuration of perpendicular lesions seen in MS (Dawson finger)
Transverse myelitis	T2 hyperintensity extended on 3 or more spinal segments with accompanying T1 hypointensity during acute attacks	Positive test for NMO-IgG/aquaporin-4 antibodies in serum or CSF	—
Exclusion of other syndromes	Sarcoidosis, Sjögren syndrome, systemic lupus erythematosus, or other syndromes	—	—

From Miller DH, Weinshenker BG, Filippi M, et al. Differential diagnosis of suspected multiple sclerosis: a consensus approach. Mult Scler 2008;14(9):1169; with permission.

pattern).[46] The size and intensity of the lesions may reduce or disappear in the chronic stages. In contrast, in MS, callosal lesions are small, nonedematous, and the intensity was homogeneous in the acute phase and located at the lower margin of the corpus callosum. Enhancement on brain MRI is not common and was seen in 13% to 36% of cases.[47] Multiple patchy enhancements with blurred margin of brain lesions (cloudlike enhancement) have been reported to be typical for NMO.[48] Pencil-like ependymal enhancement (**Fig. 1**) is another type of enhancement around the anterior horns of the lateral ventricles.[49] Brain MRI of patients experiencing a PRES episode revealed bilateral T2 hyperintensities primarily in frontal, parieto-occipital, and cerebellar regions.[50]

Kim and colleagues[51] identified brain lesions on MRI at first presentation in 24 out of 49 Korean patients (49%), and most patients (83%) showed abnormalities on brain MRI during the disease course. The localization and configuration of the lesions were unique; the characteristic brain lesions were (1) lesions involving corticospinal tracts such as the posterior limb of internal capsule and cerebral peduncle (44%); (2) extensive hemispheric lesions probably caused by vasogenic edema (29%); (3) periependymal lesions surrounding the aqueduct and the third and fourth ventricles (22%); (4) periependymal lesions surrounding the lateral ventricles (40%); and (5) medullary lesions, often contiguous with cervical lesions (31%). The extensive hemispheric lesions differed from those observed in regions of high AQP4 expression and were likely related to vasogenic edema; they sometimes looked like spilled ink and followed the white matter tracts.[51] Saiki and colleagues[52] reported a case of NMO with extensive brain lesions resembling acute disseminated encephalomyelitis without enhancement in serial scans likely caused by blood-brain barrier integrity. Magnetic

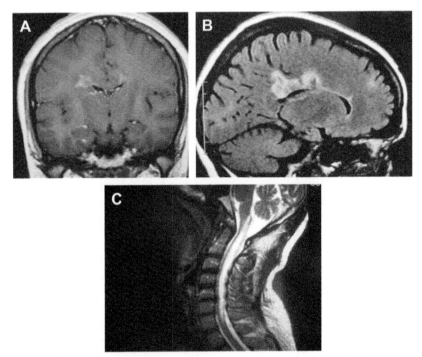

Fig. 1. MRI abnormalities specific to NMO. (*A*) Pencil-like ependymal enhancement. (*B*) Acute, large, edematous, callosal lesions, with a heterogeneous intensity. (*C*) T2 hyperintensity extended over 3 segments in spinal cord.

resonance spectroscopy studies showed normal N-acetylaspartate/creatine ratio in the normal-appearing white matter, which suggests that normal-appearing white matter is not primarily affected in NMO; this is not consistent with MS, in which normal-appearing white matter is diffusely affected.[53–55]

Imaging differences for the optic nerve in NMO and MS have not been well studied. Short-tau inversion recovery (STIR) sequence is the preferred method for evaluating the optic nerves.[56] In a Cuban study in patients with long-duration NMO, gadolinium enhancement of the optic nerve was found in 32.5%.[57]

CSF Analysis

CSF abnormalities are detected in most patients with NMO, especially if obtained during a relapse. Increased total protein levels are present in 46% to 75% of cases.[58] A prominent pleocytosis up to 50 to 1000 $\times$ 10^6 WBC/L, with a large proportion of neutrophils or eosinophils has been reported in 13% to 35% of patients.[1,59,60] Pleocytosis is a useful distinguishing feature from MS because it rarely exceeds 50 $\times$ 10^6 WBC/L in acute MS relapses and is more commonly seen in patients with LETM than in those with ON.[61,62] Oligoclonal bands are present in approximately 90% of patients with an established diagnosis of MS, and may be present in NMO. The frequency of oligoclonal bands in NMO ranges from 0% to 37% and they can be transient, in contrast with MS, which does not disappear in its presence.[1,8,11,63] The CSF content of matrix metalloproteinase-9 is greater in MS compared with NMO.[64] Jarius and colleagues[65] reported a polyspecific antiviral immune response against measles, rubella, and zoster that can help in differentiating MS from NMO. Its positive reaction, as defined by a combination of at least 2 positive antibody indices, was observed in 37/42 patients with MS, but in only 1/20 cases with NMO.[65] Although the total IgG concentrations were increased in the CSF of patients with NMO and MS, IgG1 levels and index were increased only in patients with MS. The lower CSF IgG1 level in NMO was interpreted to indicate a lesser Th1 autoimmune response than in MS.[66] The CSF content of inflammatory molecules, such as eosinophil cationic protein, interleukin (IL)-17, IL-6, IL-5, and B-cell activating factor, are increased.[67–70]

IMMUNOPATHOLOGY
Pathology

Necrosis of the spinal cord extending across multiple sections with involvement of both gray and white matter is the hallmark of NMO disorder. The necrosis may result in cavitation in the spinal cord or optic nerves. In addition to demyelination and necrosis with cavitation, eosinophils and neutrophils are commonly found in the inflammatory infiltrates of active lesions with vascular thickening and hyalinization.[71,72] Lucchinetti and colleagues[71] also described deposition of immunoglobulin and complement components in a characteristic vasculocentric rim and rosette pattern in active NMO lesions. Based on these findings, the investigators proposed that NMO was a humoral disorder targeting the perivascular region. Misu and colleagues[20] described a similar pattern of immunoglobulin deposition and complement activation in a patient with opticospinal MS (OSMS), which further supports this disorder and NMO being a single clinical entity. Postmortem pathologic studies of cavitary brain lesions confirm that these lesions have the same immunohistochemical characteristics as spinal cord and optic nerve lesions.[73]

Pathogenesis

Patients with NMO were frequently associated with multiple autoimmune disorders such as thyroiditis, systemic lupus erythematosus, or Sjögren syndrome.[1,58] A variety of autoantibodies were more frequently detected in the serum of patients with relapsing NMO or recurrent transverse myelitis.[74,75] Such observations prompted a search for a specific antibody to CNS tissues. In 2004, Lennon and colleagues[4] reported a serum autoantibody, NMO-IgG, the presence of which was 73% sensitive and 91% specific for differentiating NMO from MS. The test became commercial and its specificity validated at several international centers, and it now has a place in routine clinical practice. The antibody is produced by B cells in peripheral circulation and crosses the blood-brain barrier. The water channel aquaporin-4 (AQP4) on the foot processes of astrocytes, is the antigen target for the antibody. The binding of antibody to AQP4 results in its internalization and subsequent degeneration, which leads to glutamate excess outside the cell.[76,77] This in turn may damage the neurons and oligodenderocytes.[78] Inflammatory cells are attracted to the tissue and cause further injury.[77] Tissue injury in antibody-negative patients may be caused by unidentified antibody or cell-mediated processes.[79]

Disorders Related to NMO

NMO-IgG has also been detected in NMO-related disorders like recurrent isolated myelitis or ON. Between 25% and 60% of patients with idiopathic LETM or recurrent ON had positive NMO-IgG at presentation.[21,80–83] A prospective study showed that seropositive patients are more susceptible to developing definite NMO within 1 year.[84] Patients with symptomatic or asymptomatic brain involvement on MRI and who are seropositive for NMO-IgG are now considered to have an NMO spectrum disorder. Transverse myelitis, optic neuritis, relapsing myelitis, or NMO are well reported as complications of autoimmune diseases like systemic lupus erythematosus (SLE) or Sjögren syndrome. Myelitis and ON occurring in the context of connective tissue disease with positive serologic testing for NMO-IgG should be considered as the coexistence of 2 autoimmune disorders rather than neurologic complications of a vasculitic disease. These patients are also considered as having NMO-related disorders.[75,85] The clinical and radiological features of Asian OSMS have some similarities with recurrent NMO, and it has been suggested that OSMS and NMO may be the same entity, but traditionally they have been classified as separate entities, mainly because of the more benign course and more brain involvement.[85,86]

TREATMENT
Treatment of Acute Relapses

Intravenous (IV) corticosteroids are the preferred first-line therapy for acute attacks. IV methylprednisolone 1g daily for 3 to 5 consecutive days is the initial conventional therapy in routine clinical practice. The treatment should be initiated as soon as possible, because NMO attacks are more severe than MS exacerbations and can lead to prominent disability. Most patients (approximately 80%) respond well to IV steroids within 2 weeks.[1] Tapering with oral prednisolone has been proposed following IV steroids in NMO attacks and it has been advised to taper this drug more slowly than in MS-related attacks. Tapering for a period of 2 to 6 months has been suggested by some experts to prevent early rebounds.[86] Plasma exchange should be considered for steroid-resistant exacerbations and should be started within 5 to 10 days according to the clinical response to IV steroids.[86–88] Seven exchanges (1·0–1·5 plasma volumes per exchange) over a period of 2 weeks are typically advised. With this treatment, about 60% of patients may respond, mainly depending on the time interval between attack onset and therapy initiation.[89]

Attack Prevention

Treatments targeting relapse prevention should be considered as soon as the diagnosis of a relapsing NMO has been confirmed. It is also reasonable to start therapy after a single attack of LETM or ON in patients seropositive for NMO-IgG, because NMO-IgG is an important predictor of future relapse.[11] Treatment with immunosuppressive drugs can be postponed in seronegative patients who have experienced a single attack, especially with good recovery, to avoid long-term adverse events.[85] Several small observational studies have suggested that azathioprine (2·5–3·0 mg/kg/d) in combination with oral prednisone (1·0 mg/kg/d) may reduce the frequency of relapses.[90,91] Hematological evaluations including full blood count and liver function tests are required every 2 to 4 weeks at the initiation time, and then every 3 months when the patient has been stable for a long period.[92] In patients who do not tolerate azothioprin, alternative treatments could be chosen from other conventional immunosuppressant agents, like mycophenolate mofetil or methotrexate.[92] Sustained benefits were seen with mycophenolate (2 g/d), both in azathioprine-resistant and in treatment-naive patients.[93] Rituximab, an anti-CD20 monoclonal antibody, has been used in patients with aggressive NMO.[93,94] The recommended dose for rituximab is 375 mg/m^2 infused once per week for 4 weeks, or 1000 mg infused twice with a 2-week interval. Reinfusion should be considered after 6 to 12 months; however, optimal treatment duration is still unknown.[11] Mitoxantrone (12 mg/m^2 given every 3 months) has been successful in reducing the frequency of relapses in 4 out of 5 patients.[95] Intravenous immunoglobulin and glatiramer acetate have been studied by case reports.[69,96] β-Interferon has no proven efficacy in patients with NMO, and might even worsen the disease.[97]

SUMMARY

NMO was initially described as a severe, monophasic, necrotizing, demyelinating disease with pure involvement of optic nerves and spinal cord. During the last century, and especially the last 2 decades, understanding of the diagnosis, clinical presentation, and pathophysiology of NMO have changed greatly. The discovery of NMO-IgG in 2004 was an important step in the accurate and early recognition of NMO and its related disorders. With such improvements in diagnosis and early description of cases over the past decade, NMO is still considered a disabling disease of the CNS and future studies should be planned for better management of relapses and prevention of disability.

Case Study

The patient is a 35 year-old female who developed severe weakness of lower extremities and urinary incontinency. She had history of blurring of vision in right eye which was treated with intravenous methylprednisolone with partial recovery 18 months ago. On physical examination, she has complete paraplegia and sensory level at T4 level. Brain MRI is normal and spinal cord MRI demonstrates a cord lesion hyperintense on T2-weighted images extending from the second to the seventh thoracic vertebrae. The lesion is enhancing on T1-weighted with contrast images and occupies more than 2/3 of the spinal cord on axial views. Serum NMO IgG was positive and CSF was negative for oligoclonal bands.

REFERENCES

1. Wingerchuk DM, Hogancamp WF, O'Brien PC, et al. The clinical course of neuromyelitis optica (Devic's syndrome). Neurology 1999;53(5):1107–14.

2. Clifford Allbutt T. On the ophthalmoscopic signs of spinal disease. Lancet 1870; 95(2420):76–8.

3. Devic E. Myélite subaiguë compliquée de névrite optique. Bull Med (Paris) 1894; 8:1333.

4. Lennon VA, Wingerchuk DM, Kryzer TJ, et al. A serum autoantibody marker of neuromyelitis optica: distinction from multiple sclerosis. Lancet 2004;364(9451): 2106–12.

5. Lennon VA, Kryzer TJ, Pittock SJ, et al. IgG marker of optic-spinal multiple sclerosis binds to the aquaporin-4 water channel. J Exp Med 2005;202(4):473–7.

6. Kuroiwa Y, Igata A, Itahara K, et al. Nationwide survey of multiple sclerosis in Japan. Clinical analysis of 1,084 cases. Neurology 1975;25(9):845–51.

7. Cabrera-Gomez JA, Kurtzke JF, Gonzalez-Quevedo A, et al. An epidemiological study of neuromyelitis optica in Cuba. J Neurol 2009;256(1):35–44.

8. Asgari N, Lillevang ST, Skejoe HP, et al. A population-based study of neuromyelitis optica in Caucasians. Neurology 2011;76(18):1589–95.

9. Rivera JF, Kurtzke JF, Booth VJ, et al. Characteristics of Devic's disease (neuromyelitis optica) in Mexico. J Neurol 2008;255(5):710–5.

10. Cabre P, Heinzlef O, Merle H, et al. MS and neuromyelitis optica in Martinique (French West Indies). Neurology 2001;56(4):507–14.

11. Sellner J, Boggild M, Clanet M, et al. EFNS guidelines on diagnosis and management of neuromyelitis optica. Eur J Neurol 2010;17(8):1019–32.

12. Collongues N, Marignier R, Zephir H, et al. Neuromyelitis optica in France: a multicenter study of 125 patients. Neurology 2010;74(9):736–42.

13. Barbieri F, Buscaino GA. Neuromyelitis optica in the elderly. Acta Neurol (Napoli) 1989;11(4):247–51.

14. Banwell B, Tenembaum S, Lennon VA, et al. Neuromyelitis optica-IgG in childhood inflammatory demyelinating CNS disorders. Neurology 2008;70(5):344–52.

15. McKeon A, Lennon VA, Lotze T, et al. CNS aquaporin-4 autoimmunity in children. Neurology 2008;71(2):93–100.

16. Yamakawa K, Kuroda H, Fujihara K, et al. Familial neuromyelitis optica (Devic's syndrome) with late onset in Japan. Neurology 2000;55(2):318–20.

17. Mealy MA, Wingerchuk DM, Greenberg BM, et al. Epidemiology of neuromyelitis optica in the United States: a multicenter analysis epidemiology of NMO. Arch Neurol 2012;69(9):1176–80.

18. Wingerchuk DM, Lennon VA, Pittock SJ, et al. Revised diagnostic criteria for neuromyelitis optica. Neurology 2006;66(10):1485–9.

19. Papais-Alvarenga RM, Carellos SC, Alvarenga MP, et al. Clinical course of optic neuritis in patients with relapsing neuromyelitis optica. Arch Ophthalmol 2008; 126(1):12–6.

20. Misu T, Fujihara K, Nakashima I, et al. Intractable hiccup and nausea with periaqueductal lesions in neuromyelitis optica. Neurology 2005;65(9):1479–82.

21. Chan KH, Tse CT, Chung CP, et al. Brain involvement in neuromyelitis optica spectrum disorders. Arch Neurol 2011;68(11):1432–9.

22. Sato D, Fujihara K. Atypical presentations of neuromyelitis optica. Arq Neuropsiquiatr 2011;69(5):824–8.

23. Riphagen J, Modderman P, Verrips A. Hiccups, nausea, and vomiting: water channels under attack! Lancet 2010;375(9718):954.

24. Pittock SJ, Lennon VA, Krecke K, et al. Brain abnormalities in neuromyelitis optica. Arch Neurol 2006;63(3):390–6.

25. Kim W, Kim SH, Lee SH, et al. Brain abnormalities as an initial manifestation of neuromyelitis optica spectrum disorder. Mult Scler 2011;17(9):1107–12.

26. Mandler RN. Neuromyelitis optica - Devic's syndrome, update. Autoimmun Rev 2006;5(8):537–43.
27. Vernant JC, Cabre P, Smadja D, et al. Recurrent optic neuromyelitis with endocrinopathies: a new syndrome. Neurology 1997;48(1):58–64.
28. Uzawa A, Mori M, Muto M, et al. When is neuromyelitis optica diagnosed after disease onset? J Neurol 2012;259(8):1600–5.
29. Wingerchuk DM, Weinshenker BG. Neuromyelitis optica: clinical predictors of a relapsing course and survival. Neurology 2003;60(5):848–53.
30. Saiz A, Zuliani L, Blanco Y, et al. Revised diagnostic criteria for neuromyelitis optica (NMO). Application in a series of suspected patients. J Neurol 2007;254(9): 1233–7.
31. Argyriou AA, Makris N. Neuromyelitis optica: a distinct demyelinating disease of the central nervous system. Acta Neurol Scand 2008;118(4):209–17.
32. Miller DH, Weinshenker BG, Filippi M, et al. Differential diagnosis of suspected multiple sclerosis: a consensus approach. Mult Scler 2008;14(9):1157–74.
33. Takahashi T, Fujihara K, Nakashima I, et al. Anti-aquaporin-4 antibody is involved in the pathogenesis of NMO: a study on antibody titre. Brain 2007;130(Pt 5):1235–43.
34. Filippi M, Rocca MA, Moiola L, et al. MRI and magnetization transfer imaging changes in the brain and cervical cord of patients with Devic's neuromyelitis optica. Neurology 1999;53(8):1705–10.
35. Krampla W, Aboul-Enein F, Jecel J, et al. Spinal cord lesions in patients with neuromyelitis optica: a retrospective long-term MRI follow-up study. Eur Radiol 2009; 19(10):2535–43.
36. Bot JC, Blezer EL, Kamphorst W, et al. The spinal cord in multiple sclerosis: relationship of high-spatial-resolution quantitative MR imaging findings to histopathologic results. Radiology 2004;233(2):531–40.
37. Cruz LC Jr, Domingues RC, Gasparetto EL. Diffusion tensor imaging of the cervical spinal cord of patients with relapsing-remising multiple sclerosis: a study of 41 cases. Arq Neuropsiquiatr 2009;67(2B):391–5.
38. Pessôa FM, Lopes FC, Costa JV, et al. The cervical spinal cord in neuromyelitis optica patients: A comparative study with multiple sclerosis using diffusion tensor imaging. Eur J Radiol 2012;81:2697–701.
39. Sellner J, Luthi N, Buhler R, et al. Acute partial transverse myelitis: risk factors for conversion to multiple sclerosis. Eur J Neurol 2008;15(4):398–405.
40. Cordonnier C, de Seze J, Breteau G, et al. Prospective study of patients presenting with acute partial transverse myelopathy. J Neurol 2003;250(12):1447–52.
41. Sellner J, Luthi N, Schupbach WM, et al. Diagnostic workup of patients with acute transverse myelitis: spectrum of clinical presentation, neuroimaging and laboratory findings. Spinal Cord 2009;47(4):312–7.
42. Cabrera-Gomez J, Saiz-Hinarejos A, Graus F, et al. Brain magnetic resonance imaging findings in acute relapses of neuromyelitis optica spectrum disorders. Mult Scler 2008;14(2):248–51.
43. Li Y, Xie P, Lv F, et al. Brain magnetic resonance imaging abnormalities in neuromyelitis optica. Acta Neurol Scand 2008;118(4):218–25.
44. Dietemann JL, Beigelman C, Rumbach L, et al. Multiple sclerosis and corpus callosum atrophy: relationship of MRI findings to clinical data. Neuroradiology 1988; 30(6):478–80.
45. Friese SA, Bitzer M, Freudenstein D, et al. Classification of acquired lesions of the corpus callosum with MRI. Neuroradiology 2000;42(11):795–802.
46. Nakamura M, Misu T, Fujihara K, et al. Occurrence of acute large and edematous callosal lesions in neuromyelitis optica. Mult Scler 2009;15(6):695–700.

47. Kim JE, Kim SM, Ahn SW, et al. Brain abnormalities in neuromyelitis optica. J Neurol Sci 2011;302(1–2):43–8.
48. Ito S, Mori M, Makino T, et al. "Cloud-like enhancement" is a magnetic resonance imaging abnormality specific to neuromyelitis optica. Ann Neurol 2009;66(3):425–8.
49. Banker P, Sonni S, Kister I, et al. Pencil-thin ependymal enhancement in neuromyelitis optica spectrum disorders. Mult Scler 2012;18(7):1050–3.
50. Magana SM, Matiello M, Pittock SJ, et al. Posterior reversible encephalopathy syndrome in neuromyelitis optica spectrum disorders. Neurology 2009;72(8): 712–7.
51. Kim W, Park MS, Lee SH, et al. Characteristic brain magnetic resonance imaging abnormalities in central nervous system aquaporin-4 autoimmunity. Mult Scler 2010;16(10):1229–36.
52. Saiki S, Ueno Y, Moritani T, et al. Extensive hemispheric lesions with radiological evidence of blood-brain barrier integrity in a patient with neuromyelitis optica. J Neurol Sci 2009;284(1–2):217–9.
53. Aboul-Enein F, Krssak M, Hoftberger R, et al. Diffuse white matter damage is absent in neuromyelitis optica. AJNR Am J Neuroradiol 2010;31(1):76–9.
54. Bichuetti DB, Rivero RL, de Oliveira EM, et al. White matter spectroscopy in neuromyelitis optica: a case control study. J Neurol 2008;255(12):1895–9.
55. de Seze J, Blanc F, Kremer S, et al. Magnetic resonance spectroscopy evaluation in patients with neuromyelitis optica. J Neurol Neurosurg Psychiatry 2010;81(4): 409–11.
56. Johnson G, Miller DH, MacManus D, et al. STIR sequences in NMR imaging of the optic nerve. Neuroradiology 1987;29(3):238–45.
57. Cabrera-Gomez JA, Quevedo-Sotolongo L, Gonzalez-Quevedo A, et al. Brain magnetic resonance imaging findings in relapsing neuromyelitis optica. Mult Scler 2007;13(2):186–92.
58. O'Riordan JI, Gallagher HL, Thompson AJ, et al. Clinical, CSF, and MRI findings in Devic's neuromyelitis optica. J Neurol Neurosurg Psychiatry 1996;60(4):382–7.
59. Bichuetti DB, Rivero RL, Oliveira DM, et al. Neuromyelitis optica: brain abnormalities in a Brazilian cohort. Arq Neuropsiquiatr 2008;66(1):1–4.
60. de Seze J, Stojkovic T, Ferriby D, et al. Devic's neuromyelitis optica: clinical, laboratory, MRI and outcome profile. J Neurol Sci 2002;197(1–2):57–61.
61. Milano E, Di Sapio A, Malucchi S, et al. Neuromyelitis optica: importance of cerebrospinal fluid examination during relapse. Neurol Sci 2003;24(3):130–3.
62. Zaffaroni M, Italian Devic's Study Group. Cerebrospinal fluid findings in Devic's neuromyelitis optica. Neurol Sci 2004;25(Suppl 4):S368–70.
63. Bichuetti DB, Oliveira EM, Souza NA, et al. Neuromyelitis optica in Brazil: a study on clinical and prognostic factors. Mult Scler 2009;15(5):613–9.
64. Mandler RN, Dencoff JD, Midani F, et al. Matrix metalloproteinases and tissue inhibitors of metalloproteinases in cerebrospinal fluid differ in multiple sclerosis and Devic's neuromyelitis optica. Brain 2001;124(Pt 3):493–8.
65. Jarius S, Franciotta D, Bergamaschi R, et al. Polyspecific, antiviral immune response distinguishes multiple sclerosis and neuromyelitis optica. J Neurol Neurosurg Psychiatry 2008;79(10):1134–6.
66. Nakashima I, Fujihara K, Fujimori J, et al. Absence of IgG1 response in the cerebrospinal fluid of relapsing neuromyelitis optica. Neurology 2004;62(1):144–6.
67. Correale J, Fiol M. Activation of humoral immunity and eosinophils in neuromyelitis optica. Neurology 2004;63(12):2363–70.
68. Ishizu T, Osoegawa M, Mei FJ, et al. Intrathecal activation of the IL-17/IL-8 axis in opticospinal multiple sclerosis. Brain 2005;128(Pt 5):988–1002.

69. Okada K, Matsushita T, Kira J, et al. B-cell activating factor of the TNF family is upregulated in neuromyelitis optica. Neurology 2010;74(2):177–8.
70. Uzawa A, Mori M, Ito M, et al. Markedly increased CSF interleukin-6 levels in neuromyelitis optica, but not in multiple sclerosis. J Neurol 2009;256(12):2082–4.
71. Lucchinetti CF, Mandler RN, McGavern D, et al. A role for humoral mechanisms in the pathogenesis of Devic's neuromyelitis optica. Brain 2002;125(Pt 7):1450–61.
72. Mandler RN, Davis LE, Jeffery DR, et al. Devic's neuromyelitis optica: a clinicopathological study of 8 patients. Ann Neurol 1993;34(2):162–8.
73. Nakamura M, Endo M, Murakami K, et al. An autopsied case of neuromyelitis optica with a large cavitary cerebral lesion. Mult Scler 2005;11(6):735–8.
74. Hummers LK, Krishnan C, Casciola-Rosen L, et al. Recurrent transverse myelitis associates with anti-Ro (SSA) autoantibodies. Neurology 2004;62(1):147–9.
75. Pittock SJ, Lennon VA, de Seze J, et al. Neuromyelitis optica and non organ-specific autoimmunity. Arch Neurol 2008;65(1):78–83.
76. Saikali P, Cayrol R, Vincent T. Anti-aquaporin-4 auto-antibodies orchestrate the pathogenesis in neuromyelitis optica. Autoimmun Rev 2009;9(2):132–5.
77. Vincent T, Saikali P, Cayrol R, et al. Functional consequences of neuromyelitis optica-IgG astrocyte interactions on blood-brain barrier permeability and granulocyte recruitment. J Immunol 2008;181(8):5730–7.
78. Hinson SR, Roemer SF, Lucchinetti CF, et al. Aquaporin-4-binding autoantibodies in patients with neuromyelitis optica impair glutamate transport by down-regulating EAAT2. J Exp Med 2008;205(11):2473–81.
79. Moreh E, Gartsman I, Karussis D, et al. Seronegative neuromyelitis optica: improvement following lymphocytapheresis treatment. Mult Scler 2008;14(6):860–1.
80. Jarius S, Franciotta D, Bergamaschi R, et al. NMO-IgG in the diagnosis of neuromyelitis optica. Neurology 2007;68(13):1076–7.
81. Okai AF, Muppidi S, Bagla R, et al. Progressive necrotizing myelopathy: part of the spectrum of neuromyelitis optica? Neurol Res 2006;28(3):354–9.
82. Pirko I, Blauwet LA, Lesnick TG, et al. The natural history of recurrent optic neuritis. Arch Neurol 2004;61(9):1401–5.
83. Zuliani L, Lopez de Munain A, Ruiz Martinez J, et al. [NMO-IgG antibodies in neuromyelitis optica: a report of 2 cases]. Neurologia 2006;21(6):314–7.
84. Weinshenker BG, Wingerchuk DM, Vukusic S, et al. Neuromyelitis optica IgG predicts relapse after longitudinally extensive transverse myelitis. Ann Neurol 2006;59(3):566–9.
85. Jacob A, Matiello M, Wingerchuk DM, et al. Neuromyelitis optica: changing concepts. J Neuroimmunol 2007;187(1–2):126–38.
86. Watanabe S, Nakashima I, Miyazawa I, et al. Successful treatment of a hypothalamic lesion in neuromyelitis optica by plasma exchange. J Neurol 2007;254(5):670–1.
87. Bonnan M, Valentino R, Olindo S, et al. Plasma exchange in severe spinal attacks associated with neuromyelitis optica spectrum disorder. Mult Scler 2009;15(4):487–92.
88. Watanabe S, Nakashima I, Misu T, et al. Therapeutic efficacy of plasma exchange in NMO-IgG-positive patients with neuromyelitis optica. Mult Scler 2007;13(1):128–32.
89. Llufriu S, Castillo J, Blanco Y, et al. Plasma exchange for acute attacks of CNS demyelination: predictors of improvement at 6 months. Neurology 2009;73(12):949–53.
90. Mandler RN, Ahmed W, Dencoff JE. Devic's neuromyelitis optica: a prospective study of seven patients treated with prednisone and azathioprine. Neurology 1998;51(4):1219–20.

91. Sahraian MA, Moinfar Z, Khorramnia S, et al. Relapsing neuromyelitis optica: demographic and clinical features in Iranian patients. Eur J Neurol 2010;17(6): 794–9.
92. Palace J, Leite I, Jacob A. A practical guide to the treatment of neuromyelitis optica. Pract Neurol 2012;12(4):209–14.
93. Jacob A, Weinshenker BG, Violich I, et al. Treatment of neuromyelitis optica with rituximab: retrospective analysis of 25 patients. Arch Neurol 2008;65(11):1443–8.
94. Cree BA, Lamb S, Morgan K, et al. An open label study of the effects of rituximab in neuromyelitis optica. Neurology 2005;64(7):1270–2.
95. Weinstock-Guttman B, Ramanathan M, Lincoff N, et al. Study of mitoxantrone for the treatment of recurrent neuromyelitis optica (Devic disease). Arch Neurol 2006; 63(7):957–63.
96. Gartzen K, Limmroth V, Putzki N. Relapsing neuromyelitis optica responsive to glatiramer acetate treatment. Eur J Neurol 2007;14(6):e12–3.
97. Shimizu Y, Yokoyama K, Misu T, et al. Development of extensive brain lesions following interferon beta therapy in relapsing neuromyelitis optica and longitudinally extensive myelitis. J Neurol 2008;255(2):305–7.

Vascular Diseases of the Spinal Cord

Mark N. Rubin, MD[a], Alejandro A. Rabinstein, MD[b,c],*

KEYWORDS

- Spinal cord • Infarction • Cavernous malformation/cavernoma
- Arteriovenous malformation • Arteriovenous fistula • Epidural hematoma • Vasculitis

KEY POINTS

- Any suspicion of spinal cord infarction, particularly after aortic surgery, should prompt emergent neuroimaging and support of blood pressure (see **Fig. 1**).
- One should consider spinal dural arteriovenous fistula in a middle-aged male patient who develops a subacute progressive myelopathy, especially if worsened by Valsalva.
- Arteriovenous malformation can present acutely with hemorrhage or as a progressive myelopathy. Symptoms and prognosis are related to the complexity and location of the malformation.
- Any acute myelopathic symptoms (sensory or motor) after trauma and after surgery (especially those requiring anticoagulation and/or epidural anesthesia) should prompt emergent neuroimaging to exclude an epidural hematoma.
- There are numerous genetic syndromes associated with vascular diseases of the spinal cord including Von Hippel-Lindau disease, familial cavernomatosis (*CCM1-4*), and cutaneomeningospinal angiomatosis (Cobb syndrome).

Vascular disease affecting the spinal cord, while a relatively rare occurrence as compared with the cerebrovascular events, can cause substantial neurologic morbidity. It comprises various pathologies, including structural (*e.g.*, infarction, dural arteriovenous fistula, arteriovenous malformation (AVM), cavernous malformation (CM), compressive epidural hematoma and hematomyelia), inflammatory (*e.g.*, primary and secondary vasculitides) and genetic abnormalities. Several vascular spinal cord ailments represent neurologic emergencies. Thus, knowledge of relevant

Disclosure: The authors have nothing to disclose.
[a] Department of Neurology, Mayo Clinic, 200 First Street Southwest, Rochester, MN 55905, USA; [b] Division of Critical Care Neurology, Department of Neurology, Mayo Clinic, 200 First Street Southwest, Rochester, MN 55905, USA; [c] Division of Cerebrovascular Neurology, Department of Neurology, Mayo Clinic, 200 First Street Southwest, Rochester, MN 55905, USA
* Corresponding author. Division of Critical Care Neurology, Department of Neurology, Mayo Clinic, 200 First Street Southwest, Rochester, MN 55905.
E-mail address: rabinstein.alejandro@mayo.edu

anatomy, syndromes, pathogenesis, initial evaluation, and management is of critical importance. The aim of this article was to review the medical literature on vascular diseases of the spinal cord in adults and children and frame it in the context of our clinical experience.

SPINAL CORD ANATOMY

A detailed knowledge of spinal cord anatomy is indispensable in the evaluation of a patient with suspected spinal cord disease. Understanding the anatomy is necessary to interpret the patient's neurologic signs and symptoms, and to select appropriate diagnostic tests during initial evaluation. Therefore, it is important that the most relevant anatomic concepts are reviewed before discussing the various vascular pathologies of the spinal cord.[1–3]

Spinal Cord, Meninges, and the Epidural Space

The spinal cord is radially arranged with gray matter internally and white matter tracts peripherally. One can make a crude compartmentalization of motor function anteromedially, spinothalamic sensation (e.g., pain and temperature) anterolaterally, and proprioceptive sensation (e.g., joint position, discriminative touch, vibration) posteriorly. The spinal cord can be further simplified into the anterior two thirds, which encompass predominantly motor and spinothalamic modalities, and the posterior one third composed of the proprioceptive tracts. This dichotomization is clinically relevant owing to vascular supply, which is discussed subsequently. Thirty-one pairs of dorsal and ventral roots arise from the cervical (n = 8), thoracic (n = 12), lumbar (n = 5), sacral (n = 5), and coccygeal (n = 1) segments of the spinal cord.

The cord is immediately surrounded by the pial layer of meninges. The pia form bilaterally symmetric protrusions called denticulate ligaments, which serve to tether the cord to the next meningeal layer, the arachnoid. The dura mater is the outermost and thickest meningeal layer, and is directly adherent to the arachnoid. As in the brain, cerebrospinal fluid (CSF) is found between the pia and arachnoid layers.

The spinal epidural (or extradural) space exists within the confines of the vertebral spinal canal but outside of the dura. It extends from the foramen magnum rostrally to the sacrococcygeal membrane caudally. Spinal roots, radicular arteries, lymphatics and a valveless venous plexus traverse this space, suspended in adipose tissue.

Spinal Arteries

The anterior spinal artery, which provides the principal supply to much of the spinal cord throughout its long course, forms at the level of the craniocervical junction from the paired vertebral arteries just before they join to form the basilar artery. Sometimes the anterior spinal artery arises directly from the aorta. Paired segmental arteries (e.g., cervical, thoracic) arise from the aorta and give rise to radicular arteries that correspond with each spinal vertebral level. Radicular arteries, following nerve roots proximally, divide into radiculomedullary arteries that follow ventral roots and radiculopial arteries that align with dorsal roots. Radiculomedullary arteries branch again as they approach the spinal cord, feeding the single, midline anterior spinal artery medially and the collateral arteria vasocorona laterally. Radiculopial arteries supply paired posterior spinal arteries, which extend laterally to form a collateral network with the arteria vasocorona. The single anterior spinal artery provides the vascular supply to the anterior two thirds of the spinal cord parenchyma on both sides by branching into left and right intramedullary arteries called sulcocommissural arteries. There is a clinically relevant watershed between intramedullary and extramedullary arterial supply of the cord. Each posterior spinal artery supplies its corresponding half of the posterior one third of the cord. There is also a relative hypovascularity in the midthoracic spinal cord, with less dense anastomoses; although, the classical teaching of mid-thoracic susceptibility to hypoperfusion is not supported by the clinical findings on the most frequent locations of spinal cord infarction (SCI).[4,5]

Typically 5 to 8 of the radicular arteries become dominant during development and provide the bulk of the vascular supply to the anterior spinal artery.[6,7] In roughly 90% of people, one of the thoracolumbar radicular arteries is particularly robust and provides much of the vascular supply to the lower thoracic and lumbar spinal cord as well as the conus medullaris. This vessel is referred to as the arteria radicularis magna or its more commonly known eponym, the great artery of Adamkiewicz.[8] It arises between T8 and L3, mostly commonly at T10, and on the left side in a majority of individuals.

Spinal Veins

Radially oriented intramedullary veins drain outward and medially into the unpaired anterior and posterior median spinal veins. They also drain into an extramedullary, circumferential network of veins known as the coronal plexus. There are typically 10 to 20 radiculomedullary and radiculopial veins that arise from the anterior and posterior median spinal veins, respectively. These veins exit the dural space to form the valveless, circumferential, longitudinally continuous epidural plexus.

SPINAL CORD INFARCTION

SCI is a rare cause of acute myelopathy, frequently cited as representing only 1% of all strokes and 5 to 8% of acute myelopathies,[9] although the exact incidence and prevalence are not well known. It has been associated with myriad pathogenic mechanisms, the most significant of which have actually changed over time. Whereas syphilitic arteritis was the most common cause of SCI until the early 20th century,[10] and the cause of the first case of anterior spinal artery syndrome,[11] SCI is now most closely associated with atherosclerotic disease and surgery of the aorta.[5,12-15] Other reported causes and associations include decompression sickness (*e.g.*, "the bends"),[16] systemic hypotension,[17] spinal trauma of various degrees,[18-24] and less common iatrogenic causes such as vertebral angiography,[25] sympathectomy,[26,27] celiac plexus neurolysis,[28,29] abdominal aortography,[30] subclavian vein catheterization,[31] lumbar epidural anesthesia,[32,33] renal artery embolization,[34] single radicular artery ligation,[35] thoracoplasty,[36] intra-aortic balloon pump counterpulsation,[37] portocaval shunt placement,[38] and intrathecal injection of lidocaine[39] or phenol.[40] In addition, a substantial minority of cases have no identifiable cause.[5]

Clinical Presentation

Although many of the case series to date have relatively small cohorts, they demonstrate similarities in age, distribution of infarct localization, and clinical presentation. Range of ages affected typically span the 1st to 10th decades of life with a median age in the 6th to 7th decades. The majority of SCI are located in the thoracolumbar area (>60% in most series) and the mid-cervical region is the next most afflicted segment. Patients with SCI most typically present with acute weakness, urinary retention, and pain, in descending order of frequency across series.[5,9,12,13,15,21,30,41–47] Pain and sensory symptoms are typically the first noted by the patient, and the weakness tends to develop progressively over the coming minutes to hours. Clinical nadir is often reached within 12 hours of symptom onset. There are distinct spinal cord syndromes based on the vascular anatomy of the spinal cord. The most common is the anterior spinal artery syndrome,[11] which is clinically characterized by acute onset of symmetric motor weakness and bilateral spinothalamic sensory deficit below the level of the lesion in conjunction with autonomic sphincter dysfunction. The weakness is often flaccid and associated with absent tendon reflexes, reflecting the affliction of the anterior horns. Patients often complain of pain, either local or radicular, at the onset of symptoms. Although posterior column sensory modalities are typically spared in anterior spinal artery syndrome, it is not uncommon to see postoperative patients with SCI who have altered vibration and proprioception in the legs during the first few hours, only to recover these sensations by the following day. Coupled with this semiological caveat is that postoperative patients are also at risk of epidural hematomas owing to their exposure to anticoagulants during surgery. These are issues that must be kept in mind when evaluating postoperative patients with acute paraplegia or quadriplegia, because they underscore the need to pursue emergency imaging of the spine to rule out compression. Depending on the level of the infarct, patients might also experience respiratory distress (phrenic nerve palsy, C3–C5), orthostatic hypotension (greater splanchnic nerve palsy, T4–T9), and urologic dysfunction including detrusor hyperreflexia and sphincter dyssynergia.[48]

Patients might also sustain deficits consistent with cord hemisection, or Brown-Séquard syndrome,[49] which is defined by unilateral flaccid weakness ipsilateral to and below the lesion, with contralateral absence of spinothalamic sensation and sparing of posterior column sensory modalities. This pattern is thought to result from sulcocommissural artery occlusion. Patients rarely experience isolated lemniscal deficit, which is attributed to posterior spinal artery disruption and/or diffuse atherosclerotic disease affecting the delicate arterial collateral network. In fact, isolated posterior column dysfunction should trigger suspicion for a compressive lesion such as an epidural hematoma.

Not infrequently, there is a fair amount of overlap, as patients might present with less well anatomically delineated signs, manifesting as either partial or full transverse myelopathy. This is particularly true of venous infarction of the spinal cord. In addition to the relatively nebulous clinical presentation, a subacute decline or the presence of hemorrhage should raise suspicion of a venous infarct. Structural vascular anomalies such as dural arteriovenous fistulae and intramedullary AVMs often underlie subacute SCI with or without hematomyelia. Detailed spinal imaging including angiography is necessary in these cases.

Spinal ischemia can also manifest with intermittent attacks, as classically described by Dejerine,[50] which are commonly referred to as "spinal transient ischemic attacks." Patients present with transient weakness that is often bilateral and symmetric in the absence of other signs that might localize the process intracranially. Risk of completed stroke after spinal transient ischemic attack has not been studied. Yet, in our experience, transient ischemic symptoms from the spinal cord are rare, except for exertional claudication in patients with spinal dural arteriovenous fistulas (sdAVF).

It is important to remember that most series report roughly half of their patients' infarcts are in the immediate perioperative period. Whether the insult occurs while under anesthesia or in the postoperative period when analgesic needs are the greatest and the patient is still on bed rest, one cannot rely on the patient to notice the acute symptoms in such cases. The diagnosis of postoperative spinal cord ischemia therefore depends heavily on serial neurologic examinations, a high index of suspicion, and a low threshold to pursue further investigation.

Management: Diagnosis and Treatment

Effective treatment of SCI depends on rapid diagnosis. In the perioperative stage, particularly after relatively high-risk procedures such as open or endovascular thoracic aortic repair, management begins with serial neurologic examinations starting as soon as one awakens from general anesthesia. If SCI is suspected, particularly in the setting of recent aortic manipulation, mean arterial pressure should be maintained above 90 mm Hg, using hemodynamic augmentation with volume and/or pressors if necessary. If neurologic deficits are reversed, then the target mean arterial pressure can be gradually reduced, while continuing serial neurologic examinations to exclude recurrent deterioration.

In parallel, emergent neuroimaging of the spine should be performed to rule out spinal cord compression, most notably from epidural hematoma. Magnetic resonance imaging (MRI) is the preferred modality, although computed tomography (CT) scan can be done instead if the patient is clinically unstable or MRI facilities are unavailable. Although CT will be insensitive for SCI, a good quality CT scan should be sufficient to reveal a compressive hemorrhage. However, we have seen occasional cases in which an epidural hematoma was missed by CT because of extensive bone artifact at the level of the lesion. If a compressive lesion is found, then emergent neurosurgical consultation is warranted.

Diffusion-weighted imaging demonstrating focal restricted diffusion has become increasingly sensitive for the diagnosis of SCI,[51] but its sensitivity is not as high as in the brain. In fact, MRI can be normal when performed early (e.g., within hours); therefore, absence of abnormalities on neuroimaging during the acute phase should not dissuade a clinical diagnosis.[5] The main purpose of acute imaging is to identify a surgically treatable compressive lesion. If there is no clinical improvement within minutes of hemodynamic augmentation, one should consider placement of a lumbar drain open to 15 mm Hg or below. The goal of these combined therapies is to increase cord perfusion; analogous to cerebral hemodynamics, cord perfusion pressure is directly related to the difference between the mean arterial pressure and intradural spinal pressure. Thus, if mean arterial pressure is increased via augmentation and CSF pressure reduced via CSF drainage, then spinal cord perfusion pressure should rise.

The combination of hemodynamic augmentation and CSF drainage has been evaluated after open and endovascular thoracic and thoracoabdominal aortic surgery.[52–55] One prospective analysis[56] of routine preoperative lumbar drain placement and CSF drainage after both elective and emergent endovascular thoracic aortic repair demonstrated absence of SCI in the 56 consecutive cases studied, compared with 5 episodes of SCI among the 65 consecutive patients operated before the introduction of this practice. Of note, with implementation of hemodynamic augmentation and CSF drainage, 3 of those 5 patients with SCI showed "marked clinical improvement." The authors rightly acknowledged the ambiguity of best practice, because their data seem to support both prophylactic and symptomatic drainage.

Fig. 1 illustrates our management protocol for patients with suspected SCI. In addition, depending on the localization of the infarct, other potentially life-threatening complications may arise, such as respiratory distress with cervical spinal involvement or severe hemodynamic instability owing to a mid-thoracic lesion. These acute complications must be anticipated and close monitoring and prompt management in the intensive care unit. Over subsequent days, patients can develop additional complications, most notably venous thromboembolism, infections (especially affecting the urinary tract, or aspiration pneumonia in patients with cervical SCI), and pressure skin lesions. Autonomic dysreflexia is only seen when SCI affects the low cervical or high thoracic cord segments.

The special case of decompression sickness demands targeted therapy in the form of hyperbaric oxygenation, which has both sound physiologic basis and reports of

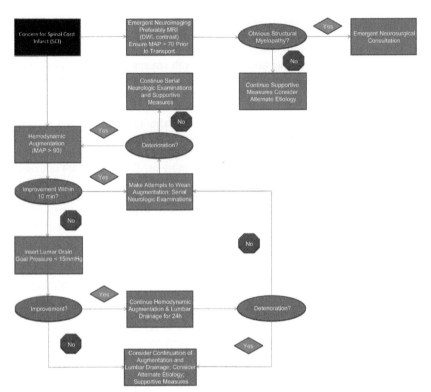

Fig. 1. Diagnostic and therapeutic algorithm for spinal cord infarction. The black box in the top left is the starting point. Blue rectangles represent management recommendations, and brown ovals clinical decision-making branch points. The first steps of hemodynamic augmentation and arrangement for emergent neuroimaging are intended to be initiated in parallel.

clinical benefit.[57] The timing of therapy is controversial,[58] but pathophysiologic considerations dictate minimization of delay.[59]

Prognosis

SCI can be functionally devastating and immediately life threatening. A summary of the 199 reported cases as of 1996, including 13 studies (with no cohort of >41 patients), demonstrated that nearly half of the patients showed some degree of recovery over a variable follow-up, whereas the other half showed no improvement or died owing to complications.[4]

The largest and most recent case series in the literature analyzes the outcome of 115 patients treated over a 17-year span at our institution.[5] Most of the patients on this cohort had severe SCI, with nearly half of the patients split evenly between the most severe categories of ASIA A and ASIA B.[59] The analysis, however, showed that 58% of survivors were walking with or without a gait aid at last follow-up (mean, 3 years). Furthermore, 41% of patients who required a wheelchair at hospital dismissal were walking and 33% of patients requiring intermittent bladder catheterization at hospital dismissal were able to void at last follow-up. Severity of neurologic impairment on initial examination was the only clinical factor associated with wheelchair and catheter use at final follow-up on multivariate logistic regression analysis.

Box 1
Spinal infarction

- SCI is strongly associated with aortic surgery.
- Most patients with SCI present with acute weakness, sensory deficit, and sphincter dysfunction.
- Diffusion-weighted MRI can be helpful, but the diagnosis is clinical.
- The mainstay of treatment is raising spinal cord perfusion pressure (see **Fig. 1**).
- SCI is often disabling, but a significant minority of severely affected patients can have a good outcome.

Still, this study confirmed that SCI decreases life expectancy. A Kaplan–Meier survival curve demonstrated a median survival of 6.1 years, a 5-year estimated survival of 55%, and a 10-year estimated survival of 42.5%. Severity of neurologic impairment and presence of peripheral vascular disease were independently associated with the risk of death after SCI on multivariate analysis (**Box 1**).[5]

Case Presentation

A 60-year-old man with a history of hypertension and substance abuse was at a party with his family when he suddenly collapsed to the ground. He was reportedly able to speak initially, but made no movements with his arms or legs and was then reported to have lost consciousness transiently and within minutes of the fall. He was transported to our emergency department where he underwent an extensive cardiopulmonary evaluation to rule out myocardial infarction, aortic dissection, and pulmonary embolism. CT angiogram of the chest showed a right-sided subsegmental pulmonary embolus. Cardiac catheterization was unremarkable. When it was noticed that the patient was not moving any limb after this procedure, an urgent neurology consultation was requested roughly 7 hours from ictus. At that time the patient was lucid, had flaccid areflexic quadriplegia, and a sensory level corresponding to the C4 dermatome. His supine mean arterial pressure was 75 mm Hg. Hemodynamic augmentation was initiated with a goal mean arterial pressure of greater than 90 mm Hg. Urgent MRI of the spine was performed (**Fig. 2**) and it demonstrated an area of focal restricted diffusion, T2 hyperintensity and cord expansion in the middle segment of the cervical spinal cord. Lumbar drainage was initiated thereafter. Unfortunately, no clinical improvement was noted during his hospitalization. Extensive evaluation, including dedicated angiography of the chest and neck and transesophageal echocardiography, failed to reveal an etiology. The documented pulmonary embolus and brief loss of consciousness triggered suspicion of thromboembolism to both the posterior cerebral circulation, causing a transient top of the basilar syndrome, and his cervical spinal arterial supply. However, no embolic source (or patent foramen ovale) was ever identified. At last follow-up, 1 year from his infarct, he remained flaccidly quadriplegic and incontinent of urine, but sensation to touch had recovered.

This case illustrates that atypical features may cause considerable delays in diagnosis. The presentation with sudden collapse and especially the initial loss of consciousness deviated attention from the quadriplegia in the emergency department.

SPINAL AVMS

An AVM is generically defined as an abnormal communication between and artery and a vein without intervening capillary architecture. These lesions occur throughout the

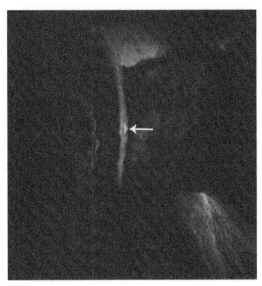

Fig. 2. Cervical spinal cord infarction. This sagittal, diffusion-weighted MRI sequence, demonstrates an area of focal restricted diffusion and cord expansion in the mid-cervical spinal cord (*arrow*).

central nervous system (CNS), including the spinal cord, and further classification of spinal lesions is stratified by localization and morphology.[60] Spinal AVMs are a rare clinical phenomenon, although precise estimations of incidence are lacking for all but a specific subset called sdAVF, which is reported to affect 5 to 10 patients per million population annually.[61] These represent upwards of 70% of all spinal AVMs. For the rest of the AVMs, namely those of the peri- and intramedullary variety, there is a lack of sound epidemiologic data.

Both sdAVFs and AVMs are predominantly thoracolumbar, but all levels of the spinal cord may be affected. They cause symptoms primarily from venous hypertension, which produces cord edema and eventually infarction. The clinical presentation of peri- and intramedullary AVMs is characteristically in the third decade, whereas sdAVF typically present in the fifth and sixth decades.[62] Prompt recognition can be challenging because of the lack of pathognomonic signs and symptoms, but it is crucial. These vascular anomalies are eminently treatable, especially sdAVF, but can produce irreparably disabling spinal cord damage if left untreated or treated too late.

Clinical Presentation

The symptoms caused by sdAVF are nonspecific and the disease is often misdiagnosed as spinal stenosis, demyelinating disease, transverse myelitis, or a spinal cord tumor. As a consequence, diagnosis is delayed by an average of 11 to 18 months from onset of symptoms.[63,64] The majority of patients are middle-aged men (roughly 9:1 male-to-female predominance) who develop subacute myelopathic symptoms including gait disturbance, various sensory abnormalities in the legs, and leg weakness, occasionally precipitated by maneuvers that increase venous pressure, such as Valsalva.[63] By the time of diagnosis, most patients have appreciable sensory deficits, sphincter dysfunction, and weakness.[64–66] Pain in the lower back is present in roughly 25 to 50% of patients, and may or may not radiate in a radicular pattern, contributing to diagnostic confusion with spondylotic disease. In one large series, the most common sensory level was L1, and sensory level did not correlate well with sdAVF location.[65] Some variations in clinical presentation are important to consider. These include stepwise or acute decline in roughly 25% and 5% of cases, respectively.[64,67] The pattern of weakness is also variable, with roughly half of cases demonstrating bilateral but asymmetric weakness, and a substantial minority (16% in one series[65]) having unilateral weakness. Tetraparesis has also been reported with craniocervical sdAVF, but this presentation is particularly rare.[67–69]

Peri- and intramedullary AVMs can also present with a syndrome similar to that of sdAVFs depending on the anatomy and location, but possess the distinct pathophysiologic tendency to cause hemorrhage when compared with their dural counterparts.[70] Hemorrhages have been reported in both the extradural[71] and intradural[72] regions, producing different clinical presentations. An extradural hemorrhage presents as rapid-onset compressive myelopathy, whereas an intradural hemorrhage can have variable presentations ranging from headache and meningismus to catastrophic cord transection depending on and the precise location of the hemorrhage. Spinal subarachnoid hemorrhage (SAH) can be clinically indistinct from intracranial SAH, and thus requires a high index of suspicion in patients with thunderclap headache with meningismus and no abnormalities on head CT. In case series with more than 10 patients, the reported rates of spinal SAH have ranged between 31 and 58% with perimedullary[73–75] and 23 and 70% with intramedullary[76–80] AVMs.

Management: Diagnosis and Treatment

Spinal MRI and angiography are essential in establishing a diagnosis of spinal AVMs. Spinal MRI has excellent sensitivity and specificity for the detection of spinal AVMs and sdAVF as long as it includes all necessary sequences and is interpreted by experienced neuroradiologists.[81,82] MRI of the entire spine should be performed, be it in the setting of a progressive myelopathy or spinal SAH, because neurologic signs and symptoms do not correspond well with the level of the vascular lesion. The MRI characteristics of the myelopathy associated with sdAVF—longitudinally extensive T2 hyperintensity within the central aspect of the spinal cord—involves the conus medullaris in as many as 95% of patients. Spinal cord enlargement and dilated perimedullary veins can also be noted, most prominently on sagittal T2 sequences (**Fig. 3**).[65] Spinal cord MRI characteristics of peri- and intramedullary AVMs can be similar to those with sdAVF, although the abnormal vessels, indicated by large serpentine flow voids, are distinctly within or just apposed to the spinal cord parenchyma (**Fig. 4**).

MR angiography can identify the presence of abnormal vessels and help to guide superselective catheter angiography[83]; however, the latter is still necessary for treatment planning. Digital subtraction angiography can localize the nidus of the fistula, its feeding arteries, and draining vein. When angiography fails to localize the AVM, MRI with myelographic sequences (e.g., fast imaging employing steady-state acquisition, or FIESTA) can be of assistance.[84]

Both open surgery[85] and endovascular occlusion[86,87] have been established as safe and effective treatments for sdAVF. With both techniques, the treatment goal is to occlude the most proximal portion of the arterialized draining vein. Surgery has proven durable and safe, with reported long-term shunt occlusion in 98% of cases and a morbidity rate of less than 2%.[83] Endovascular therapy may achieve comparable results, but complex and tortuous lesions may not be amenable to this modality. Although complete occlusion can be achieved in more than 95% of sdAVF with open surgery, rates are lower with endovascular therapy,[83] and continuously improving. Furthermore, the long-term durability of occlusion after endovascular

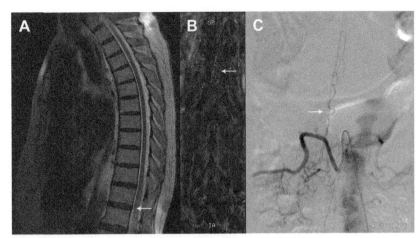

Fig. 3. sdAVF. A triptych of key radiographic features of sdAVF in a single patient. (*A*) Sagittal T2-weighted image of the lumbar spine demonstrates the longitudinally-extensive T2 signal abnormality corresponding to the myelopathy (*arrow*). (*B*) Coronal magnetic resonance angiography demonstrating the abnormal vasculature (*arrow*). (*C*) Selective spinal digital subtraction angiography which shows the abnormal vessel (*arrow*) extending rostrally from a thoracic radicular artery.

embolization has been questioned.[64,83,88] Treatment must be pursued as soon as the diagnosis of sdAVF is confirmed.

The other varieties of spinal AVM are also mostly managed by open surgery, endovascular embolization, or a staged combination of the two.[60] However, owing to the complex vascularity and intramedullary components of the AVMs, treatment of these anomalies is often technically difficult. Identification and obliteration of feeding vessels

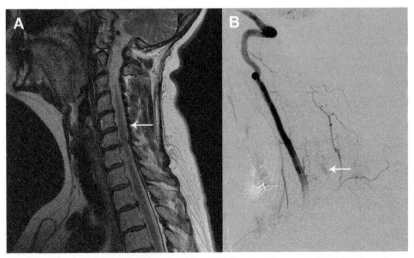

Fig. 4. Spinal AVM. (*A*) T2-weighted cervical spinal MRI shows T2 hypointense abnormal "flow void" near the dorsal aspect of the mid-cervical cord (*arrow*). (*B*) Digital subtraction angiography in the same patient, which demonstrates an abnormal "blush" (*arrow*) in a region that corresponds to the perimedullary cervical cord and the MRI abnormality.

is still the operative goal, but the presence of multiple feeding vessels, connections with anterior and posterior spinal arteries or the artery of Adamkiewicz, and intraparenchymal loops create greater risk for operative harm. Thus, surgical expectations need to be realistically adjusted, and sometimes a partial resolution of the disorder should be considered satisfactory. Despite the increased technical difficulty, surgery for obliteration of feeding vessels and excision or occlusion of the AVM nidus remains standard. Different approaches and combinations of endovascular and open microsurgical techniques are recommended based on the newer, anatomically based classification of AVMs.[60] If a lesion is not considered amenable to open or endovascular surgery, owing to a primarily intraparenchymal or critical location (*e.g.*, brainstem), stereotactic radiosurgery can be a useful alternative.[89,90]

Prognosis

Although there are no large, comprehensive studies on the natural history of spinal AVMs and sdAVF, the ischemic myelopathy caused by these anomalies is progressive. The largest series to date of open surgery for sdAVF,[85] which included 154 patients at a single institution, demonstrated a 96.6% rate of motor improvement (82.2%) or stability (14.4%) after surgery. There were no perioperative deaths or major neurologic complications, although 6% of patients developed subjective or objective worsening of symptoms before hospital discharge which persisted at follow-up. In a meta-analysis of 9 studies – including open surgical and endovascular series—the observed postoperative outcomes were improvement in 55% of cases and stability in 34%.[83] Nonmotor symptoms (*e.g.*, numbness, pain, sphincter dysfunction) typically do not improve as consistently or only partially after surgery. There is a strong association between postoperative recanalization of the spinal AVM and neurologic deterioration.[91]

Peri- and intramedullary AVMs can cause progressive disability from ischemia and rapid decline owing to hemorrhage. Operative outcomes can be favorable in a majority of patients at discharge and improvement or stability can be maintained over time.[60,87] Stereotactic radiosurgery may afford significant reductions in AVM volumes even if the malformation is still visible on angiography.[92] The risk of hemorrhage and radiation damage after radiosurgical treatment of spinal AVMs seems to be low, but more studies are needed.

The prognosis of patients with sdAVF after treatment depends primarily on the severity of preoperative deficits (as measured by the Aminoff-Logue disability scale).[65,92–95] In one series, postoperative improvement was seen in 78% of patients with mild disability (score 0–3), 29% of patients with moderate disability (score 4–5), and only 11% of patients with severe preoperative disability (score 6–8).[94] Notwithstanding, clinical recovery is possible, even with paraplegia, and treatment should not be withheld owing to perceived futility.[65,96,97] We have observed that the absence of a sensory level to pinprick preoperatively is independently associated with a greater chance of independent ambulation after surgery, whereas its presence portends a lower likelihood of postoperative improvement, suggesting that the presence of a sensory level might indicate irreversible spinal cord ischemia.[65]

Radiographic changes noted pre- and postoperatively have been studied as prognostic biomarkers, but associations remain limited to single studies and, in general, the extent of pre- or postoperative spinal cord signal abnormalities do not correspond to postoperative disability, at least in the case of sdAVF.[65,98] Single studies have shown that lower thoracic lesions (*e.g.*, between T9 and T12) portend a better rate of symptomatic improvement[99] and that spinal cord atrophy may predict unfavorable outcome (**Box 2**).[100]

> **Box 2**
> **Spinal AVM**
>
> - Spinal AVMs can be clinically dichotomized into the more common sdAVF (~70%) and all other AVMs.
> - sdAVF typically occur in middle-aged men, cause a progressive myelopathy, and often mimic other nonvascular spinal cord pathology.
> - Other AVM symptomatology depends on the complexity of the vascular lesion and the surrounding neurologic and vascular structures.
> - MRI and MRA are essential for making the diagnosis of sdAVF or AVM.
> - Surgery, open or endovascular, is recommended for sdAVF and AVM.

Spinal CM

CMs, also referred to as "cavernomas," "cavernous hemangiomas," and "cavernous angiomas," are hamartomatous sinusoidal collections of abnormal vascular loops that have little or no intervening parenchyma. They can be found in most regions of the body but most commonly in skin, viscera, and the CNS.[101] Intracerebral CMs are more common than spinal lesions, with an estimated prevalence in the general population of 0.4 to 0.8%,[102,103] whereas spinal CMs are thought to represent only 5% of all CMs of the CNS.[104] In fact, the literature on spinal CMs was limited to case reports and small series for much of the 20th century until relatively large series[105,106] and comprehensive reviews became available more recently.[107]

Although most spinal CMs are solitary, spontaneous lesions, CMs of the CNS have an association with known genetic abnormalities[108,109] as well as radiation exposure.[110–113] Familial spinal CM, variably defined in studies as the presence of known genetic abnormalities or simply as one family member with at least one known CM of their own, represents a substantial minority of CMs, ranging from 8 to 12% of all cases with spinal CM in some of the larger series.[105,114] Familial cases are much more common among patients with multiple CMs throughout the nervous system, accounting for almost 50% of those patients.[105,107] One study of six non-related families, five of which were Hispanic in descent, suggests average age of diagnosis is substantially younger in familial CM (e.g., 25 years) but this likely reflects referral bias. There are no histologic differences between familial and non-familial CMs.[115] There are four genes in two different chromosomes that have been associated with familial CM, called CCM 1 (7q11–22),[116,117] CCM2 (7p13),[118,119] CCM3 (3q26.1),[120] and CCM4 (3q26.3–27.2)[121]; all seem to be transmitted in an autosomal-dominant pattern of inheritance.[108]

The rare reported cases of post-radiation spinal CM have occurred in children who received radiation for various primary tumors and presented with neurologic symptoms referable to a spinal CM 5 to 29 years after radiation exposure.[111–113] With so few recognized cases of spinal CM after radiation, it is difficult to draw conclusions, but the increasingly more common reports of cerebral CM after cranial radiation suggest that the association is pathogenic.[110]

Clinical Presentation

The average age at presentation was 42 and men and women are affected in equal proportions.[115] CMs are predominantly thoracic (57%), with the majority of the remainder in the cervical cord (38%).[115] Coexistent intracranial CMs can be found in a quarter of cases and even more frequently in familial cases.[122–127]

Roughly two thirds of patients present with motor weakness and sensory deficit, whereas only 27% have pain and 11% bowel or bladder dysfunction.[115] The temporal profile is variable. Progressive neurologic decline is most common, but acute presentations and stepwise worsening with recurrent acute episodes of neurologic deficits can also occur. The degree of neurologic impairment is typically categorized using the McCormick grades[128] (actually published in an article concerning operative outcomes after resection of spinal cord ependymomas), which range from I to IV, with higher scores corresponding with greater disability. In one relatively large surgical series, the average McCormick grade preoperatively was below II (McCormick II = "presence of sensorimotor deficit affecting function of involved limb; mild to moderate gait difficulty; severe pain or dysesthetic syndrome impairing patient's quality of life; still functions and ambulates independently") and the average duration of symptoms before intervention was 7 months.[129]

Management: Diagnosis and Treatment

The diagnosis of spinal CM requires MRI.[130,131] The typical imaging characteristics include a single lobular mass, often in the range of 1 cm in diameter, with heterogenous signal intensity within the lesion itself and a perilesional rim of hypointensity on both T1- and T2-weighted imaging. The nature of these findings are thought to be related to blood degradation products of varying ages within the body of the lesion surrounded by hemosiderin and gliosis. The appearance is often likened in both the medical literature and clinical vernacular to that of "popcorn" (**Fig. 5**) Gradient-echo and susceptibility-weighted imaging are particularly sensitive for CMs given the degree of hemosiderin associated with the lesions.[132,133] Calcification can be noted,

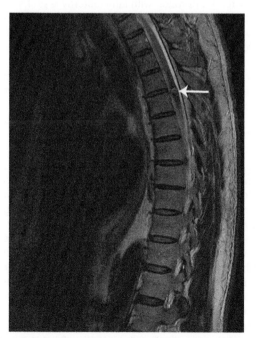

Fig. 5. Spinal CM. CM of the cervical spinal cord. Note the characteristically lobular borders, which give it the appearance of "popcorn" (*arrow*). The signal changes in and around the cord correspond to heme degradation products of varying chronicity.

but less frequently than in cerebral CMs. There is typically little or no perilesional edema unless a recent hemorrhage has occurred. Contrast enhancement is usually minimal or absent, and CMs are angiographically occult. In the setting of acute hemorrhage, however, angiography might need to be performed to exclude an AVM. Other conditions commonly considered in the differential diagnosis include multiple sclerosis, inflammatory transverse myelitis, metastasis, ependymoma, hemangioblastoma, and astrocytoma. In roughly one third of patients with spinal CM, a venous malformation is noted in the proximity of the CM, which may assist in discerning a CM from other spinal cord abnormalities.[122,125,126,134–136] When spinal CM is expected, it is also recommended that imaging of the remainder of the neuraxis be performed given the high rate of lesion multiplicity affecting other remote areas of the CNS. In addition, the finding of multiple CMs assists in clarifying the diagnosis.[107]

Whether or not it is best to perform surgery on spinal CMs, asymptomatic or not, is unclear.[137] The natural history of asymptomatic or minimally symptomatic spinal CMs has been reported to be quite benign.[105,138,139] Cohen-Gadol and colleagues[105] reported on 42 patients with spinal CM who were followed for an average of nearly 10 years (mean, 9.7) and only 5 patients experienced a "neurologic event" (with only 4 having documented hemorrhage on neuroimaging), making for a calculated annual hemorrhage risk of 1.6% per patient per year. Kharkar and colleagues[138] followed 10 patients with symptomatic spinal CM (mean McCormick grade, II) expectantly for an average of nearly 7 years. There were no acute deteriorations throughout the follow-up period and McCormick grade was the same or better at last follow-up in 9 of 10 patients. Liang and colleagues[139] followed 11 patients with small, ventral spinal CMs for an average of only 32 months, and found that 5 of 11 improved by last follow-up and the other 6 remained neurologically stable. Meanwhile surgery can produce good results in well-selected cases. A posterior approach with laminectomy is preferred for dorsal lesions and radical facetectomy with dentate ligament release is necessary for ventral lesions.[114,129] Intraoperative ultrasound can assist in real-time localization and to help avoid the potential for false localization with MRI (likely owing to the "blooming artifact" caused by the ferromagnetic properties of hemosiderin).[126,132,133,136]

We advocate an individualized approach to treatment based on clinical presentation and lesion characteristics. Observation is most prudent for asymptomatic or only mildly symptomatic patients with deep intramedullary lesions. Instead, we favor a carefully planned surgical excision for exophytic lesions that abut the pial surface and are causing progressive neurologic decline.[107]

Prognosis

There have been only limited studies that have focused on prognostication.[140] Mitha and colleagues[114] found that greater anteroposterior dimension was associated with worse long-term clinical outcome; however, the functional grading scale used in this study is more heavily weighted by motor symptoms than other functional scales, and anterior encroachment of a lesion might be expected to cause motor deficit. In a study of patients with familial CM, Zabramski and colleagues[115] characterized cerebral CMs by their T1 and T2 MRI characteristics and, by inference, their blood product composition. They found that lesions with hyperintensity or mixed intensity (types I and II) were more common in the most symptomatic patients. The hypointense lesions (types III and IV), corresponding pathologically to chronic heme degradation, were most often asymptomatic. Another series using the same radiologic classification found that type I lesions (e.g., primarily subacute blood) led to a symptomatic hemorrhage in 33% of patients, whereas type II lesions (e.g., mixed signal intensity, less active bleeding by inference) did so in only 14% of patients.[106] The caveat with these

---

Box 3
Spinal CM

- Spinal CM is very rare, and often familial and/or concomitant with other CMs in the CNS.
- Presents in early middle age as progressive myelopathy, although can present acutely with hemorrhage.
- MRI is diagnostic; CMs are angiographically occult.
- Surgery for CM is controversial because natural history data is lacking, but it can produce stabilization or improvement in a reasonable number of patients.

---

studies is that they focused on cerebral CMs. Spinal CMs are pathologically indistinct from cerebral CMs[101]; thus, it is reasonable to infer that the same radiologic categorization can be extrapolated to spinal CMs, but confirmatory studies are lacking.

Surgical outcomes can be favorable in well-selected patients. A review of available series reported postoperative neurologic improvement in 61%, stability in 27%, and decline in 12% at long-term follow-up, but results were variable across individual series.[107] The uncertainty surrounding the natural history of spinal CMs makes it difficult to determine whether achieving postoperative stabilization is an operative success or not, and further studies are needed.

When surgery is considered, it should be mentioned during preoperative counseling that immediate postoperative worsening is not rare, occurring in 11 to 50% of patients.[114,126,141,142] Patients should be reassured, however, that such postoperative decline is typically transient and followed by gradual and sustained improvement (**Box 3**).

Spinal epidural hematoma

Spinal epidural hematoma (SEH) is a rare but potentially devastating form of acute compressive myelopathy. It often arises postoperatively (especially after anticoagulation), or after trauma (including regional anesthesia),[143] but can occur spontaneously.[144] The pathophysiologic mechanism of the hemorrhage is not very well understood in any of these settings, outside of direct trauma to vascular structures. Upwards of two thirds of patients with spontaneous SEH have no identifiable mechanism or underlying vascular anomaly (such as AVM or CM).[144] The exact incidence of SEH after spinal or epidural anesthesia is unknown; some large series have estimated an incidence below 1 in 150,000 to 220,000 spinal anesthesia procedures,[145,146] but more recent studies suggest that these numbers may be an underestimation.[147,148] Incidence figures for spontaneous SEH are lacking owing to their rarity.

We have encountered acute postoperative SEH particularly after surgeries requiring systemic anticoagulation, most notably cardiovascular surgery and cardiac interventions. Although SCI should be strongly considered in these cases, immediate neuroimaging of the spinal must be performed to exclude a surgically treatable complication such as SEH (see **Fig. 1**).

Clinical Presentation

In one of the larger series[148] comprising 61 patients, 68% manifested their SEH via progressive "motor or sensory block." Only 8% had bowel or bladder dysfunction and none presented with radicular back pain. Thirty of the patients had received intravenous or subcutaneous (unfractionated or low-molecular-weight) heparin. In addition, 12 patients had evidence of coagulopathy or thrombocytopenia or were treated with antiplatelet medications, oral anticoagulants, or thrombolytics immediately before or after the spinal or epidural anesthetic. Needle and catheter placement was reported to be difficult in 15 (25%) or bloody in 15 patients (25%). Overall, in 53 (87%) of the 61 cases, either a clotting abnormality or needle placement difficulty was present. A spinal anesthetic was administered in 15 patients. The remaining 46 patients received an epidural anesthetic, including 32 patients with an indwelling catheter. In 15 of these 32 patients, the spinal hematoma occurred immediately after the removal of the epidural catheter. Nine of these catheters were removed during therapeutic levels of heparinization. In 2 smaller series reporting SEH after catheter placement and removal, the lesion was located above the site of needle stick, leading authors to suggest that the possibility of traumatic hemorrhage was less likely.[149,150]

Management: Diagnosis and Treatment

Diagnosis of SEH, as discussed in the SCI section, is made by emergent neuroimaging of the spine. MRI is the preferred modality because of its sensitivity for localizing a SEH and distinguishing it from other etiologies, but noncontrast CT has acceptable sensitivity. We recommend imaging of the entire spine (see **Fig. 1**) because examination features, in particular sensory level, may be unreliable for localization of the level of the lesion during the hyperacute phase.[65]

Prognosis

In the aforementioned large series of intervention-related SEH, only 38% of the 61 patients had a "partial or good neurologic recovery." Patients who had emergency surgery (i.e., <8 hours from onset of neurologic decline) were more likely to recover (**Box 4**).[148]

SPINAL VASCULITIS

Spinal cord involvement from systemic vasculitis[151–156] or primary vasculitis of the CNS[157] (PCNSV) is exceedingly rare. Furthermore, several of the cases reported as likely systemic vasculitides are without true diagnoses in the absence of documented clinical or laboratory evidence of a vasculitic syndrome.[152,155,156] Infectious vasculitis affecting the vasa nervosa, characteristic of syphilitic arteritis,[11] is a vasculitis per se, but has been included in the SCI section of this review.

Clinical Presentation

The clinical presentation of spinal vasculitis is variable but demonstrates a key stratification: All 6 of the cases attributed to a systemic vasculitis presented with spinal SAH,[151–156] whereas the 5 cases reported as PCNSV did not.[157] The cases with SAH demonstrated spinal artery aneurysm(s) on angiography, which are otherwise exceptionally rare.[158] Spinal aneurysms were not reported in the PCNSV vasculitis cohort, although dedicated angiography was not performed. The 6 patients with spinal

---

Box 4
SEH

- Should be suspected in cases of acute myelopathy, especially postoperative.
- Emergent MRI is preferred, CT acceptable.
- Can develop in the absence of trauma in anticoagulated patients.
- Perioperative risk may be increased with epidural anesthesia and anticoagulation.
- Emergent surgical decompression is required; outcomes are worse with delay.

SAH had acute-onset myelopathic symptoms in association with their back pain and meningismus. The 5 patients with PCNSV developed progressive myelopathies before, during, or after cerebral involvement with nearly equal frequency.

Management: Diagnosis and Treatment

The diagnosis was unclear in all but 2 of the 6 systemic vasculitis cases. The two with proven diagnoses demonstrated clinical and laboratory evidence of polyarteritis nodosa.[151,154] In the other cases, despite extensive rheumatologic evaluations, no specific or nonspecific markers of inflammation were noted. In the PCNSV cohort, serum erythrocyte sedimentation rate was elevated in 3 of the 5 patients and normal in the other two. No other serum laboratory assessments were specifically reported. CSF findings were reported in in 4 of the 5 patients, showing marked proteinorhacia (98–1034 mg/dL) and pleocytosis (59–535 cells/mm^3).

Patients with suspected spinal vasculitis should be evaluated with MRI of the entire spine and selective catheter angiography. MRI can show extramedullary hemorrhage or intramedullary, longitudinally extensive T2 hyperintensity with contrast enhancement in the thoracic cord and/or the conus medullaris.[157] Digital subtraction angiography can show intercostal arteritis.[156] In all cases, variable courses of corticosteroids (pulse and/or high-dose maintenance) and immunosuppressants (including cyclophosphamide, azathioprine, and mycophenolate mofetil) were used with mostly beneficial clinical result. However, two of the reported patients, one with no diagnosis but presumed systemic vasculitis and one with PCNSV, had catastrophic courses and died.

Prognosis

Of course, with so few patients, no broad statements can be made regarding prognosis. However, in general, patients responded well to immunomodulation, especially those affected by PCNSV. Typically, patients had very mild to only moderate dysfunction at follow-up, although relapses did occur (**Box 5**).[157]

Box 5
Spinal vasculitis

- Can be from primary CNS or systemic vasculitides.
- Systemic vasculitis (*e.g.*, polyarteritis nodosa) seems to be associated with spinal SAH and spinal artery aneurysm and presents acutely.
- Primary vasculitis typically occurs with concomitant cerebral vascular abnormalities and presents progressively.
- PCNSV: Diagnosis can be made with history, CSF, MRI and angiography.
- Systemic vasculitis: Diagnosis via history, serology, and angiography.
- Both primary and secondary vasculitides are amenable to immunotherapy.

Box 6
Spinal genetic and neurocutaneous syndromes

- CMs can be associated with von Hippel-Lindau disease.
- Familial CMs associated with 4 distinct genes (*CCM1-4*).
- Cutaneomeningospinal angiomatosis (Cobb syndrome) is a disorder characterized by a complex AVM that involves the spinal cord, meninges, and related dermatomal skin segment.

Table 1
Clinical features of vascular diseases of the spinal cord

Spinal Cord Condition	Epidemiology	MRI Findings	Temporal Profile	Clinical Presentation	Pathogenesis
SCI	Age = 60s, aortic surgery, mostly thoracolumbar	Focal cord swelling ± T2 hyperintensity ± restricted diffusion; can be normal	Acute	Weakness (mostly bilateral, flaccid), myelopathic sensory level, urinary retention; often postoperative aortic surgery	Many: postoperative, iatrogenic, often idiopathic
sdAVF	Age = 60s, ~9:1 male:female, mostly low thoracic	MRI/MRA can detect abnormal vessels, ± T2 hyperintensity in cord, radiographic changes may not correspond with degree of debility	Variable: subacute (70%), stepwise (25%), acute (5%)	Weakness (variable, often bilateral asymmetric or unilateral), ± sensory level (can falsely localize), often pain, often bowel/bladder dysfunction; difficult to diagnose	Thought to be acquired; symptoms often precipitated or made worse by Valsalva
AVM	Peri-/intramedullary: age = 20s, mostly thoracolumbar	MRI, MRA can detect abnormal vessels, T2 hyperintensity in spinal cord, ± blood products from hemorrhage	Often acute, can be subacute	Myelopathic weakness/sensory/ bladder ± spinal SAH depending on acuity, location of hemorrhage	Thought to be sporadic/congenital; can also be made worse by Valsalva and mechanical stressors
CM	Age = 40s; mostly thoracic, but cervical in ~40%, significant minority have intracranial as well ± family history of CM	MRI demonstrates "popcorn" with T1/T2 hypointense rim; MRA = angiographically occult	Subacute (~55%), stepwise (~30%), acute (~15%)	~66% have weakness and sensory level, ~25% have pain, ~10% have bladder dysfunction	Some Sporadic/ congenital, substantial minority familial, radiation (perhaps ~10%) induced (rare)

Epidural hematoma	Age variable	Acute	MRI (or CT) can show acute blood; MRI may show focal cord T2 hyperintensity and/or restricted diffusion at site of compression	Myelopathic weakness/ sensory/bladder, back pain	Trauma, postoperative (including regional anesthesia) ± recent anticoagulation, spontaneous after anticoagulation
Vasculitis	Age variable, only adults studied; PCNSV or associated with systemic vasculitis	Mostly subacute, can be acute (hemorrhage)	PCNSV: longitudinally extensive T2 hyperintensity in cord w/contrast enhancement; systemic vasculitis: spinal artery aneurysm, focal T2 hyperintensity, acute blood products	Variable. PCNSV: myelopathic signs before/during/after cerebral signs; systemic vasculitis: myelopathic signs weeks to months after systemic signs, spinal SAH	Polyarteritis nodosa, "mixed" anti-neutrophil cytoplasmic antibodies/ myeloperoxidase vasculitis; PCNSV patients all had cerebral symptoms at some point
Genetic and neurocutaneous vascular syndromes	Variable; often young adults	Mostly subacute, can be acute (hemorrhage)	MRI/MRA can demonstrate abnormal vessels in Cobb; MRI will show hemangioblastoma ± heme products in von Hippel-Lindau disease	Cobb: myelopathy from spinal AVM with cutaneous angioma in same distribution; von Hippel-Lindau disease: myelopathy from hemangioblastoma	Genetic

Abbreviation: MRA, magnetic resonance angiography.

Table 2
Prognostic indicators in vascular diseases of the spinal cord

Spinal Cord Condition	Poor Prognostic Indicator
SCI	Degree of neurologic impairment at onset
sdAVF	Degree of neurologic impairment preoperatively; presence of sensory level to pinprick preoperatively
AVM	None that are evidence-based; higher grade (*e.g.*, more anatomically complex), proximity to vital neurologic/vascular structures
CM	Acute/subacute heme products (grade I or II)
Epidural hematoma	Surgery >8 h from symptom onset
Vasculitis	None that are evidence based
Genetic and neurocutaneous vascular syndromes	None that are evidence based

SPINAL GENETIC AND NEUROCUTANEOUS VASCULAR SYNDROMES

Von Hippel-Lindau disease is a genetic disorder that predisposes to the development of hemangioblastomas of the CNS, retina, and abdominal viscera.[159] The cerebrum and cerebellum are primarily affected, but the spinal cord can be involved. In one pathologic report of five cases of Von Hippel-Lindau disease, two patients had spinal cord hemangioblastomas.[160] Of note, in one of those patients, there were two relatively small hemangioblastomas, one each in the cervical and lower thoracic cord, that caused the patient to have a syrinx that extended for almost the entirety of the spinal cord.

Genetic abnormalities predisposing to familial CMs can also be associated with systemic cavernomatosis. In one report of a 12-member family with known *CCM1* mutation, CMs were noted in the retina, skin, liver, and vertebral bodies in addition to brain and spinal cord.[161]

Cutaneomeningospinal angiomatosis, or Cobb syndrome, is an exceedingly rare sporadic disorder characterized by spinal segmental AVM and corresponding cutaneous angioma in the same metamere.[162] The condition often involves extensive spinal AVMs, causing the same progressive myelopathic symptoms associated with nonsyndromic AVM. Treatment series to date are small and recommend open

Table 3
Recommended diagnostics in vascular diseases of the spinal cord

Spinal Cord Condition	Recommended Diagnostics
SCI	Emergent MRI w/DWI
sdAVF	MRI, MRA
AVM	MRI (FIESTA), MRA, DSA
CM	MRI
Epidural hematoma	Emergent MRI, CT
Vasculitis	MRI, MRA, DSA
Genetic and neurocutaneous vascular syndromes	MRI, MRA, DSA

Abbreviations: DSA, digital subtraction angiography; FIESTA, fast imaging employing steady-state acquisition; MRA, magnetic resonance angiography.

Table 4
Recommended therapies and associated outcomes in vascular diseases of the spinal cord

Spinal Cord Condition	Recommended Therapy	Outcome
SCI	See **Fig. 1**: imaging, mean arterial pressure > 90 mm Hg, lumbar drainage	Occasionally frank improvement with early treatment. Otherwise, disabling but gradual late recovery is possible
sdAVF	Surgery: open or endovascular	Very good (especially motor symptoms) with timely surgery
AVM	Surgery: open, endovascular, both (*e.g.*, staged), radiosurgery	Good, case dependent
CM	Asymptomatic, deep: observation Exophytic, progressive: excision	Good, case dependent
Epidural hematoma	Emergent evacuation	Good recovery possible with immediate evacuation Poor outcome if delayed evacuation (especially if >8 h)
Vasculitis	Immunotherapy	Good, case dependent
Genetic and neurocutaneous vascular syndromes	CM/von Hippel-Lindau disease: same as non-hereditary CM; Cobb: open or endovascular surgery	Case dependent

microsurgical, endovascular, and/or corticosteroid therapy. The extent of the lesions often precludes cure, but minimization of symptoms is a reasonable outcome.[162–165]

Another syndrome often associated with spinal AVM in the medical literature is Klippel-Trenaunay, which is a mostly sporadic limb overgrowth syndrome associated with cutaneous angiomas and venous anomalies. Although there are numerous reports of associations with spinal AVM, a recent review questioned this clinical connection (**Box 6, Tables 1–4**).[166]

ACKNOWLEDGMENTS

Many thanks to our esteemed neuroradiologist colleagues, T. Kaufmann and J. Morris, for providing several of the images in this manuscript.

REFERENCES

1. Krauss WE. Vascular anatomy of the spinal cord. Neurosurg Clin N Am 1999; 10(1):9–15.
2. Gillilan LA. Veins of the spinal cord. Anatomic details; suggested clinical applications. Neurology 1970;20(9):860–8.
3. Gillilan LA. The arterial blood supply of the human spinal cord. J Comp Neurol 1958;110(1):75–103.
4. Cheshire WP, Santos CC, Massey EW, et al. Spinal cord infarction: etiology and outcome. Neurology 1996;47(2):321–30.
5. Robertson CE, Brown RD Jr, Wijdicks EF, et al. Recovery after spinal cord infarcts: long-term outcome in 115 patients. Neurology 2012;78(2):114–21.

6. Romanes GJ. The arterial blood supply of the human spinal cord. Paraplegia 1965;2:199–207.
7. Suh TH, Alexander L. Vascular system of the human spinal cord. Paraplegia 1939;41:659–77.
8. Adamkiewicz AA. Die Blutgefasse des menschlichen Riickenmarkes. I1 Theil. Die Gefasse der Ruckenmarksoberflache. S B Heidelberg Akad Wiss 1882; 85:101–30.
9. Sandson TA, Friedman JH. Spinal cord infarction. Report of 8 cases and review of the literature. Medicine 1989;68(5):282–92.
10. Spiller WG. Thrombosis of the cervical anterior median spinal artery: syphilitic acute anterior poliomyelitis. J Nerv Ment Dis 1909;36:601–13.
11. Preobrashenski PA. Syphilitic paraplegia with dissociation disturbance of sensation. J Nevropat i Psikhiat 1904;4:394–433.
12. Adams HD, Van Geertruyden HH. Neurologic complications of aortic surgery. Ann Surg 1956;144(4):574–610.
13. Picone AL, Green RM, Ricotta JR, et al. Spinal cord ischemia following operations on the abdominal aorta. J Vasc Surg 1986;3(1):94–103.
14. Ross RT. Spinal cord infarction in disease and surgery of the aorta. Can J Neurol Sci 1985;12(4):289–95.
15. Steegmann AT. Syndrome of the anterior spinal artery. Neurology 1952;2(1): 15–35.
16. Hallenbeck JM, Bove AA, Elliott DH. Mechanisms underlying spinal cord damage in decompression sickness. Neurology 1975;25(4):308–16.
17. Marcus ML, Heistad DD, Ehrhardt JC, et al. Regulation of total and regional spinal cord blood flow. Circ Res 1977;41(1):128–34.
18. Lee C, Woodring JH, Walsh JW. Carotid and vertebral artery injury in survivors of atlanto-occipital dislocation: case reports and literature review. J Trauma 1991; 31(3):401–7.
19. Hughes JT, Brownell B. Cervical spondylosis complicated by anterior spinal artery thrombosis. Neurology 1964;14:1073–7.
20. Schneider RC, Schemm GW. Vertebral artery insufficiency in acute and chronic spinal trauma, with special reference to the syndrome of acute central cervical spinal cord injury. J Neurosurg 1961;18:348–60.
21. Foo D, Rossier AB, Cochran TP. Complete sensory and motor recovery from anterior spinal artery syndrome after sprain of the cervical spine. A case report. Eur Neurol 1984;23(2):119–23.
22. Hanus SH, Homer TD, Harter DH. Vertebral artery occlusion complicating yoga exercises. Arch Neurol 1977;34(9):574–5.
23. Ahmann PA, Smith SA, Schwartz JF, et al. Spinal cord infarction due to minor trauma in children. Neurology 1975;25(4):301–7.
24. Novy J, Carruzzo A, Maeder P, et al. Spinal cord ischemia: clinical and imaging patterns, pathogenesis, and outcomes in 27 patients. Arch Neurol 2006;63(8): 1113–20.
25. El-Toraei I, Juler G. Ischemic myelopathy. Angiology 1979;30(2):81–94.
26. Hughes JT, Macintyre AG. Spinal cord infarction occurring during thoracolumbar sympathectomy. J Neurol Neurosurg Psychiatr 1963;26:418–21.
27. Mosberg WH Jr, Voris HC, Duffy J. Paraplegia as a complication of sympathectomy for hypertension. Ann Surg 1954;139(3):330–4.
28. Mittal MK, Rabinstein AA, Wijdicks EF. Pearls & oy-sters: acute spinal cord infarction following endoscopic ultrasound-guided celiac plexus neurolysis. Neurology 2012;78(9):e57–9.

29. Cherry DA, Lamberty J. Paraplegia following coeliac plexus block. Anaesth Intensive Care 1984;12(1):59–61.
30. Szilagyi DE, Hageman JH, Smith RF, et al. Spinal cord damage in surgery of the abdominal aorta. Surgery 1978;83(1):38–56.
31. Koehler PJ, Wijngaard PR. Brown-Sequard syndrome due to spinal cord infarction after subclavian vein catheterisation. Lancet 1986;2(8512):914–5.
32. Kane RE. Neurologic deficits following epidural or spinal anesthesia. Anesth Analg 1981;60(3):150–61.
33. Ackerman WE, Juneja MM, Knapp RK. Maternal paraparesis after epidural anesthesia and cesarean section. South Med J 1990;83(6):695–7.
34. Gang DL, Dole KB, Adelman LS. Spinal cord infarction following therapeutic renal artery embolization. JAMA 1977;237(26):2841–2.
35. Azzarelli B, Roessmann U. Diffuse "anoxic" myelopathy. Neurology 1977;27(11): 1049–52.
36. Rouques L, Passelecq A. Brown-Sequard syndrome after thoracoplasty. Rev Neurol (Paris) 1957;97(2):146–7 [in French].
37. Singh BM, Fass AE, Pooley RW, et al. Paraplegia associated with intraaortic balloon pump counterpulsation. Stroke 1983;14(6):983–6.
38. Giangaspero F, Dondi C, Scarani P, et al. Degeneration of the corticospinal tract following portosystemic shunt associated with spinal cord infarction. Virchows Arch A Pathol Anat Histopathol 1985;406(4):475–81.
39. Phillips OC, Ebner H, Nelson AT, et al. Neurologic complications following spinal anesthesia with lidocaine: a prospective review of 10,440 cases. Anesthesiology 1969;30(3):284–9.
40. Hughes JT. Thrombosis of the posterior spinal arteries. A complication of an intrathecal injection of phenol. Neurology 1970;20(7):659–64.
41. Anderson NE, Willoughby EW. Infarction of the conus medullaris. Ann Neurol 1987;21(5):470–4.
42. Garland H, Greenberg J, Harriman DG. Infarction of the spinal cord. Brain 1966; 89(4):645–62.
43. Henson RA, Parsons M. Ischaemic lesions of the spinal cord: an illustrated review. Q J Med 1967;36(142):205–22.
44. Kim SW, Kim RC, Choi BH, et al. Non-traumatic ischaemic myelopathy: a review of 25 cases. Paraplegia 1988;26(4):262–72.
45. Silver JR, Buxton PH. Spinal stroke. Brain 1974;97(3):539–50.
46. Zull DN, Cydulka R. Acute paraplegia: a presenting manifestation of aortic dissection. Am J Med 1988;84(4):765–70.
47. Cheng MY, Lyu RK, Chang YJ, et al. Spinal cord infarction in Chinese patients. Clinical features, risk factors, imaging and prognosis. Cerebrovasc Dis 2008; 26(5):502–8.
48. Kaplan SA, Chancellor MB, Blaivas JG. Bladder and sphincter behavior in patients with spinal cord lesions. J Urol 1991;146(1):113–7.
49. Brown-Séquard CE. De la transmission croisée des impressions sensitives par la moelle épinière. C R Soc Biol (Paris) 1850;2:70.
50. Dejerine J. La claudication intermittente de la moelle épinière. Presse Med 1911; 19:981–4.
51. Thurnher MM, Bammer R. Diffusion-weighted MR imaging (DWI) in spinal cord ischemia. Neuroradiology 2006;48(11):795–801.
52. Cheung AT, Pochettino A, McGarvey ML, et al. Strategies to manage paraplegia risk after endovascular stent repair of descending thoracic aortic aneurysms. Ann Thorac Surg 2005;80(4):1280–8.

53. Cheung AT, Weiss SJ, McGarvey ML, et al. Interventions for reversing delayed-onset postoperative paraplegia after thoracic aortic reconstruction. Ann Thorac Surg 2002;74(2):413–9.

54. McGarvey ML, Cheung AT, Szeto W, et al. Management of neurologic complications of thoracic aortic surgery. J Clin Neurophysiol 2007;24(4):336–43.

55. McGarvey ML, Mullen MT, Woo EY, et al. The treatment of spinal cord ischemia following thoracic endovascular aortic repair. Neurocrit Care 2007;6(1):35–9.

56. Hnath JC, Mehta M, Taggert JB, et al. Strategies to improve spinal cord ischemia in endovascular thoracic aortic repair: outcomes of a prospective cerebrospinal fluid drainage protocol. J Vasc Surg 2008;48(4):836–40.

57. Thalmann ED. Principles of US Navy recompression treatments for decompression sickness. Bethesda (MD): Undersea and Hyperbaric Medical Society; 1996.

58. Gempp E, Blatteau JE. Risk factors and treatment outcome in scuba divers with spinal cord decompression sickness. J Crit Care 2010;25(2):236–42.

59. Wilson CM, Ross JA, Sayer M. Saturation treatment in shore-based chambers for divers with deteriorating cerebro-spinal decompression sickness. Diving Hyperb Med 2009;39(3):170–4.

60. Kim LJ, Spetzler RF. Classification and surgical management of spinal arteriovenous lesions: arteriovenous fistulae and arteriovenous malformations. Neurosurgery 2006;59(5 Suppl 3):S195–201.

61. Koch C. Spinal dural arteriovenous fistula. Curr Opin Neurol 2006;19(1):69–75.

62. Rosenblum B, Oldfield EH, Doppman JL, et al. Spinal arteriovenous malformations: a comparison of dural arteriovenous fistulas and intradural AVM's in 81 patients. J Neurosurg 1987;67(6):795–802.

63. Fugate JE, Lanzino G, Rabinstein AA. Clinical presentation and prognostic factors of spinal dural arteriovenous fistulas: an overview. Neurosurg Focus 2012;32(5):E17.

64. Van Dijk JM, TerBrugge KG, Willinsky RA, et al. Multidisciplinary management of spinal dural arteriovenous fistulas: clinical presentation and long-term follow-up in 49 patients. Stroke 2002;33(6):1578–83.

65. Muralidharan R, Saladino A, Lanzino G, et al. The clinical and radiological presentation of spinal dural arteriovenous fistula. Spine 2011;36(25):E1641–7.

66. Jellema K, Canta LR, Tijssen CC, et al. Spinal dural arteriovenous fistulas: clinical features in 80 patients. J Neurol Neurosurg Psychiatr 2003;74(10):1438–40.

67. Hurst RW, Bagley LJ, Scanlon M, et al. Dural arteriovenous fistulas of the craniocervical junction. Skull Base Surg 1999;9(1):1–7.

68. Symon L, Kuyama H, Kendall B. Dural arteriovenous malformations of the spine. Clinical features and surgical results in 55 cases. J Neurosurg 1984;60(2):238–47.

69. Atkinson JL, Miller GM, Krauss WE, et al. Clinical and radiographic features of dural arteriovenous fistula, a treatable cause of myelopathy. Mayo Clin Proc 2001;76(11):1120–30.

70. Lv X, Li Y, Yang X, et al. Endovascular embolization for symptomatic perimedullary AVF and intramedullary AVM: a series and a literature review. Neuroradiology 2012;54(4):349–59.

71. Olivero WC, Hanigan WC, McCluney KW. Angiographic demonstration of a spinal epidural arteriovenous malformation. Case report. J Neurosurg 1993;79(1):119–20.

72. Veerapen RJ, Sbeih IA, O'Laoire SA. Surgical treatment of cryptic AVM's and associated hematoma in the brain stem and spinal cord. J Neurosurg 1986;65(2):188–93.

73. Meng X, Zhang H, Wang Y, et al. Perimedullary arteriovenous fistulas in pediatric patients: clinical, angiographical, and therapeutic experiences in a series of 19 cases. Childs Nerv Syst 2010;26(7):889–96.

74. Cho KT, Lee DY, Chung CK, et al. Treatment of spinal cord perimedullary arteriovenous fistula: embolization versus surgery. Neurosurgery 2005;56(2):232–41.

75. Rodesch G, Hurth M, Alvarez H, et al. Spinal cord intradural arteriovenous fistulae: anatomic, clinical, and therapeutic considerations in a series of 32 consecutive patients seen between 1981 and 2000 with emphasis on endovascular therapy. Neurosurgery 2005;57(5):973–83.

76. Corkill RA, Mitsos AP, Molyneux AJ. Embolization of spinal intramedullary arteriovenous malformations using the liquid embolic agent, Onyx: a single-center experience in a series of 17 patients. J Neurosurg Spine 2007;7(5):478–85.

77. Cullen S, Alvarez H, Rodesch G, et al. Spinal arteriovenous shunts presenting before 2 years of age: analysis of 13 cases. Childs Nerv Syst 2006;22(9):1103–10.

78. Donner C, Shahabi S, Thomas D, et al. Selective feticide by embolization in twin-twin transfusion syndrome. A report of two cases. J Reprod Med 1997;42(11):747–50.

79. Niimi Y, Sala F, Deletis V, et al. Neurophysiologic monitoring and pharmacologic provocative testing for embolization of spinal cord arteriovenous malformations. AJNR Am J Neuroradiol 2004;25(7):1131–8.

80. Rodesch G, Pongpech S, Alvarez H, et al. Spinal cord arteriovenous malformations in a pediatric population children below 15 years of age the place of endovascular management. Intervent Neuroradiol 1995;1(1):29–42.

81. Toossi S, Josephson SA, Hetts SW, et al. Utility of MRI in spinal arteriovenous fistula. Neurology 2012;79(1):25–30.

82. Hartman J, Rabinstein AA. Can we rule out a spinal arteriovenous fistula using only MRI? Yes, we can. Neurology 2012;79(1):15–6.

83. Steinmetz MP, Chow MM, Krishnaney AA, et al. Outcome after the treatment of spinal dural arteriovenous fistulae: a contemporary single-institution series and meta-analysis. Neurosurgery 2004;55(1):77–87.

84. Morris JM, Kaufmann TJ, Campeau NG, et al. Volumetric myelographic magnetic resonance imaging to localize difficult-to-find spinal dural arteriovenous fistulas. J Neurosurg Spine 2011;14(3):398–404.

85. Saladino A, Atkinson JL, Rabinstein AA, et al. Surgical treatment of spinal dural arteriovenous fistulae: a consecutive series of 154 patients. Neurosurgery 2010;67(5):1350–7.

86. Andres RH, Barth A, Guzman R, et al. Endovascular and surgical treatment of spinal dural arteriovenous fistulas. Neuroradiology 2008;50(10):869–76.

87. Detweiler PW, Porter RW, Spetzler RF. Spinal arteriovenous malformations. Neurosurg Clin N Am 1999;10(1):89–100.

88. Niimi Y, Berenstein A, Setton A, et al. Embolization of spinal dural arteriovenous fistulae: results and follow-up. Neurosurgery 1997;40(4):675–82.

89. Sinclair J, Chang SD, Gibbs IC, et al. Multisession CyberKnife radiosurgery for intramedullary spinal cord arteriovenous malformations. Neurosurgery 2006;58(6):1081–9.

90. Avanzo M, Romanelli P. Spinal radiosurgery: technology and clinical outcomes. Neurosurg Rev 2009;32(1):1–12.

91. Guillevin R, Vallee JN, Cormier E, et al. N-butyl 2-cyanoacrylate embolization of spinal dural arteriovenous fistulae: CT evaluation, technical features, and outcome prognosis in 26 cases. AJNR Am J Neuroradiol 2005;26(4):929–35.

92. Behrens S, Thron A. Long-term follow-up and outcome in patients treated for spinal dural arteriovenous fistula. J Neurol 1999;246(3):181–5.
93. Aminoff MJ, Logue V. The prognosis of patients with spinal vascular malformations. Brain 1974;97(1):211–8.
94. Cecchi PC, Musumeci A, Faccioli F, et al. Surgical treatment of spinal dural arterio-venous fistulae: long-term results and analysis of prognostic factors. Acta Neurochir 2008;150(6):563–70.
95. Nagata S, Morioka T, Natori Y, et al. Factors that affect the surgical outcomes of spinal dural arteriovenous fistulas. Surg Neurol 2006;65(6):563–8.
96. Narvid J, Hetts SW, Larsen D, et al. Spinal dural arteriovenous fistulae: clinical features and long-term results. Neurosurgery 2008;62(1):159–66.
97. Tacconi L, Lopez Izquierdo BC, Symon L. Outcome and prognostic factors in the surgical treatment of spinal dural arteriovenous fistulas. A long-term study. Br J Neurosurg 1997;11(4):298–305.
98. Kaufmann TJ, Morris JM, Saladino A, et al. Magnetic resonance imaging findings in treated spinal dural arteriovenous fistulas: lack of correlation with clinical outcomes. J Neurosurg Spine 2011;14(4):548–54.
99. Cenzato M, Versari P, Righi C, et al. Spinal dural arteriovenous fistulae: analysis of outcome in relation to pretreatment indicators. Neurosurgery 2004;55(4): 815–22.
100. Shinoyama M, Endo T, Takahash T, et al. Long-term outcome of cervical and thoracolumbar dural arteriovenous fistulas with emphasis on sensory disturbance and neuropathic pain. World Neurosurg 2010;73(4):401–8.
101. McCormick WF. The pathology of vascular ("arteriovenous") malformations. J Neurosurg 1966;24(4):807–16.
102. Del Curling O Jr, Kelly DL Jr, Elster AD, et al. An analysis of the natural history of cavernous angiomas. J Neurosurg 1991;75(5):702–8.
103. Rigamonti D, Drayer BP, Johnson PC, et al. The MRI appearance of cavernous malformations (angiomas). J Neurosurg 1987;67(4):518–24.
104. Deutsch H, Jallo GI, Faktorovich A, et al. Spinal intramedullary cavernoma: clinical presentation and surgical outcome. J Neurosurg 2000;93(Suppl 1): 65–70.
105. Cohen-Gadol AA, Jacob JT, Edwards DA, et al. Coexistence of intracranial and spinal cavernous malformations: a study of prevalence and natural history. J Neurosurg 2006;104(3):376–81.
106. Labauge P, Bouly S, Parker F, et al. Outcome in 53 patients with spinal cord cavernomas. Surg Neurol 2008;70(2):176–81.
107. Gross BA, Du R, Popp AJ, et al. Intramedullary spinal cord cavernous malformations. Neurosurg Focus 2010;29(3):E14.
108. Brouillard P, Vikkula M. Genetic causes of vascular malformations. Hum Mol Genet 2007;16:R140–9.
109. Dashti SR, Hoffer A, Hu YC, et al. Molecular genetics of familial cerebral cavernous malformations. Neurosurg Focus 2006;21(1):e2.
110. Nimjee SM, Powers CJ, Bulsara KR. Review of the literature on de novo formation of cavernous malformations of the central nervous system after radiation therapy. Neurosurg Focus 2006;21(1):e4.
111. Maraire JN, Abdulrauf SI, Berger S, et al. De novo development of a cavernous malformation of the spinal cord following spinal axis radiation. Case report. J Neurosurg 1999;90(Suppl 2):234–8.
112. Yoshino M, Morita A, Shibahara J, et al. Radiation-induced spinal cord cavernous malformation. Case report. J Neurosurg 2005;102(Suppl 1):101–4.

113. Jabbour P, Gault J, Murk SE, et al. Multiple spinal cavernous malformations with atypical phenotype after prior irradiation: case report. Neurosurgery 2004;55(6): 1431.
114. Mitha AP, Turner JD, Abla AA, et al. Outcomes following resection of intramedullary spinal cord cavernous malformations: a 25-year experience. J Neurosurg Spine 2011;14(5):605–11.
115. Zabramski JM, Wascher TM, Spetzler RF, et al. The natural history of familial cavernous malformations: results of an ongoing study. J Neurosurg 1994; 80(3):422–32.
116. Laberge-le Couteulx S, Jung HH, Labauge P, et al. Truncating mutations in CCM1, encoding KRIT1, cause hereditary cavernous angiomas. Nat Genet 1999;23(2):189–93.
117. Sahoo T, Johnson EW, Thomas JW, et al. Mutations in the gene encoding KRIT1, a Krev-1/rap1a binding protein, cause cerebral cavernous malformations (CCM1). Hum Mol Genet 1999;8(12):2325–33.
118. Denier C, Goutagny S, Labauge P, et al. Mutations within the MGC4607 gene cause cerebral cavernous malformations. Am J Hum Genet 2004;74(2): 326–37.
119. Liquori CL, Berg MJ, Siegel AM, et al. Mutations in a gene encoding a novel protein containing a phosphotyrosine-binding domain cause type 2 cerebral cavernous malformations. Am J Hum Genet 2003;73(6):1459–64.
120. Bergametti F, Denier C, Labauge P, et al. Mutations within the programmed cell death 10 gene cause cerebral cavernous malformations. Am J Hum Genet 2005;76(1):42–51.
121. Liquori CL, Berg MJ, Squitieri F, et al. Low frequency of PDCD10 mutations in a panel of CCM3 probands: potential for a fourth CCM locus. Hum Mutat 2006;27(1):118.
122. Bian LG, Bertalanffy H, Sun QF, et al. Intramedullary cavernous malformations: clinical features and surgical technique via hemilaminectomy. Clin Neurol Neurosurg 2009;111(6):511–7.
123. Chabert E, Morandi X, Carney MP, et al. Intramedullary cavernous malformations. J Neuroradiol 1999;26(4):262–8.
124. Lunardi P, Acqui M, Ferrante L, et al. The role of intraoperative ultrasound imaging in the surgical removal of intramedullary cavernous angiomas. Neurosurgery 1994;34(3):520–3.
125. Sandalcioglu IE, Wiedemayer H, Gasser T, et al. Intramedullary spinal cord cavernous malformations: clinical features and risk of hemorrhage. Neurosurg Rev 2003;26(4):253–6.
126. Vishteh AG, Sankhla S, Anson JA, et al. Surgical resection of intramedullary spinal cord cavernous malformations: delayed complications, long-term outcomes, and association with cryptic venous malformations. Neurosurgery 1997;41(5):1094–100.
127. Zevgaridis D, Medele RJ, Hamburger C, et al. Cavernous haemangiomas of the spinal cord. A review of 117 cases. Acta Neurochir (Wien) 1999;141(3):237–45.
128. McCormick PC, Torres R, Post KD, et al. Intramedullary ependymoma of the spinal cord. J Neurosurg 1990;72(4):523–32.
129. Lu DC, Lawton MT. Clinical presentation and surgical management of intramedullary spinal cord cavernous malformations. Neurosurg Focus 2010;29(3):E12.
130. Do-Dai DD, Brooks MK, Goldkamp A, et al. Magnetic resonance imaging of intramedullary spinal cord lesions: a pictorial review. Curr Probl Diagn Radiol 2010;39(4):160–85.

131. Hegde AN, Mohan S, Lim CC. CNS cavernous haemangioma: "popcorn" in the brain and spinal cord. Clin Radiol 2012;67(4):380–8.
132. Ross JS, editor. Cavernous malformation, spinal cord. Salt Lake City (UT): Amirsys & Elsevier; 2007. Ross JS, B-ZM, Moore KR, et al, editors. Diagnostic Imaging: Spine; No. 2.
133. Chen MZ, editor. Idiopathic acute transverse myelitis. Salt Lake City (UT): Amirsys & Elsevier; 2007. Ross JS, B-ZM, Moore KR, et al, editors. Diagnostic Imaging: Spine; No. 2.
134. Cosgrove GR, Bertrand G, Fontaine S, et al. Cavernous angiomas of the spinal cord. J Neurosurg 1988;68(1):31–6.
135. Santoro A, Piccirilli M, Frati A, et al. Intramedullary spinal cord cavernous malformations: report of ten new cases. Neurosurg Rev 2004;27(2):93–8.
136. Weinzierl MR, Krings T, Korinth MC, et al. MRI and intraoperative findings in cavernous haemangiomas of the spinal cord. Neuroradiology 2004;46(1):65–71.
137. Kondziella D, Brodersen P, Laursen H, et al. Cavernous hemangioma of the spinal cord - conservative or operative management? Acta Neurol Scand 2006;114(4):287–90.
138. Kharkar S, Shuck J, Conway J, et al. The natural history of conservatively managed symptomatic intramedullary spinal cord cavernomas. Neurosurgery 2007;60(5):865–72.
139. Liang JT, Bao YH, Zhang HQ, et al. Management and prognosis of symptomatic patients with intramedullary spinal cord cavernoma: clinical article. J Neurosurg Spine 2011;15(4):447–56.
140. Steiger HJ, Turowski B, Hanggi D. Prognostic factors for the outcome of surgical and conservative treatment of symptomatic spinal cord cavernous malformations: a review of a series of 20 patients. Neurosurg Focus 2010;29(3):E13.
141. Jallo GI, Freed D, Zareck M, et al. Clinical presentation and optimal management for intramedullary cavernous malformations. Neurosurg Focus 2006;21(1):e10.
142. Matsuyama Y, Sakai Y, Katayama Y, et al. Surgical results of intramedullary spinal cord tumor with spinal cord monitoring to guide extent of resection. J Neurosurg Spine 2009;10(5):404–13.
143. Horlocker TT, Wedel DJ, Rowlingson JC, et al. Regional anesthesia in the patient receiving antithrombotic or thrombolytic therapy: American Society of Regional Anesthesia and Pain Medicine Evidence-Based Guidelines (Third Edition). Reg Anesth Pain Med 2010;35(1):64–101.
144. Foo D, Rossier AB. Preoperative neurological status in predicting surgical outcome of spinal epidural hematomas. Surg Neurol 1981;15(5):389–401.
145. Tryba M. Epidural regional anesthesia and low molecular heparin: Pro. Anasthesiol Intensivmed Notfallmed Schmerzther 1993;28(3):179–81 [in German].
146. Horlocker TT, Wedel DJ. Anticoagulation and neuraxial block: historical perspective, anesthetic implications, and risk management. Reg Anesth Pain Med 1998;23(6 Suppl 2):129–34.
147. Moen V, Dahlgren N, Irestedt L. Severe neurological complications after central neuraxial blockades in Sweden 1990-1999. Anesthesiology 2004;101(4):950–9.
148. Vandermeulen EP, Van Aken H, Vermylen J. Anticoagulants and spinal-epidural anesthesia. Anesth Analg 1994;79(6):1165–77.
149. Kaneda T, Suzuki T, Takeda J. A case of acute spinal epidural hematoma after abdominal aortic aneurysm operation. Tokai J Exp Clin Med 2006;31(1):45–8.
150. Zeyneloglu P, Gulsen S, Camkiran A, et al. An epidural hematoma after epidural anesthesia for endovascular aortic aneurysm repair. J Cardiothorac Vasc Anesth 2009;23(4):580–2.

151. Oomura M, Yamawaki T, Naritomi H, et al. Polyarteritis nodosa in association with subarachnoid hemorrhage. Intern Med 2006;45(9):655–8.
152. Rengachary SS, Duke DA, Tsai FY, et al. Spinal arterial aneurysm: case report. Neurosurgery 1993;33(1):125–9.
153. Torralba KD, Colletti PM, Quismorio FP Jr. Spinal subarachnoid hemorrhage in necrotizing vasculitis. J Rheumatol 2008;35(1):180–2.
154. Thompson B, Burns A. Subarachnoid hemorrhages in vasculitis. Am J Kidney Dis 2003;42(3):582–5.
155. Garcia CA, Dulcey S, Dulcey J. Ruptured aneurysm of the spinal artery of Adamkiewicz during pregnancy. Neurology 1979;29(3):394–8.
156. Jacob JT, Tanaka S, Wood CP, et al. Acute epidural spinal hemorrhage from vasculitis: resolution with immunosuppression. Neurocrit Care 2012;16(2):311–5.
157. Salvarani C, Brown RD Jr, Calamia KT, et al. Primary CNS vasculitis with spinal cord involvement. Neurology 2008;70(24 Pt 2):2394–400.
158. Gonzalez LF, Zabramski JM, Tabrizi P, et al. Spontaneous spinal subarachnoid hemorrhage secondary to spinal aneurysms: diagnosis and treatment paradigm. Neurosurgery 2005;57(6):1127–31.
159. Lindau A. Capillary angiomatosis of the central nervous system. Acta Genet Stat Med 1957;7(2):338–40.
160. Rho YM. Von Hippel-Lindau's disease: a report of five cases. Can Med Assoc J 1969;101(3):135–42.
161. Toldo I, Drigo P, Mammi I, et al. Vertebral and spinal cavernous angiomas associated with familial cerebral cavernous malformation. Surg Neurol 2009;71(2):167–71.
162. Maramattom BV, Cohen-Gadol AA, Wijdicks EF, et al. Segmental cutaneous hemangioma and spinal arteriovenous malformation (Cobb syndrome). Case report and historical perspective. J Neurosurg Spine 2005;3(3):249–52.
163. Clark MT, Brooks EL, Chong W, et al. Cobb syndrome: a case report and systematic review of the literature. Pediatr Neurol 2008;39(6):423–5.
164. Miyatake S, Kikuchi H, Koide T, et al. Cobb's syndrome and its treatment with embolization. Case report. J Neurosurg 1990;72(3):497–9.
165. Veznedaroglu E, Nelson PK, Jabbour PM, et al. Endovascular treatment of spinal cord arteriovenous malformations. Neurosurgery 2006;59(5 Suppl 3):S202–9.
166. Alomari AI, Orbach DB, Mulliken JB, et al. Klippel-Trenaunay syndrome and spinal arteriovenous malformations: an erroneous association. AJNR Am J Neuroradiol 2010;31(9):1608–12.

Spine and Spinal Cord Trauma
Diagnosis and Management

Shihao Zhang, MD, Rishi Wadhwa, MD, Justin Haydel, MD,
Jamie Toms, BS, Kendrick Johnson, BS, Bharat Guthikonda, MD*

KEYWORDS

• Spine • Trauma • Spinal cord • Spinal cord injuries

KEY POINTS

- Spine trauma is a devastating clinical condition that affects many people annually on a worldwide basis.
- Management of spinal trauma has become much more surgically oriented with advances in stabilization techniques over the past two decades.
- The degree of injury to the spinal cord dictates the prognosis of the patient in cervical and thoracolumbar trauma.
- Traumatic spinal cord injury is a major area of socioeconomic burden and, as such, is a burgeoning area of ongoing research interest.

Traumatic spinal cord injury (SCI) can cause dramatic impairments to health, social, emotional, and economic well-being; this injury can also predispose the victims to a range of secondary medical conditions later in life.[1] To fully appreciate the diverse problems associated with these debilitating insults it is imperative to review the epidemiology and demographics of SCI.

In 2012, the United States is estimated to have approximately 270,000 living individuals suffering from a SCI.[2] There are 11.5 to 53.4 new cases per million people per year in developed countries with 12,000 new cases per million people per year occurring in the United States.[3] Most traumatic spinal cord trauma (80.6%) occurs in males and most cases are among whites (66%), followed by African Americans (26.2%) and Hispanics (8.3%).[2] Most involve young adults,[1–3] with the median age at injury being 27 years old.[3] The average age at injury has increased since the 1970s from 28.7 years old[3,4] to 41 years old[2] because of a decrease in childhood trauma and an increase in injury in those older than 65 years old (**Table 1**).[4] There are many different causes of traumatic SCI (**Fig. 1**).[2] The predominant sources of spinal cord trauma results from

Department of Neurosurgery, LSU HSC, 1501 Kings Highway, Shreveport, LA 71103, USA
* Corresponding author.
E-mail address: bguthi@lsuhsc.edu

Neurol Clin 31 (2013) 183–206
http://dx.doi.org/10.1016/j.ncl.2012.09.012
0733-8619/13/$ – see front matter © 2013 Elsevier Inc. All rights reserved.

Table 1 Age changes over time at onset of SCI		
Characteristic	1973–1979	2000–Present
Average age in years at injury	28.7	41[a]
Percentage of people >60 y old at injury	4.7	10.9

[a] This number was updated with current data from Reference 2.

Data from Ho CH, Wuermser LA, Priebe MM, et al. Spinal cord injury medicine. 1. Epidemiology and classification. Arch Phys Med Rehabil 2007;88(Suppl 1):S49–S54.

motor vehicle crashes (39.2%); falls (28.3%); violence or gunshot (14.6%); and sports related (8.2%).[2] Not surprisingly, alcohol abuse plays a key role in about 25% of all traumatic spinal cord injuries.[3]

The level at which SCI occurs can have dramatic effects on the overall prognosis; quadriplegia can result from injury to the cervical regions and paraplegia can result from damage to the thoracic, lumbar, or sacral regions.[2] Cervical injuries occur more often than thoracic and lumbar.[4] Cervical injuries (C1 to C7-T1) account for approximately 55% of all traumatic SCI. Thoracic (T1-T11), thoracolumbar (T11-T12 to L1-L2), and lumbosacral (L2-S5) account for 15% of cases each.[3] Despite medical intervention, less than 1% of patients have full neurologic recovery at hospital discharge; most patients experience incomplete quadriplegia (40.8%), complete paraplegia (21.6%), incomplete paraplegia (21.4%), or complete quadriplegia (15.8%).[2]

The life expectancy of those with SCI increases every year, but it is still significantly lower than the general population.[2] Many individuals die on their way from the site of trauma to the hospital, and death after hospitalization ranges from 4.4% to 16.7%.[3] After this initial time frame, mortality rates are higher during the first year after injury than during the subsequent year (**Table 2**).[2]

Most individuals with SCI suffer from multisystem injuries and their spinal injury,[3] and in the past, the lead culprit that caused death in these people was renal failure.

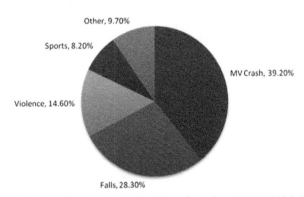

Fig. 1. Causes of spinal cord injury since 2005. (*Data from* the NSCISC 2012 Spinal Cord injury Facts and Figures at a Glance. Spinal Cord Injury Facts and figures at a Glance. (February 2012) National Spinal Cord Injury Statistical Center. https://www.nscisc.uab.edu. Accessed June 9, 2012.)

Table 2
Life expectancy after SCI

		For persons who survive the first 24 h					For persons surviving at least 1 y postinjury				
Age at Injury	No SCI	AIS D – Motor Functional at Any Level	Para	Low Quadra	High Quadra	Ventilator-dependent Any Level	AIS D – Motor Functional at Any Level	Para	Low Tetra	High Tetra	Ventilator-dependent Any Level
20	58.8	52.1	44.8	39.6	35.3	16.8	52.5	45.4	40.5	36.9	24.8
40	39.9	33.8	27.4	23.2	19.7	7.5	34.1	27.9	23.9	21	12.3
60	22.5	17.5	12.8	10	7.8	1.6	17.7	13.2	10.4	8.6	3.8

Data from the NSCISC 2012 Spinal cord injury facts and figures at a glance. Spinal cord injury facts and figures at a glance. (February 2012) National Spinal Cord Injury Statistical Center. https://www.nscisc.uab.edu. Accessed June 9, 2012.

Now, in most SCI cases, respiratory complications are the leading causes of death.[1-3] Other reasons for death include nonischemic heart disease, septicemia, pulmonary emboli, ischemic heart disease, suicide, and unintentional injury.[1,3]

The economic burden and length of hospitalization in individuals with spinal cord trauma can be drastic. It was estimated in 1990 that in the United States the annual cost of all SCI management was $4 billion[3] and that the average cost of the initial hospitalization was more than $95,000 per patient with SCI.[5] Recent figures have placed the total lifetime expense per 25-year-old patient to be anywhere from $1.5 million to more than $4.5 million depending on the level of injury and severity (Table 3).[2] Hospitalization for individuals with traumatic SCI has a median duration of 11 days with 37 days of rehabilitation, but it should be understood that the overall hospitalization increases with the severity of the neurologic injury.[2] Other costs include the cost of drugs and equipment. It is estimated that 82% of all patients with SCI are on one to four different prescription drugs. Individuals who are complete quadriplegics have the highest economic burden regarding prescription drugs, followed by incomplete paraplegics, complete paraplegics, and finally incomplete quadriplegics. This distribution is mostly caused by incomplete paraplegics spending more money on pain medicines. Other than these concerns, nonprescription medication costs, adaptive equipment costs,[5] and loss of productivity or complete inability to maintain employment play a major role in the economic health of these patients.[2]

BRIEF REVIEW OF SPINAL ANATOMY
Vertebral Column

The normal mature spinal column consists of 33 vertebrae, specifically 7 cervical, 12 thoracic, 5 lumbar, 5 fused sacral, and 4 fused coccygeal vertebrae. The primary curvatures of the spine are in the thoracic and sacral regions. In the sagittal plane, the normal cervical and lumbar spines have a degree of lordotic curvature, and the thoracic and sacral spines have kyphotic curvature.[6-8] In general, each vertebra is composed of a body and vertebral arch (Fig. 2).

The vertebral arch consists of paired pedicles and laminae. The vertebral arch provides protection for the spinal cord and provides conduits for passage of neurovascular structures emerging from the spinal canal.

Table 3
Lifetime cost after SCI

Severity of Injury	Average Yearly Expenses (in February 2012 Dollars)		Estimated Lifetime Costs by Age At Injury (Discounted at 2%)	
	First Year	Each Subsequent Year	25 y old	50 y old
High tetraplegia (C1-C4) AIS ABC	$1,023,924	$177,808	$4,543,182	$2,496,856
Low tetraplegia (C5-C8) AIS ABC	$739,874	$109,077	$3,319,533	$2,041,809
Paraplegia AIS ABC	$499,023	$66,106	$2,221,596	$1,457,967
Incomplete motor-functional at any level AIS D	$334,170	$40,589	$1,517,806	$1,071,309

Data from American Spinal Injury Association. Standard for neurologic classification of spinal injured patients. Chicago (IL): American Spinal Injury Association; 1982; and Bridwell KH, DeWald RL. The textbook of spinal surgery. 3rd edition. philadelphia: Lippincott, Williams and Wilkins, 2011.

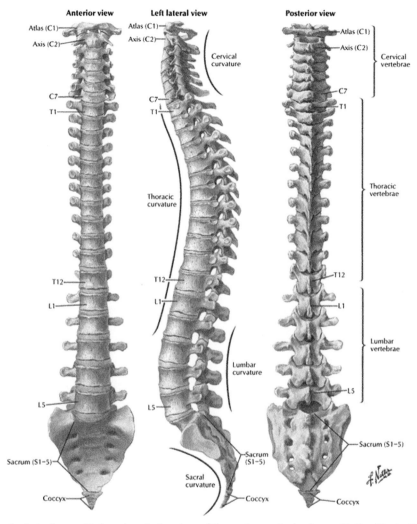

Fig. 2. Anterior, sagittal, and posterior view of the mature spinal column. (Netter illustration from www.netterimages.com. © Elsevier, Inc. All rights reserved.)

Spinal Cord

The spinal cord is a tubular complex of nervous tissue that extends from the brain ending in the conus medullaris at approximately the level of L1-L2. The spinal cord functions as the primary transit of neuronal signal between the brain and the rest of the body through its 31 pairs of spinal nerves (**Figs. 3** and **4**).

The spinal cord is organized into systems of ascending and descending neuronal pathways. Bundles of fibers with similar functionality are commonly termed "tracts." The ascending pathways carry sensory information from the body to the brain and the descending pathways convey motor impulses to the body. This high level of organization coupled with an understanding of clinical neuroanatomy, allows the clinician to accurately localize lesions of the spinal cord (**Figs. 5** and **6**).

Spinal nerves

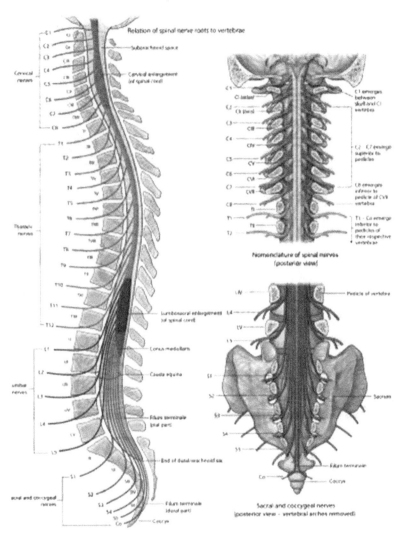

Fig. 3. Spinal cord, spinal nerves, and their exit in relation to corresponding vertebral bodies. (*From* Drake RL, Vogl AW. Gray's Atlas of Anatomy. 1st edition. Philadelphia: Churchill Livingstone, 2007; with permission.)

Descending tracts from the brain are classified into two basic groups: pyramidal and extrapyramidal tracts. The pyramidal tract, also know as corticospinal tract, is a descending motor pathway located primarily in the anterior spinal cord. The corticospinal tract is the major motor pathway in the human brain.[6,9] Most of these fibers cross in the medulla at the pyramidal decussation, and subsequently travel in the lateral corticospinal tracts of the spinal cord. A smaller proportion of corticospinal

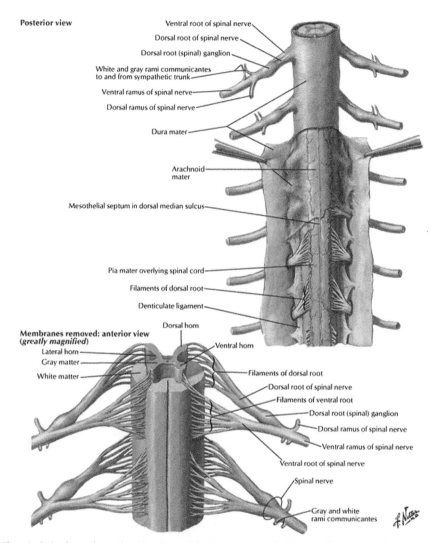

Fig. 4. Spinal cord section in situ with Dura opened. (Netter illustration from www. netterimages.com. © Elsevier, Inc. All rights reserved.)

fibers descend uncrossed in the anterior corticospinal tract.[5] Other descending tracts are highlighted in **Table 4**.

Ascending tracts from the body leading to the brain convey many forms of sensory input. The dorsal column pathway is composed of two discrete tracts know as the fasciculus gracilis and the fasciculus cuneatus. The fasciculus gracilis and the fasciculus cuneatus are responsible for sensory input from the lower body and upper body, respectively. The dorsal columns convey fine touch, proprioception, point-to-point discrimination, and vibratory sensation; these fibers ascend, uncrossed, in the posterior columns to the lower brainstem.[10]

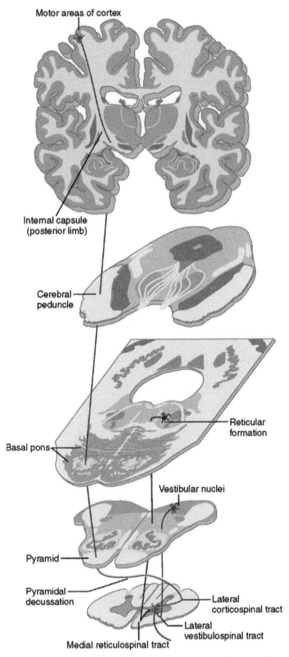

Fig. 5. Descending Tracts. (*From* Nolte J. Elsevier's Integrated Neuroscience. Philadelphia: Mosby, 2007; with permission.)

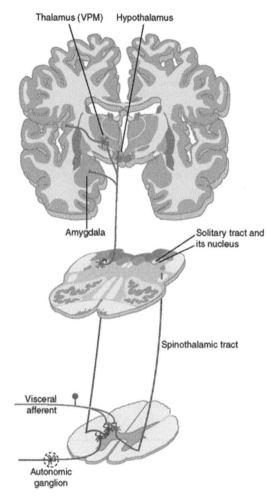

Fig. 6. Ascending fibers. (*From* Nolte J. Elsevier's Integrated Neuroscience. Philadelphia: Mosby, 2007; with permission.)

The spinothalamic tract is responsible for sensation of pain, temperature, and crude touch. The spinothalamic tract is essentially composed of two pathways: the lateral and anterior spinothalamic tracts. The lateral spinothalamic tract is responsible for conveying pain and temperature sensation upward from the body and the anterior spinothalamic tract is responsible for conveying light touch. Other ascending tracts are highlighted in **Table 5**.

The vertebral arteries arise from the subclavian arteries bilaterally. Arising from the vertebral arteries, a midline convergence of two branches forms the anterior spinal artery. The anterior spinal artery travels along the ventral surface of the spinal cord. The anterior spinal artery is supplied by segmental medullary arteries, the most prominent of which, the artery of Adamkiewicz, helps to supply the lower two-thirds of the spinal cord.[11] The anterior spinal artery provides blood supply to most of the spinal cord (**Fig. 7**).

Table 4
Descending spinal cord tracts

System	Function	Origin	Ending	Location in Cord
Lateral corticospinal tract	Fine motor function (controls distal musculature) Modulation of sensory functions	Motor and premotor cortex	Anterior horn cells	Lateral column crosses at the level of medulla
Anterior corticospinal tract	Gross and postural motor function proximal and axial musculature	Motor and premotor cortex	Anterior horn neurons	Anterior column uncrossed
Vestibulospinal tract	Postural reflexes	Lateral and medial vestibular nucleus	Anterior horn inter-neurons and motor neurons	Ventral column
Rubrospinal	Motor control	Red nucleus	Ventral horn interneurons	Lateral column
Reticulospinal	Modulation of sensory transmission Modulation of spinal reflexes	Brain stem reticular formation	Dorsal and ventral horn	Anterior column
Tectospinal	Reflex head turning	Midbrain	Ventral horn inter-neurons	Ventral column
Medial longitudinal fasciculus	Head and eye movements coordination	Vestibular nuclei	Cervical gray	Ventral column

DIAGNOSIS AND MANAGEMENT
Examination

Patients with acute spinal cord trauma often present with confounding injuries making an accurate diagnosis difficult. In addition to this, 20% of patients with a major spine injury at one level have an additional injury at another level.[12] Because patients can present without any significant symptoms, a systematic approach is necessary to rapidly identify and prevent potential spinal injuries.

The clinical approach to a patient with SCI begins with the basic neurologic examination. If the patient is awake and oriented, such information as the mechanism of injury and loss of consciousness should be evaluated. Assess whether the patient is able to move extremities passively. A detailed motor examination should follow. Sensation can be examined with pinprick, light touch, and proprioception. Presence of rectal tone and bulbocavernosus reflex should be noted.

To develop guidelines and recommendations for SCI the American Spinal Injury Association (ASIA) created a systematic method for rapidly classifying spine injuries.[13] The motor component of this method breaks the skeletal system into 10 key muscle groups. Each muscle group is scored from 0 to 5 for the left and for right for a total score of 100 (**Fig. 8**). The sensory component includes 28 points that are

Table 5
Ascending spinal cord tracts

Name	Function	Origin	Ending	Location in Cord
Dorsal column	Fine touch, proprioception, two-point discrimination	Skin, joints, tendons	Dorsal column nuclei. Second-order neurons project to contralateral thalamus	Dorsal column cross at the level of medulla
Spinothalamic tracts	Sharp pain, temperature, crude touch	Skin	Dorsal horn. Second-order neurons project to contralateral thalamus	Ventrolateral column cross at two levels above the entry into the spinal cord
Dorsal spinocerebellar tract	Movement and position mechanisms	Golgi tendon organs, Muscle spindles, touch and pressure receptors	Cerebellar paleocortex	Lateral column
Ventral spinocerebellar	Movement and position mechanisms	Golgi tendon organs, Muscle spindles, touch and pressure receptors	Cerebellar paleocortex	Lateral column
Spinoreticular pathway	Deep and chronic pain	Deep somatic structures	Reticular formation of brain stem	Diffuse pathway in ventrolateral column

scored separately for light and pinprick for a maximum score of 224 (see **Fig. 8**). The patient can be classified into Class A to E under the ASIA impairment scale. Using this information predictions can be made regarding patients' overall outcome and can guide clinicians in developing potential treatments and useful rehabilitation programs.[14]

Diagnostic

Diagnostic evaluation begins with plain radiograph films of the area in question. Overall alignment and bony integrity can be assessed. Plain films are particularly beneficial when evaluating the lumbar and cervical spine. The lower cervical and thoracic spine is often difficult to evaluate using plain films secondary to overlying bony anatomy.

If plain films are unable to provide adequate visualization or if the patient is unable to give a detailed physical examination, computed tomography (CT) scans with three-dimensional reconstructions should be ordered. CT can image the entire spinal axis and is useful in identifying fractures or malalignment. CT cannot evaluate soft tissue or possible ligamentous injury.[15] To identify a possible ligamentous or soft

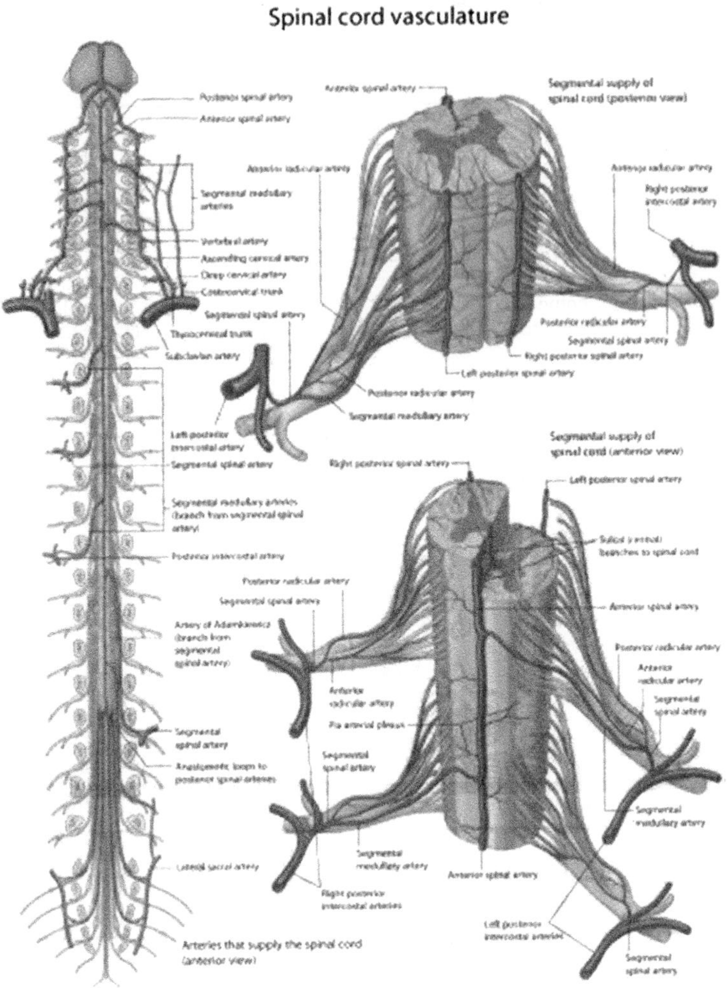

Spinal cord vasculature

Fig. 7. Spinal cord circulation. (*From* Drake RL, Vogl AW. Gray's Atlas of Anatomy. 1st edition. Philadelphia: Churchill Livingstone, 2007; with permission.)

tissue injury, flexion-extension films or magnetic resonance imaging (MRI) can be ordered.

Often with acute trauma it is impractical and unsafe to obtain MRI emergently. Distinction must be made for patients for whom emergent MRI is necessary. Emergent MRI is indicated in patients with incomplete SCI where neurologic findings are not explained by radiologic findings.[12] MRI on an urgent basis is also indicated in patients who experience a progressive neurologic deterioration after injury. MRI on a nonemergent basis is recommended within 72 hours after injury in patients where ligamentous injury is suspected.[16]

Steroids

The use of methylprednisone in the setting of acute SCI remains highly controversial. There are no uniform recommendations as to its use in the setting of acute SCI. It

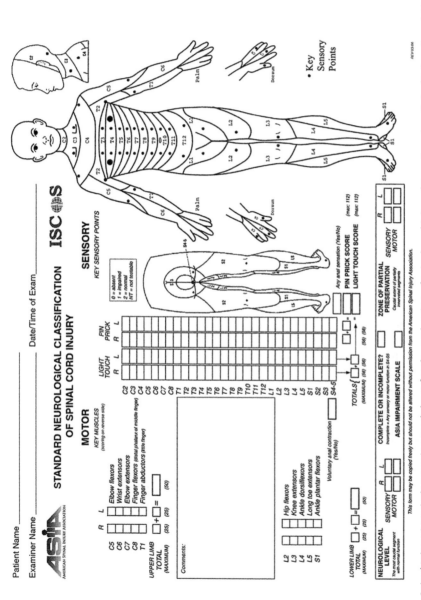

Fig. 8. American Spinal Injury Association scoring worksheet for the evaluation of spinal cord injury. (*From* American Spinal Injury Association. Standard for neurologic classification of spinal injured patients. Chicago (IL): American Spinal Injury Association; 1982.)

has been published that patients who received methylpredisone intravenous bolus, 30 mg/kg, followed by 5.4 mg/kg/h for 23 hours within 8 hours of initial injury did slightly better in motor and sensory deficits at 6 weeks, 6 months, and 1 year after an acute injury.[17,18] Exclusionary criteria for this study include patients age less than 13, cauda equina syndrome, gunshot wounds, pregnancy, and patients with life-threatening morbidities. Additionally, patients receiving high-dose steroids are at an increased risk for pneumonia, sepsis, hyperglycemia, and acute corticosteroid myopathy. More recent data indicate a trend away from the routine use of methylprednisolone for acute SCI because of the risks of complications outweighing the potential benefits.[19]

CERVICAL SPINE INJURIES
Classification

There are numerous classifications for spinal injuries in the literature. Mizra and colleagues[20] have described multiple attributes of a quality classification system. They include the following: injury description, mechanism and treatment guidelines, account for neurologic injury, include bony and ligamentous injury, allow differentiation from other injuries, and finally prognosis. Although several systems have been proposed, each seems to be missing an important element; thus, no gold standard has been established. **Table 6** provides a concise description of subaxial cervical injuries.[21] Modern classification systems of cervical spinal injuries include the Cervical Spine Injury Severity Score and the Subaxial Cervical Injury Classification. An algorithm is provided for the two classification systems in **Table 7**.[21]

Surgical Management of Cervical Spine Fractures

Spinal cord injuries commonly involve the cervical spine. They mostly occur in males aged 16 to 32. Most commonly they are secondary to motor vehicle accidents and falls. Interestingly, the age of patients with cervical spine injuries has increased to 39 from 28 over the past 35 years. The elderly also have a 10% increase in SCI in

Table 6 Subaxial cervical injury classification systems		
System	**Strengths**	**Weaknesses**
Nicoll	Functional outcomes	Retrospective Lacks Details No neurological assessment
Holdsworth	Posterior ligament complex	Limited descriptors Ignores anterior soft tissues No neurological assessment
Louis	Conceptually simple	Anatomic description only Ignores soft tissures No neurological assessment
White and Panjabi	Neurological assessment Point based	Intricate radiographic criteria Stretch test Limited assessment of soft tissues
Allen et al	Comprehensive	Mechanistic-inferred description and assessment of stability
Harris et al	Organized by severity	Large number of subgroups

Data from Bridwell KH, DeWald RL. The Textbook of Spinal Surgery. 3rd edition. Philadelphia: Lippincott, Williams and Wilkins, 2011.

Table 7 Subaxial injury classification (SLIC) and severity scale		
		Points
Morphology	No Abnormality	0
	Compression	1
	Burst	+1=2
	Distraction	3
	Rotation/translation	4
Discoligamentous complex	Intact	0
	Indeterminate	1
	Disrupted	2
Neurological status	Intact	0
	Root injury	1
	Complete cord injury	2
	Incomplete cord injury	3
	Continuous cord compression	+1

Data from Bridwell KH, DeWald RL. The Textbook of Spinal Surgery. 3rd edition. Philadelphia: Lippincott, Williams and Wilkins, 2011.

that time period.[22] In children, however, injuries tend to occur less often than in adults, most likely secondary to their ligamentous laxity.[12] The major causes of death in SCI are aspiration pneumonia and shock.[23] Management of cervical spine injuries includes (1) immobilization of the patient and neck, (2) maintenance of blood pressure, (3) maintenance of oxygenation, and (4) a brief motor examination. Management in the hospital includes theses steps with the addition of nasogastric tubes to prevent aspiration, Foley catheter to observe for urinary retention, temperature regulation, electrolytes, and a more detailed neurologic examination. Evaluation begins with a detailed history and physical examination. It is important to immobilize the cervical spine to prevent a new or worsening neurologic injury, especially in the comatose patient. The ASIA published guidelines for neurologic classification of spinal cord injuries. Proper use of the form can assess any neurologic improvement or decline in a patient (see **Fig. 8**).[24]

Clearance of the cervical spine includes a nonintoxicated neurologically intact patient without distracting injury. Films traditionally included a three-view cervical spine radiograph (to the C7-T1 junction), but now most patients have a CT scan of the cervical spine with axial, coronal, and sagittal reconstructions. Several cervical spine clearance injury algorithms have been proposed. One of the most widely used, the Canadian C-Spine rule, is shown in **Fig. 9**.[25]

It has been estimated that 30% of patients with cervical spine injuries are between the occiput and C2. Common injuries of C2 include Hangman fractures (bilateral pars interarticularis) (types 1–3) (**Fig. 10**) and odontoid fractures (types 1–3) (**Fig. 11**).[12,21] Common fractures of C1 include ring fractures (Jefferson fractures). Atlanto-occipital dislocations are caused by high-energy trauma and often result in high morbidity.[26] The other 70% of cervical spine injuries are subaxial (C3-7). These can include compression fractures, burst fractures, and dislocated facets. These often require reduction and fixation.

Indications for surgical treatment include need for spinal canal decompression and restoration of spinal stability. The goal of the latter is to prevent chronic pain from either abnormal motion or static deformity. Decompression of neural elements

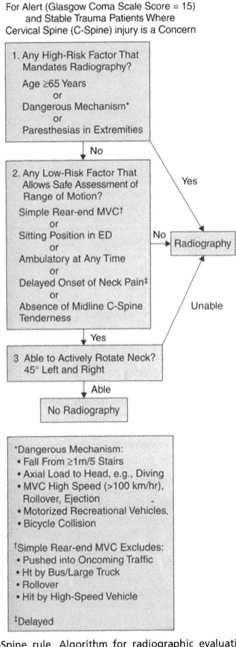

Fig. 9. Canadian C-Spine rule. Algorithm for radiographic evaluation of stable trauma patients with potential cervical spine injury. (*Courtesy of* Professor Ian G. Stiell, MD, University of Ottawa, Ottawa, ON; with permission.)

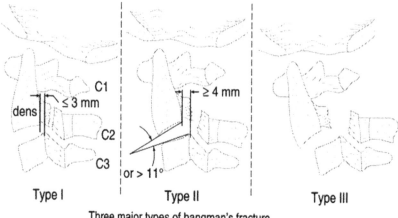

Type I   Type II   Type III

Three major types of hangman's fracture

Fig. 10. Classification of traumatic spondylolisthesis of the axis. (*A*) Type I fracture through the neural arch, no angulation, as much as 3 mm of displacement. (*B*) Type II fracture has significant angulation and displacement. (*C*) Type IIa fracture has minimal displacement but severe angulation. (*D*) Type III axial fractures include fracture of the neural arch and bilateral facet dislocation between the second and third cervical vertebrae. (*From* Bridwell KH, DeWald RL. The Textbook of Spinal Surgery, 3rd edition. Philadelphia: Lippincott, Williams and Wilkins, 2011; with permission.)

is vital and in cases of incomplete motor dysfunction, spinal cord decompression can result in improvement in neurologic function. Schneider and coworkers[27] have recommended the following as indications for emergency decompressive surgery: progression of neurologic signs, complete subarachnoid block, bone or soft tissue fragments in the canal discovered radiographically, necessity for decompression of a vital cervical root, compound fracture or penetrating trauma to the spine, acute anterior spinal cord syndrome, and nonreducible fracture dislocations from locked facets causing spinal cord compression. Contraindications to emergent operation include complete SCI for more than 24 hours and a medically unstable patient.[21]

The key features of central cord syndrome include disproportionately greater motor deficit in the upper extremities than the lower; it usually results from the hyperextension of the cervical cord over bony osteophytes. Decompressive surgery is often helpful to improve neurologic function.[28,29] Anterior spinal artery syndrome, otherwise known as anterior cord syndrome, may result from a traumatic herniated disk or bony fragment or by occlusion of the anterior spinal artery. Its key features include paraplegia secondary to the descending motor tract compromise and dissociated pain loss below the lesion (ie, loss of pain and temperature; spinothalamic tract lesion) and preserved proprioception and deep pressure sensation (posterior column function.)[12,30]

SCI without Radiographic Abnormality

Some young patients with increased elasticity of the spinous ligaments and perivertebral soft tissue present with SCI without radiographic abnormality. This mostly occurs in children younger than 9 years of age. In this particular subset of spinal cord injuries that includes contusions and stretch injuries, there is no radiographic evidence of

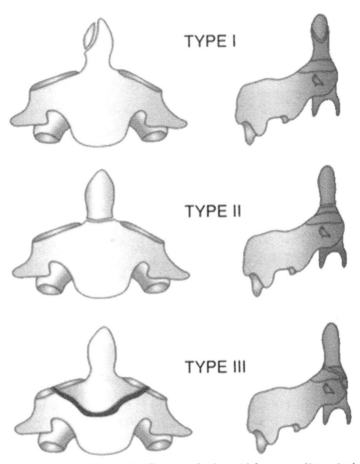

Fig. 11. Anderson and D'Alonzo classification of odontoid fractures. (*From* Anderson LD, D'Alonzo RT. Fractures of the odontoid process of the axis. J Bone Joint Surg Am 1974;56:1663–74; with permission.)

injury. The modified treatment protocol includes hospital admission, MRI of the cervical spine, immobilization of the cervical spine for up to 3 months, and prohibition of sports until the patient shows good recovery.[31,32]

TRAUMATIC THORACOLUMBAR SPINE TRAUMA

One of the most frequent types of injuries seen by spine surgeons is fractures of the thoracolumbar spine. This area transitions from the rigid, kyphotic thoracic spine to the more mobile, lordotic lumbar spine. Up to 75% of thoracic or lumbar fracture occurs between T12 and L2.[33]

Classification

Spinal fracture classification remains controversial despite the vast amount of available literature on this topic.[34–39] Historically, the classification system has focused on mechanism of injury and does not offer any clinical applications. Denis[35] introduced the three-column model in 1983. The anterior column extends from the anterior longitudinal ligament to the anterior half of the vertebral body and disk. The middle column is composed of the posterior half of the vertebral body and disk to the posterior longitudinal ligament. The posterior column involves the posterior bony arch and interposed posterior ligaments including facet joints, capsule, and ligamentum flavum. In this model, fractures were divided into four categories: (1) compression, (2) burst, (3) seat-belt type, and (4) fracture dislocation.[33,34]

The McAfee classification modified the three column model by placing more emphasis on the mechanism of injury.[38] These categories were expanded to six groups: (1) wedge-compression, (2) stable burst, (3) unstable burst, (4) Chance fractures, (5) flexion-distraction injuries, and (6) translational injuries. Compression fracture is caused by a failure of the anterior column. Burst fracture usually involves the anterior and the middle column with or without retropulsion. Flexion-distraction is failure of middle and posterior columns. Chance fractures are caused by flexion injury with a fracture horizontally thorough the bone.[33,34]

The Modified Comprehensive Classification is currently the most commonly used classification system. Fractures are described as three types: (1) compression, (2) distraction, or (3) translation injuries. This system is quite complicated with 27 subtypes and is difficult to remember or to use in a clinical setting. Some structures are hard to visualize on imaging, thus making the diagnosis somewhat subjective.[37]

A new classification system called the Thoracolumbar Injury Classification and Severity Score (TLICS) was created to provide universal language to describe fractures and guide clinical management.[34,39] The morphology of the injury, integrity of the posterior ligamentous complex, and neurologic status were identified as critical in determining a diagnosis and treatment of these fractures.

Morphology: Fracture Pattern

Three types of fracture pattern described are (1) compression, (2) translation and rotation, and (3) distraction.

Compression

Compression is described as when an axial load causes vertebral body failure. Less severe compression occurs when there is bucking of the anterior wall of the vertebrae. Burst fracture is a more severe compression fracture with failure of the posterior cortex of the vertebral body with associated retropulsion.[34,39]

Rotation and Translation

Rotation or translation spinal column failure is usually caused by torsional and shear forces. Thoracolumbar spine is designed to move in flexion and extension and resist rotation and translation. More significant force than is needed to cause compression fractures is necessary for rotation and translation injury to occur and leads to greater instability. Horizontal separation of the spinous processes or acutely altered alignment of the pedicle above and below the level of injury on anteroposterior radiograph indicates rotational injury. Sagittal CT provides details on facet jump or fracture. A shift in midline across the injury site on axial CT could indicate a translation injury.[34,39]

Distraction

Distraction injury is caused by severe forces that lead to separation of the spinal column. Both anterior and posterior ligaments and bony elements are disrupted. It is essential to recognize that the rostral component is separated from the caudal component; therefore, distraction is usually an unstable fracture.[34,39]

A combination of the three primary morphologies could be used to describe more complex spinal column fractures.

Neurologic Status

Neurologic function is an important indication of the severity of injury. Incomplete injury is generally accepted as an indication for more urgent surgical decompression.[33,34] ASIA score is used to classify the degree of injury with ASIA A as complete injury, whereas ASIA B, C, and D are incomplete injury. In the TLICS systems, neurologic status is described in increased order of urgency as follows: neurologically intact, nerve root injury, complete spinal cord, and incomplete spinal cord or cauda equine injury. All of these combine for an injury severity score (**Table 8**).[39]

Injury Severity Score

A total score higher than five suggests strong consideration for surgical treatment, whereas a score less than three advocates nonoperative management. TLICS system attempts to be inclusive, but it cannot anticipate all potential patient variables that may be used to determine specific treatment.[39]

Surgical Fracture Management

The goal of surgery is to reduce the fracture, stabilize the spinal column, and decompress the neural canal. The surgical approaches can be divided as anterior, posterior, or anteroposterior combined instrumentation. Posterior approach is usually favored

Table 8
Injury severity score

Type	Qualifiers	Points
Compression		1
	Burst	1
Translational/rotational		3
Distraction		4

Posterior Ligamentous Complex Disrupted in Tension, Rotation, or Translation	Points
Intact	0
Suspected or indeterminate	2
Injured	3

Involvement	Qualifiers	Points
Intact		0
Nerve root		2
Cord, conus medullaris	Complete	2
	Incomplete	3
Cauda equina		3

Data from Vaccaro AR, Lehman RA, Hurlbert RJ, et al. A new classification of thoracolumbar injuries: the importance of injury morphology, the integrity of the posterior ligamentous complex, and neurologic status. Spine 2005;30(20):232–33.

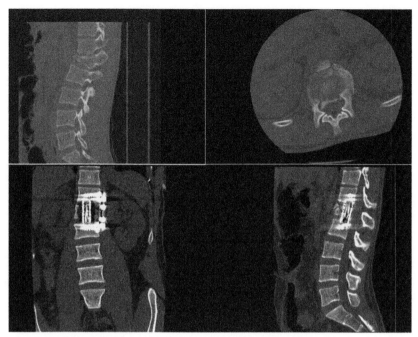

Fig. 12. Preoperative CT showing L1 burst fracture and postoperative CT showing L1 corpectomy with insertion of cage and T12-L2 anterior fusion and plating.

when there is disruption of the posterior ligamentous complex. Anterior approach is preferred with severe kyphosis or incomplete neurologic injury with obvious anterior thecal sac compression.[34,40] For patients with incomplete injuries and canal compromise, early decompression is usually advocated.[33,34]

Case report

The patient is a 29-year-old woman taken to the emergency room after a motor vehicle accident. This was a head-on collision at high speed. Patient complained of severe back pain and difficulty moving her proximal lower extremities because of pain. She states there is no radicular pain or numbness down her legs. No loss of bladder or bowel control. On physical examination, she is four-fifths in bilateral lower extremities. Weakness is symmetric. No saddle anesthesia or clonus reflex. CT scan showed an L1 burst fracture with canal compromise. She was taken to the operating room for L1 corpectomy with cage reconstruction and T12-L2 anterior fusion and plating (**Fig. 12**).

SUMMARY

Spine trauma is a devastating clinical condition that affects many people annually on a worldwide basis. Management of spinal trauma has become much more surgically oriented with advances in stabilization techniques over the past two decades. The degree of injury to the spinal cord dictates the prognosis of the patient in cervical and thoracolumbar trauma. Traumatic SCI is a major area of socioeconomic burden and, as such, is a burgeoning area of ongoing research interest.

REFERENCES

1. van den Berg ME, Castellote JM, de Pedro-Cuesta J, et al. Survival after spinal cord injury: a systematic review. J Neurotrauma 2010;27(8):1517–28.
2. Spinal Cord Injury Facts and figures at a Glance. (February 2012) National Spinal Cord Injury Statistical Center. Available at: https://www.nscisc.uab.edu. Accessed June 9, 2012.
3. Sekhon LH, Fehlings MG. Epidemiology, demographics, and pathophysiology of acute spinal cord injury. Spine 2001;26(Suppl 24):S2–12.
4. Ho CH, Wuermser LA, Priebe MM, et al. Spinal cord injury medicine. 1. Epidemiology and classification. Arch Phys Med Rehabil 2007;88(3 Suppl 1):S49–54.
5. Harvey C, Wilson SE, Greene CG, et al. New estimates of the direct costs of traumatic spinal cord injuries: results of a nationwide survey. Paraplegia 1992;30(12): 834–50.
6. Bae JS, Jang JS, Lee SH, et al. A comparison study on the change in lumbar lordosis when standing, sitting on a chair, and sitting on the floor in normal individuals. J Korean Neurosurg Soc 2012;51(1):20–3.
7. Fon GT, Pitt MJ, Thies AC Jr. Thoracic kyphosis: range in normal subjects. AJR Am J Roentgenol 1980;134(5):979–83.
8. Grob D, Frauenfelder H, Mannion AF. The association between cervical spine curvature and neck pain. Eur Spine J 2007;16(5):669–78.
9. Jang SH. Somatotopic arrangement and location of the corticospinal tract in the brainstem of the human brain. Yonsei Med J 2011;52(4):553–7.
10. Waxman SG. The spinal cord. In: Clinical neuroanatomy. 26th edition. New York: McGraw-Hill; 2010. p. 45–69.
11. Waxman SG. The vertebral column and other structures surrounding the spinal cord. In: Clinical neuroanatomy. 26th edition. New York: McGraw-Hill; 2010. p. 70–80.
12. Greenberg M. Spine injuries. In: Greenberg, editor. Handbook of neurosurgery. edition. New York: Thieme Medical Publishers; 2010. p. 930–10006.
13. Kirshblum SC, Burns SP, Biering-Sorensen F, et al. International standards for neurological classification of spinal cord injury (revised 2011). J Spinal Cord Med 2011;34(6):535–46.
14. Spiess MR, Müller RM, Rupp R, et al. Conversion in ASIA impairment scale during the first year after traumatic spinal cord injury. J Neurotrauma 2009;26(11): 2027–36.
15. Tehranzadeh J, Bonk RT, Ansari A, et al. Efficacy of limited CT for nonvisualized lower cervical spine in patients with blunt trauma. Skeletal Radiol 1994;23(5): 349–52.
16. Benzel EC, Hart BL, Ball PA, et al. Magnetic resonance imaging for the evaluation of patients with occult cervical spine injury. J Neurosurg 1996;85(5):824–9.
17. Bracken MB, Shepard MJ, Collins WF, et al. A randomized, controlled trial of methylprednisolone or naloxone in the treatment of acute spinal-cord injury. Results of the second national acute spinal cord injury study. N Engl J Med 1990;322(20):1405–11.
18. Bracken MB, Shepard MJ, Collins WF Jr, et al. Methylprednisolone or naloxone treatment after acute spinal cord injury: 1-year follow-up data. Results of the second national acute spinal cord injury study. J Neurosurg 1992; 76(1):23–31.
19. Ito Y, Sugimoto Y, Tomioka M, et al. Does high dose methylprednisolone sodium succinate really improve neurological status in patient with acute cervical cord

injury? A prospective study about neurological recovery and early complications. Spine 2009;34(20):2121–4.

20. Mirza SK, Mirza AJ, Chapman JR, et al. Classifications of thoracic and lumbar fractures: rationale and supporting data. J Am Acad Orthop Surg 2002;10(5): 364–77.

21. Patel AA, Vaccaro AR, Anderson PA. Classification of cervical spinal injury. In: Bridwell, editor. The textbook of spinal surgery. 3rd edition. Philadelphia: Lippinoctt Williams and Wilkins; 2011. p. 1381–9.

22. Vaccaro AR, Hulbert RJ, Patel AA, et al. The subaxial cervical spine injury classification system: a novel approach to recognize the importance of morphology, neurology, and integrity of the disco-ligamentous complex. Spine 2007;32(21): 2365–74.

23. Chestnut RM. Emergency management of spinal cord injury. In: Chestnut, editor. Neurotrauma. New York: McGraw-Hill; 1996. p. 1121–38.

24. American Spinal Injury Association. Standard for neurological classification of spinal injured patients. Chicago: American Spinal Injury Association; 1982.

25. Stiell IG, Wells GA, Vandemheen KL, et al. The Canadian C-spine rule for radiography in alert and stable trauma patients. JAMA 2001;286(15):1841–8.

26. Labler L, Eid K, Platz A, et al. Atlanto-occipital dislocation: four case reports of survival in adults and review of the literature. Eur Spine J 2004;13(2):172–80.

27. Schneider RC, Crosby EC, Russo RH, et al. Chapter 32. Traumatic spinal cord syndromes and their management. Clin Neurosurg 1973;20:424–92.

28. Epstein N, Epstein JA, Benjamin V, et al. Traumatic myelopathy in patients with cervical spinal stenosis without fracture or dislocation: methods of diagnosis, management, and prognosis. Spine 1980;5(6):489–96.

29. Lenehan B, Fisher CG, Vaccaro A, et al. The urgency of surgical decompression in acute central cord injuries with spondylosis and without instability. Spine 2010; 35(Suppl 21):S180–6.

30. Schneider RC. The syndrome of acute anterior spinal cord injury. J Neurosurg 1955;12(2):95–122.

31. Hamilton MG, Myles ST. Pediatric spinal injury: review of 174 hospital admissions. J Neurosurg 1992;77(5):700–4.

32. Pollack IF, Pang D, Sclabassi R. Recurrent spinal cord injury without radiographic abnormalities in children. J Neurosurg 1988;69(2):177–82.

33. Rengachary S, Ellenbogen R. Thoracolumbar spine fractures. In: Ellenbogen, editor. Principles of neurosurgery. 2nd edition. London: Elsevier Mosby; 2005. p. 381–6.

34. Lehman RA, Bessey JT, Vaccaro AR. Classification of thoracic and lumbar fractures. In: Bridwell, editor. The textbook of spinal surgery. 3rd edition. Philadelphia: Lippincott Williams and Wilkins; 2011. p. 1390–8.

35. Denis F. The three column spine and its significance in the classification of acute thoracolumbar spinal injuries. Spine 1983;8(8):817–31.

36. Gertzbein SD. Spine update. Classification of thoracic and lumbar fractures. Spine 1994;19(5):626–8.

37. Magerl F, Aebi M, Gertzbein SD, et al. A comprehensive classification of thoracic and lumbar injuries. Eur Spine J 1994;3(4):184–201.

38. McAfee PC, Yuan HA, Fredrickson BE, et al. The value of computed tomography in thoracolumbar fractures. An analysis of one hundred consecutive cases and a new classification. J Bone Joint Surg Am 1983;65(4):461–73.

39. Vaccaro AR, Lehman RA Jr, Hurlbert RJ, et al. A new classification of thoracolumbar injuries: the importance of injury morphology, the integrity of the

posterior ligamentous complex, and neurologic status. Spine 2005;30(20): 2325–33.

40. Oprel P, Tuinebreijer WE, Patka P, et al. Combined anterior-posterior surgery versus posterior surgery for thoracolumbar burst fractures: a systematic review of the literature. Open Orthop J 2010;4:93–100.

Metabolic, Nutritional, and Toxic Myelopathies

Robert N. Schwendimann, MD

KEYWORDS

- Myelopathy • Myeloneuropathy • Cobalamin • Methylmalonic acid • Homocysteine
- Copper deficiency • Lathyrism • Konzo

KEY POINTS

- Vitamin B12 deficiency can result in symptoms that may involve the nervous system at different levels, including the cerebral hemispheres, spinal cord, and peripheral nerve.
- Laboratory evaluation of vitamin B12 deficiency includes measurement of vitamin B12, homocysteine, and methylmalonic acid levels.
- Copper deficiency can produce clinical symptoms that are almost identical to those caused by vitamin B12 deficiency.
- Vitamin E deficiency may result in clinical symptoms that are similar to those seen in various hereditary spinocerebellar ataxias.
- MRI of the spinal cord may reveal abnormalities that are somewhat typical of metabolic and nutritional myelopathies.

INTRODUCTION

Disorders affecting the spinal cord can occur acutely or can be insidious in onset. In any case, they must be recognized as early as possible to prevent progression that can lead to permanent disability. Compressive lesions from neoplasms, degenerative disc disease, acute spinal cord trauma, or infection may have to be managed surgically to relieve the cord compression in hopes of restoring normal function. Other primary neurologic diseases, such as multiple sclerosis, neuromyelitis optica, idiopathic transverse myelitis, and effects of infectious processes, may not be amenable to surgical intervention. This article concerns various metabolic, nutritional, and toxic causes that cause myelopathy and myeloneuropathy and that may require a totally different approach to diagnosis and treatment.

Disclosures: None.
Conflict of interest: None.
Department of Neurology, LSU Health-Shreveport, 1501 Kings Highway, Shreveport, LA 71130-3932, USA
E-mail address: rschwe@lsuhsc.edu

Neurol Clin 31 (2013) 207–218
http://dx.doi.org/10.1016/j.ncl.2012.09.002   neurologic.theclinics.com

VITAMIN B12 DEFICIENCY

Leichtenstern[1] and Lichtheim[2] described pathologic abnormalities in the dorsal and lateral columns of the spinal cord in patients with megaloblastic anemia in the late nineteenth century. In 1900, Russell and colleagues[3] termed these changes subacute combined degeneration (SCD). The neurologic effects of pernicious anemia were well known at the time and included SCD and peripheral neuropathy, as well as cognitive symptoms and dementia. At that time the diagnosis of pernicious anemia depended on demonstration of the absence of acid in the stomach (achlorhydria), though Kinnear Wilson[4] demonstrated that up to 25% of patients with SCD and other neurologic symptoms had stomach acid present.

Folic acid was synthesized in 1945 and, 3 years later, vitamin B12 (cobalamin) was isolated. Folic acid was used for treatment of pernicious anemia and seemed to have positive effects on the anemia, but deleterious effects on the neurologic problems associated with pernicious anemia. Later, when vitamin B12 was isolated and added to the therapy, there were positive effects on both the anemia and the neurologic manifestations of the disease.

Vitamin B12 deficiency can produce overlapping clinical syndromes of peripheral neuropathy, SCD, autonomic abnormality, optic atrophy, mood and behavior changes, psychosis, and dementia. Major neurologic symptoms are typically insidious in onset and consist of only vague complaints, such as fatigue and generalized weakness. Autonomic symptoms include urinary frequency, constipation, or erectile dysfunction in men (**Box 1**). These symptoms may occur early in the course of the disease and are suggestive of spinal cord involvement. The presence of gait abnormalities may indicate a sensory ataxia. This may occur in association with hyperreflexia, spasticity, loss of position and vibratory sensation, and evidence of pathologic reflexes. Distal paresthesias are present when the myelopathy is associated with peripheral neuropathy. Cognitive problems associated with vitamin B12 deficiency may also be present. SCD can also be associated with megaloblastic anemia with increased mean corpuscular volumes and hypersegmented polymorphonuclear leukocytes.[5,6]

Box 1
Clinical manifestations of vitamin B12 deficiency

- Hematologic manifestations
  - Megaloblastic anemia
  - Pancytopenia (leukopenia, thrombocytopenia)
- Psychiatric manifestations
  - Dementia, memory impairment
  - Personality changes
  - Depression
  - Psychosis
- Cardiovascular manifestations
  - Increased risk of stroke and myocardial infarction
- Other neurologic manifestations
  - Peripheral neuropathy
  - Paresthesias

The diagnosis of SCD depends on a high index of suspicion. Low serum cobalamin levels may be all that is needed to make a diagnosis; however, when these levels are borderline or normal, measurement of homocysteine and methylmalonic acid levels may lead to a diagnosis of cobalamin deficiency. In this situation, homocysteine and methylmalonic acid levels may be elevated. Homocysteine and methylmalonic acid levels are elevated in about one-third of patients with normal assays of cobalamin. Intrinsic factor and parietal cell antibodies are useful studies when there is associated anemia. Nerve conduction studies and electromyography may be needed when there seems to be an associated peripheral neuropathy. These studies may demonstrate evidence of an axonal type of peripheral neuropathy.[7]

MRI has proven to be extremely useful in the diagnosis of myelopathy related to cobalamin deficiency. Imaging of the lower cervical and thoracic spinal cord may show increased T2-weighted signal in the posterior and lateral columns of the spinal cord. There can also be enhancement of these same areas on T1-weighted images performed with contrast (**Figs. 1** and **2**).[8,9]

Deficiencies of cobalamin may occur in conditions such as pernicious anemia, but often are related to malabsorption syndromes, gastric surgery, drugs such as H2 antagonists and metformin, nitrous oxide (N2O) use and abuse, and parasitic infestation by fish tapeworm (*Diphyllobothrium latum*). The standard treatment for neurologic problems associated with cobalamin deficiency, including myelopathy, is replacement with high doses of cobalamin given intramuscularly. A common treatment

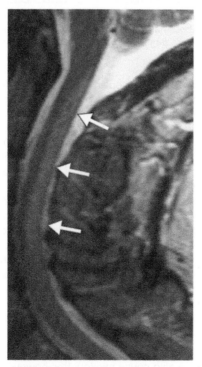

Fig. 1. Sagittal T2-weighted MRI of the cervical spinal cord shows hyperintensity (*arrows*) in the dorsal of the cord spinal, extending from the level of C2 to the level of C5. This is the typical appearance in vitamin B12 and many other myelopathies described in this article. (*From* Naidich MJ, Ho SU. Subacute combined cord degeneration. Radiology 2005;237:101–5; with permission.)

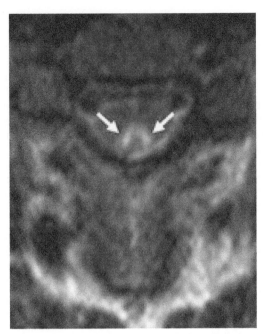

Fig. 2. Transverse T2-weighted MRI obtained through the cervical spinal cord. Bilateral symmetric signal intensity abnormality within the dorsal columns (*arrows*). (*From* Naidich MJ, Ho SU. Subacute combined cord degeneration. Radiology 2005;237:101–5; with permission.)

plan is 1000 μg of cobalamin intramuscularly daily for 2 weeks, followed by 1000 μg monthly. Some improvement of neurologic symptoms may occur in the first 6 months of therapy; however, significant improvement may be delayed and is often incomplete.

Exposure to N2O can lead to an acute to subacute myelopathic picture in individuals that may have a subclinical cobalamin deficiency.[10] N2O is an anesthetic agent, also known as laughing gas, used in many surgical and dental surgical procedures. It can also be used as a recreational drug because of its euphoria-producing effects. The myelopathy associated with N2O exposure can develop after single or multiple exposures to N2O. The term "anesthesia paresthetica" has been used to describe this condition.[11] N2O interferes with the metabolic pathway that produces methionine synthase, which is vitamin B12 dependent. This leads to loss of myelin cohesion and vacuolization of the spinal cord.[12] N2O toxicity can produce symptoms identical to those seen in cobalamin deficiency. T2 hyperintensities in the posterior and lateral columns may be seen on MRI. Treatment is with large doses of cobalamin. Cobalamin can be given prophylactically to individuals with low levels of cobalamin who are having anesthesia using N2O.

FOLATE DEFICIENCY

Folate deficiency alone can also cause myelopathy; however, this occurs much less often than cobalamin deficiency and is often seen with other nutritional deficiencies. Other neurologic manifestations of folate deficiency include peripheral neuropathy, optic atrophy, and cognitive problems. Folate deficiencies are known to be associated with neural tube defects. Folate deficiency can occur as a result of alcoholism, gastrointestinal disease, and drugs such as methotrexate and trimethoprim. Homo-cysteine levels are typically elevated in patients with clinically significant folate deficiency.[12]

COPPER DEFICIENCY

In 2001, Schleper and Stuerenburg[13] reported a postgastrectomy patient with myelop-athy that was associated with copper deficiency. In 2003, Kumar and colleagues[14] subsequently reported a patient who had myelopathy secondary to copper deficiency in the face of zinc toxicity. Over the next several years, numerous articles described patients with symptoms and signs of myelopathy and myeloneuropathy that were asso-ciated with copper deficiency.[15,16] Since then, copper deficiency has become well-recognized as a frequent cause of myelopathy and myeloneuropathy.

Copper is a trace metal that is essential in various metalloenzymes. It is important in mitochondrial metabolism and in the function of the bone marrow and nervous system. The hematological manifestations of copper deficiency have been known and described for many years and include a megaloblastic anemia similar to that seen in pernicious anemia.[17]

Neurologic manifestations of copper deficiency had previously been described in the veterinary literature. Deficiency of copper was known to produce a condition known as swayback in various animals, particularly ruminants.[14] In humans, the neurologic clinical picture in humans is very similar to SCD. Patients typically present with gait abnormalities related to a sensory ataxia and spasticity due to posterior and lateral column dysfunction. Paresthesias in the hands and feet are not uncommon and there may be an associated axonal peripheral neuropathy. The neurologic examina-tion shows presence of a spastic paraparesis or quadriparesis and evidence of a sensory ataxia. Reflexes may be increased or depressed, depending on whether neuropathy is present. Extensor plantar responses are not uncommon.

The diagnosis of myelopathy related to copper deficiency depends on demonstra-tion of low serum copper and low serum ceruloplasmin levels. Zinc levels may also be elevated in many patients with copper deficiency. MRI shows abnormalities on T2-weighted images of the spinal cord with increased signal in the posterior and lateral columns. These abnormalities typically are seen in the cervical spinal cord and are similar to those seen in cobalamin deficiency and SCD.[18]

The causes of copper deficiency are varied. The most common cause seems to be related to abnormalities of copper absorption. Copper is an essential dietary nutrient and the daily requirements are quite low. It is absorbed in the duodenum and, to a lesser degree, the stomach. Many patients who develop copper deficiency have had previous gastric surgery, particularly bariatric surgery for the treatment of morbid obesity. Deficiency of copper has also been noted following other types of gastric surgery. Malabsorption secondary to celiac disease may lead to copper deficiency.[17]

Another interesting cause is related to excessive intake of zinc. Zinc upregulates the expression of the chelator, metallothionein, but affinity for metallothionein is higher in copper than zinc. Copper displaces zinc from metallothionein and remains in the enterocytes in the wall of the gut that are later sloughed off and eliminated in the feces. This leads to a reduction of absorbed copper and often an elevated serum level of zinc. Zinc is available as an over-the-counter dietary supplement and is incorporated into various over-the-counter medications to prevent the common cold. Zinc is also used in various dental adhesives. Zinc toxicity leading to copper deficiency has been reported due to excessive use of these commercially available products. Most of these products are now packaged with a warning about excessive zinc intake.[19]

Treatment of copper deficiency, and the neurologic problems associated with it, is supplementation of elemental copper that is given orally beginning with 8 mg/d for 1 week, 6 mg/d for 1 week, 4 mg/d for a week, and maintenance thereafter on 2 mg/d. It can also be treated with intravenous supplementation of copper. Limiting excessive intake of zinc alone may lead to improvement in myelopathic symptoms related to zinc toxicity.

VITAMIN E DEFICIENCY

Vitamin E is absorbed in the intestine as alpha-tocopherol and is bound to the alpha-tocopherol transport protein. It subsequently is incorporated into very low-density lipoproteins. Vitamin E is an antioxidant that prevents peroxidation of membrane fatty acids.

In adults, deficiency of vitamin E is most often associated with malabsorption syndromes such as celiac disease, cystic fibrosis, cholestasis, and various other intestinal disorders. Deficiency may also be a result of genetic defects in alpha-tocopherol transfer protein, abetalipoproteinemia, or defects in chylomicron synthesis and secretion.[20]

Neurologic manifestations of vitamin E deficiency vary and include spinocerebellar syndromes and neuropathy resulting in gait abnormalities, decreased or absent tendon reflexes, impairment of position and vibratory sensation, movement disorders, gaze palsies, and retinopathy. Clinical findings in vitamin E deficiency are somewhat similar to those seen in Friedreich ataxia.[21]

The diagnosis in adult patients is based on demonstration of low vitamin E levels. MRI findings include hyperintensities in the posterior columns. Genetic testing may be helpful in childhood cases.[22]

Replacement of vitamin E is the treatment of choice. In adults, 800 to 1200 mg of vitamin E daily results in normalization of plasma levels and stopping progression; however, improvement of neurologic symptoms and signs in severe cases may not usually occur.[23]

TOXIC MYELOPATHIES

Exposure to a variety of toxins can result in myelopathy. Some of these are very unlikely to be seen in the United States and are much more likely to occur in other geographic areas. They cause pathologic conditions that are generally thought to be preventable. Two of these likely to occur in less well-developed countries are lathyrism and Konzo. Lathyrism is one of the oldest types of neurotoxicity. It is believed that Hippocrates may have known about this condition as late as 460 BC. An Italian physician described "lathyrismo" in 1873 and Kessler described the condition occurring in Romanian prisoners of war in 1947.[24] This condition is more common in India, Bangladesh, and Ethiopia.

Lathyrism is caused by exposure to a toxic amino acid, beta-N-oxalylamino-L-alanine contained in the grass (chickling) pea, *Lathyrus sativus*. This toxin causes an irreversible, but nonprogressive spastic paraparesis associated with degenerative changes in the spinal cord. The onset is often sudden and the acute phase of the disease may last for a month. Examination shows evidence of an upper motor neuron type of weakness with spasticity and hyperreflexia that causes a spastic gait disorder. Autonomic symptoms may be present with bladder and bowel dysfunction. Subjective sensory symptoms may be present, although objective sensory findings are unusual. The condition can be prevented by avoiding consumption of the pure grass (chickling) pea and combining it with other cereals. The toxin can also be leached out by removing the husks and boiling the peas.[25]

Konzo was described in 1936 by Trolli.[26] Konzo means "tired legs" in the native language. It is caused by consumption of poorly processed cassava that contains cyanide. It most often occurs in various parts of Africa. The onset of symptoms is abrupt with initial complaints of muscle cramps and weakness in the legs. There is evidence of damage to upper motor neurons that result in a spastic paraparesis or quadriparesis. The condition, like lathyrism, is irreversible and nonprogressive. The gait may be affected, leading to frequent falls. There may be visual problems, speech difficulties, and sensory symptoms in the legs. Optic neuropathy occurs in about half of the patients. A smaller number of patients may have ocular motility impairments also.[27]

Diagnosis is based on a history of exposure and measurement of serum thiocyanate levels that serve as a marker for dietary exposure. MRI studies generally have been reported as negative. Somatosensory evoked potentials, however, may show abnormalities, which indicate poor conduction through the spinal cord.[28]

CUBAN MYELONEUROPATHY

An unusual epidemic of optic neuropathy occurred in Cuba between 1992 and 1993 and affected more than 50,000 people. About one-third of those affected developed evidence of peripheral neuropathy, ataxia, hearing loss and dorsal myelopathy. The cause of this epidemic was attributed to malnutrition, although smoking, alcohol, and excessive sugar consumption were identified as risks. Many patients improved with treatment with cobalamin and folate and other B complex vitamins.[29,30]

MYELOPATHY RELATED TO MEDICATIONS, OTHER TOXINS

Various drugs and chemical agents have been described as causative agents for myelopathy and myeloneuropathy. Clioquinol was finally found to be the cause of subacute myelo-optic neuropathy, which was seen primarily in Japan from 1955 to 1970. This drug was used to treat intestinal parasitic diseases. The clinical picture was one of subacute onset of paresthesias in the legs, spastic paraparesis, and optic neuropathy. Examination findings included hyperreflexia and extensor plantar responses. How the drug caused these symptoms is not known; however, because the drug is a copper chelator, it is possible that it induced myelopathy similar to that seen in copper deficiency.[31,32]

Organophosphate poisoning has been reported as a cause of myelopathy and myeloneuropathy.[33] The organophosphates are common components of various pesticides and are available in many home settings. A major chemical that causes these clinical symptoms is triorthocresyl phosphate. This compound has been found as an adulterant in various cooking oils and was also a major contributor to the clinical syndrome caused by exposure to Jamaican ginger that led to an epidemic of toxic neuropathy decades ago.[34] Although this toxin seemed to more commonly cause a neuropathy, it is clear that myelopathic symptoms also occur late in the course of the pathologic state. The nicotinic and muscarinic effects of the acetylcholinesterase inhibitor cause signs and symptoms of acute organophosphate poisoning. These include pinpoint pupils, excessive salivation, generalized weakness, and respiratory collapse. These acute symptoms are best treated with pralidoxime and atropine. Acute intoxication is followed by a latent period of several weeks. A progressive phase may follow, during which patients develop signs and symptoms of motor-sensory neuropathy in the extremities. A stationary phase follows with improvement in neuropathic symptoms. During this phase, there is evidence of spasticity with paraparesis and quadriparesis. MRI at this phase of exposure may reveal evidence of spinal cord atrophy. Somatosensory evoked potentials are often abnormal. Exposure to these toxins results in progressive weakness in the legs that may be associated with sensory symptoms. There can also be involvement of the upper extremities. There is usually some delay in onset after exposure to organophosphates. Measurement of cholinesterase activity in the red blood cells is used to help confirm the diagnosis.[35]

Various cancer chemotherapeutic agents are known to cause myelopathy and neuropathy. Drugs include cisplatin, cladarabine, doxorubicin, vincristine, cytosine arabinoside, and intrathecal methotrexate. Twenty to forty percent of patients treated with cisplatin develop a Lhermitte sign but do not subsequently develop signs of myelopathy. Administration of chemotherapeutic agents intrathecally may increase the incidence of myelopathy related to the agent itself or to preservatives and diluents used in the agents. Radiation myelopathy can be considered as another toxic type of myelopathy. It may occur months to years following irradiation that involves the spinal cord.[36]

Hepatic myelopathy occurs rarely and is characterized by a spastic paraparesis and occasionally sensory symptoms, particularly in those with portosystemic shunts (surgically created or spontaneous).[37] The pathophysiology is unknown but may be related to ammonia or other metabolites bypassing the liver. The myelopathy may also be related to elevated manganese levels. Pathologically, there is evidence of myelin loss in the lateral columns of the spinal cord. There is no particular effective treatment, although some patients seem to improve following liver transplantation.[38]

Myelopathy is known to occur with heroin abuse, by either inhalation or intravenous use.[39] The onset is acute and there is evidence of spinal cord T2-weighted hyperintensities resembling those seen in transverse myelitis.[40] The pathophysiologic mechanism

Table 1
MRI findings of clinical conditions

Clinical Condition	MRI Findings
Vitamin B12 Deficiency Myelopathy	T2 hyperintensities involving posterior and lateral columns, especially cervical and upper thoracic cord, extending over several segments
N2O Intoxication	Very similar to vitamin B12 deficiency
Copper Deficiency Myelopathy	T2 hyperintensities involving posterior columns cervical > thoracic > lumbar. Spinal cord atrophy in severe cases. Brainstem lesions have also been reported
Vitamin E Deficiency	T2-hyperintensitie in posterior columns ± cerebellar atrophy
Heroin-Induced Myelopathy	Cord hyperintensities on T2 and FLAIR affecting posterior and lateral columns, similar lesions in pontomedullary region and in ventral pons; evidence of cord swelling with GAD enhancement resembling transverse myelitis
Organophosphate Poisoning	Atrophy of spinal cord
Hepatic Myelopathy	Increased pallidal signal on T1-weighted cranial MRI; symmetric demyelination of lateral corticospinal tracts, posterior columns and spinocerebellar tracts
Lathyrism, Konzo	No typical MRI findings. SSEPs may be helpful in evaluation

Abbreviations: FLAIR, Fluid-attenuated inversion recovery; GAD, Gadolinium; SSEP, Somatosensory evoked potentials.

Table 2
Causes, tests, and treatments of clinical conditions

Condition	Causes	Useful Tests	Treatment
Vitamin B12	Pernicious anemia, aging, gastric surgery, malabsorption, N2O toxicity, fish tapeworm	Vitamin B12 levels, methylmalonic acid and homocysteine level, hematologic studies, Schilling test, parietal cell antibodies	Intramuscular cobalamin 1000 μg daily × 5 d, monthly afterward
Folate	GI disease, folate antagonists, alcoholism, association with other nutritional deficiencies	Serum folate, RBC folate, plasma total homocysteine	Folate po 1 mg tid for several days followed by 1 mg daily; increase dietary intake of green, leafy vegetables and citrus fruits
Copper	GI surgery especially bariatric surgery, malabsorption, zinc toxicity	Serum and urinary copper, serum ceruloplasmin, zinc levels, hematological tests	Oral copper 8 mg/d × 1 wk, 6 mg/d × 1 wk, 4 mg/d × 1 wk then 2 mg/d
Vitamin E	Chronic cholestasis, pancreatic insufficiency, hypobetalipoproteinemia, abetalipoproteinemia, chylomicron retention disease	Serum vitamin E, ratio of vitamin E to serum cholesterol and triglycerides	Vitamin E 200 mg–1000 mg/d

Abbreviations: GI, gastrointestinal; RBC, red blood cell.

is not known but may be related to vasculitis, direct toxicity, or hypersensitivity reaction. Hypotension related to the drug may possibly result in border-zone infarction in the cord.[41]

SUMMARY

Myelopathy and myeloneuropathy related to metabolic, nutritional, and toxic causes are not rare clinical conditions. Identification of causative deficiencies or excesses and toxic conditions may lead to treatment decisions that will cure, if not arrest the symptoms of these disabling conditions (**Tables 1** and **2**).

Case Report

A 61-year-old woman was seen for evaluation of weakness in her legs for several years by an outside neurologist in 2001. She noted problems with episodic weakness, more in her proximal limbs. At initial neurological evaluation, she had no sensory symptoms. She denied problems affecting her hands and arms. She reported mild pain in her legs that she related to a diagnosis of fibromyalgia. Her health was generally good. She was taking fluoxetine and alprazolam because of a history of bipolar disorder and anxiety. History was important in that she had undergone gastric by-pass surgery twenty years before that evaluation. She had been treated with Vitamin B12 since that surgery along with several other vitamins and supplements. She denied tobacco or alcohol use, exposure to poisons or toxins, and family history of neuromuscular problems. Initially, the results of her neurological examination were normal. She underwent numerous studies including MRI of her entire spinal cord and brain, nerve conduction studies with electromyography, somatosensory-evoked potentials and laboratory studies, the results of which were all reported as normal. No diagnosis was given at that time.

Two years later, she was evaluated at our University neurology clinic, describing progression of her symptoms with worsening of weakness and onset of distal sensory symptoms in her toes and feet. At that time, her gait was unsteady with negative Romberg. Motor and sensory examination results were normal. Reflexes were present, including ankle jerks and plantar responses were flexor. Laboratory studies showed hemoglobin level of 10.6 g, hematocrit of 31.5% and mean corpuscular volume of 105 cubic mm. Vitamin B12 and folate levels were normal. Nerve conduction studies showed evidence of a mild axonal polyneuropathy. Subsequently other laboratory studies, including serum protein electrophoresis with immunofixation, also showed normal results. She underwent marrow biopsy, the results of which showed decreased level of iron stores and she began treatment with iron.

The clinical course showed slow progression with increased difficulties in walking and frequent falls. MRI of her brain and cervical spinal cord were repeated and appeared normal. The result of cerebrospinal fluid examination was normal. She continued to progress as far as her sensory ataxia was concernedwith no demonstrable weakness. Her reflexes remained present and she developed extensor plantar responses.

Repeat laboratory studies failed to show abnormalities. Finally, serum copper and ceruloplasmin levels were measured at 5 μg/dl (N 70-155) and 2.9 μg/dl (N16.2-35.6), respectively. Serum Zinc level was 116 μg/dl (N 70-150). She was treated with supplement copper. Serum copper and ceruloplasmin levels have normalized; however, she continues to have significant sensory ataxia although she no longer is falling.

Comment: This patient was evaluated before the descriptions of SCD caused by copper deficiency. Copper deficiency as a cause of this clinical picture is now well known and measurements of serum copper, ceruloplasmin, and serum zinc levels are often performed routinely.

REFERENCES

1. Leichtenstern O. Progressive perniciose anamie bei tabeskranken. Dtsch Med Wochenschr 1884;10:849–50 [in German].
2. Lichtheim L. Zur kenntniss der perniosen anamie. Munch Med Wochenschr 1887; 34:301–6 [in German].
3. Russell JSR, Batten FE, Collier J. Subacute combined degeneration of the spinal cord. Brain 1900;23:39–110.
4. Kinnier Wilson SA. Neurology. London: Arnold; 1941. p. 1339–58.
5. Healton EB, Savage DG, Brust JC, et al. Neurologic aspects of cobalamin deficiency. Medicine (Baltimore) 1991;70:229–45.
6. Carmel R, Green R, Rosenblatt, et al. Update on cobalamin, folate, and homocysteine. Hematology Am Soc Hematol Educ Program 2003;63:62–81.
7. Green R, Kinsella LJ. Current concepts in the diagnosis of cobalamin deficiency. Neurology 1995;45:1435–40.
8. Larner AJ, Zeman AZ, Allen CM. MRI appearances in subacute combined degeneration of the spinal cord due to vitamin B12 deficiency. J Neurol Neurosurg Psychiatry 1997;62:99–100.
9. Ravina B, Loevner LA, Bank W. MR findings in subacute combined degeneration of the spinal cord: a case of reversible cervical myelopathy. AJR Am J Roentgenol 2000;174:863–5.
10. Layzer RB. Myeloneuropathy after prolonged exposure to nitrous oxide. Lancet 1978;2:1227–30.

11. Kinsella LJ, Green R. "Anesthesia paresthetica:" nitrous oxide-induced cobalamin deficiency. Neurology 1995;45:1608–10.
12. Reynolds EH. Benefits and risks of folic acid to the nervous system. J Neurol Neurosurg Psychiatry 2002;72:567–71.
13. Schleper B, Stuerenburg HJ. Copper deficiency-associated myelopathy in a 46-year-old woman. J Neurol 2001;248:705–6.
14. Kumar N, McEvoy KM, Ahlskog E. Myelopathy due to copper deficiency following gastrointestinal surgery. Arch Neurol 2003;60:1782–5.
15. Greenberg SA, Briemberg HR. A neurological and hematological syndrome associated with zinc excess and copper deficiency. J Neurol 2003;251:111–4.
16. Kumar N, Gross JB, Ahlskog JE. Copper deficiency myelopathy produces a clinical picture like subacute combined degeneration. Neurology 2004;63:33–9.
17. Jaiser SR, Winston GP. Copper deficiency myelopathy. J Neurol 2010;257:869–81.
18. Kumar N, Ahlskog JE, Klein CJ, et al. Imaging features of copper deficiency myelopathy: a study of 25 cases. Neuroradiology 2006;48:78–83.
19. Nations SP, Boyer PJ, Love LA, et al. Denture cream: an unusual source of excess zinc, leading to hypocupremia and neurologic disease. Neurology 2008;71:639–43.
20. Sokol RJ. Vitamin E deficiency and neurologic disease. Annu Rev Nutr 1988;8:351–73.
21. Muller DPR. Vitamin E and neurological function. Mol Nutr Food Res 2010;54:710–8.
22. Vorgerd M, Tegenthoff M, Kuhne D, et al. Spinal MRI in progressive myeloneuropathy associated with vitamin E deficiency. Neuroradiology 1996;38:S111–3.
23. Sokol RJ, Guggenheim MA, Iannaccone ST, et al. Improved neurologic function after long-term correction of vitamin E deficiency in children with chronic cholestasis. N Engl J Med 1985;313:1580–6.
24. Kessler A. Lathrismus. Monatsschrift fur Psychiatre und Neurolgie 1947;113:76–92 [in German].
25. Ludolph AC, Hugon J, Dwivedi MP, et al. Studies on the aetiology and pathogenesis of motor neuron diseases. 1.Lathyrism:clinical findings in established cases. Brain 1987;110:149–65.
26. Trolli G. Paralplegie spastique epidemique., Syndrome aed wmateux, cutane et dyschrimique. Medecins du Foreami 1936;112:1–38 [in French].
27. Howlett WP, Brubaker GR, Mlingi N, et al. Konzo, an epidemic upper motor neuron disease studied in Tanzania. Brain 1990;113:223–35.
28. Nzwalo H, Cliff J. Konzo: from poverty, cassava, and cyanogen intake to toxico-nutritional neurological disease. PLoS Negl Trop Dis 2011;5:e1051.
29. Roman GC. An epidemic in Cuba of optic neuropathy, sensorineural deafness, peripheral sensory neuropathy and dorsolateral myeloneuropathy. J Neurol Sci 1994;127:11–28.
30. Sadun AA, Martone JF, Muci-Mendoza R, et al. Epidemic optic neuropathy in Cuba. Arch Ophthalmol 1994;112:691–9.
31. Mao X, Schimmer AD. The toxicology of clioquinol. Toxicol Lett 2008;182:1–6.
32. Kongaya M, Matsumoto A, Takase S, et al. Clinical analysis of longstanding subacute myelo-optico-neuropathy: sequelae of clioquinol at 32 years after 85-90.y.
33. Thivakaran T, Gamage R, Gunarathne KS, et al. Chlorpyrifos-induced delayed myelopathy and pure motor neuropathy. Neurologist 2012;18:226–8.
34. Morgan JP, Penovich P. Jamaica ginger paralysis: forty-seven year follow-up. Arch Neurol 1978;35:530–2.

35. Chuang CC, Lin TS, Tsai MC. Delayed neuropathy and myelopathy after organo-phosphate intoxication. N Engl J Med 2002;347:1119–21.
36. Schiff D, Wen P. Central nervous system toxicity from cancer therapies. Hematol Oncol Clin North Am 2006;20:1377–98.
37. Campellone JV, Lacomis D, Giuliani MJ, et al. Hepatic myelopathy: a case report with review of the literature. Clin Neurol Neurosurg 1996;98:242–6.
38. Troisi R, Debruyne J, deHemptinne B. Improvement of hepatic myelopathy after liver transplantation. N Engl J Med 1999;340:151.
39. McCreary M, Emerman C, Hanna J, et al. Acute myelopathy following intranasal insufflation of heroin: a case report. Neurology 2000;55:316–7.
40. Nyffeler T, Stabba A, Sturzenegger M. Progressive myelopathy with selective involvement of the lateral and posterior columns after inhalation of heroin vapour. J Neurol 2003;250:496–8.
41. Papadakis SA, Bambourda EC, Papadakis S, et al. Incomplete paraplegia following the use of heroin: a case report and review of the literature. Eur J Orthop Surg Traumatol 2004;14:169–71.

Spinal Cord: Motor Neuron Diseases

Kourosh Rezania, MD*, Raymond P. Roos, MD

KEYWORDS

- Motor neuron diseases • Amyotrophic lateral sclerosis • Spinal cord
- Familial amyotrophic lateral sclerosis

KEY POINTS

- Amyotrophic lateral sclerosis (ALS), which targets upper and lower motor neurons (MNs), is the most common motor neuron disease.
- Clinicians need to be able to differentiate ALS from motor neuron disease mimics by means of the clinical examination, electromyography, imaging, and appropriate laboratory studies.
- ALS is not just a disease of MNs because non-MN cells can have pathological changes (as in the case of frontotemporal dementia) and can also influence disease.
- Approximately 10% of cases of ALS cases are familial (FALS) with mutations in several different genes, including *SOD1, TDP-43, FUS,* and *C9ORF72.*
- An expanded hexanucleotide repeat in *C9ORF72* is the most common cause of FALS and some cases thought to be sporadic ALS.

INTRODUCTION

Motor neuron disease (MND) represents a group of genetic or neurodegenerative diseases that primarily affect the motor neurons (MNs), resulting in progressive paralysis and death. This article starts with an overview of the anatomy of the anterior horn of the spinal cord, followed by the epidemiology, genetics, clinical aspects, pathogenesis, and treatment of MNDs that affect the lower motor neurons (LMNs) of the spinal cord. The focus of the article is amyotrophic lateral sclerosis (ALS), which is the most common type of MND.

ANATOMY OF THE VENTRAL HORN OF THE SPINAL CORD

MNs that innervate the skeletal muscles are located in the ventral horn (lamina IX) of the spinal cord.[1] These neurons are more abundant in the cervical and lumbar cord expansions, where they localize in sharply demarcated regions. The number of MNs

Department of Neurology, University of Chicago Medical Center, 5841 South Maryland Avenue, MC 2030, Chicago, IL 60637, USA
* Corresponding author.
E-mail address: krezania@neurology.bsd.uchicago.edu

Neurol Clin 31 (2013) 219–239
http://dx.doi.org/10.1016/j.ncl.2012.09.014　　　**neurologic.theclinics.com**

decreases significantly after the age of 60.[2] The axial and truncal muscles are innervated by MNs located in the medial part of the ventral horn, whereas the upper and lower limb muscles are innervated by MNs located more laterally.[1] The most posterolaterally located MNs supply the distal hand and foot muscles (**Fig. 1**). Onuf nucleus refers to a group of MNs in the most ventral aspect of the sacral spinal cord (S2-4) that innervate muscles of the pelvic floor, including the striated muscles of the sphincters, through the pudendal nerves. MNs are divided based on the type of cell they innervate: α MNs, which supply the extrafusal myofibers, are larger in size than the neighboring cells (soma size of α MNs is generally >37 μm); γ MNs, which innervate the intrafusal myofibers involved in maintaining muscle tone,[3] are larger in number but smaller in size.

Other cells that reside in the ventral horns and play an important role in the function and viability of MNs include interneurons and glial cells. Renshaw cells are inhibitory interneurons that receive collaterals from adjacent α MNs. They mediate "recurrent inhibition" for the activated α MN they supply and for adjacent MNs through their high-frequency burst discharges.[4,5] Descending pathways of the spinal cord project on to Renshaw cells and affect their firing rate, thus adjusting the sensitivity of MNs to descending inputs. Renshaw cells also make inhibitory connections with inhibitory Ia interneurons, which act on the antagonistic MNs.[6] Glial cells outnumber neurons 10 to 50 times in vertebrates.[7] Astrocytes are involved in the housekeeping and health of MNs, including clearance of potentially excitotoxic glutamate from the synaptic space.[8] Reactive astrocytes are generated in neurodegenerative and inflammatory states and are thought to be involved in limiting inflammation, clearing central nervous system (CNS) debris, and maintaining the blood-brain barrier. Microglial cells are the main immune effector cells of the CNS. Besides being involved in immune surveillance,

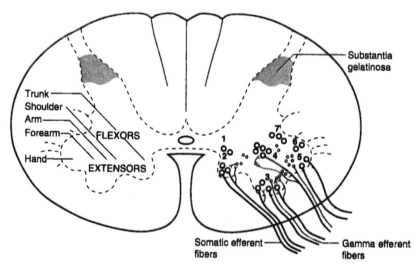

Fig. 1. Cervical spinal cord cross section. On the left side of the figure the location of MNs in the anterior horn innervating different muscle groups of the upper limb and trunk is demonstrated. The MNs innervating the flexors are dorsal to those innervating the extensors. On the right side of the figure, demarcated areas with populations of MNs are shown: 1-posteromedial, 2-anteromedial, 3-anterior, 4-central, 5-anterolateral, and 6-posterolateral. Also note the somatic efferent fibers from MNs have collaterals that innervate Renshaw cells. The efferent fibers innervate the intrafusal fibers. (*From* Parent A, Carpenter MB. Carpenter's human neuroanatomy. 9th edition. Baltimore (MD): Williams & Wilkins; 1996. p. 344, Fig. 10.19; with permission.)

they secrete cytokines and neurotrophins that can have neuroprotective or neurotoxic effects. An important role for oligodendrocytes in the health of MNs has been recently identified.[9]

OVERVIEW OF MNDS

The term MND refers to a group of neurodegenerative diseases that target the LMNs and upper motor neurons (UMNs). MND is either sporadic (ie, secondary to idiopathic degeneration of MNs) or familial, in which case the progressive loss of MNs is caused by a pathogenic mutation. ALS is the most common subtype of MND. At times, ALS is genetic and known as familial ALS (FALS). ALS should be considered a heterogeneous disease from the clinical and pathologic standpoint because involvement of parts of the CNS besides the motor system is not infrequently encountered.

Progressive muscular atrophy (PMA) is characterized by predominantly LMN involvement. It should be noted, however, that pathologic evidence of involvement of the UMNs with corticospinal tract degeneration may be found in patients with PMA, which suggests that PMA may be a subtype of ALS without clinical evidence of UMN involvement.[10,11] Spinal muscular atrophy (SMA) and spinal and bulbar muscular atrophy (SBMA), or Kennedy disease, are two inherited MNDs with pure LMN degeneration. Monomelic amyotrophy (Hirayama disease) is a monophasic illness affecting the LMNs innervating one or both upper extremities, usually in C7/T1 distribution. Primary lateral sclerosis (PLS), which is not discussed further in this article because of its emphasis on spinal cord LMN disorders, is a subtype of MND characterized by pure UMN degeneration.

EPIDEMIOLOGY OF SELECTED MNDS

Sporadic ALS has an incidence of 2 to 3 and prevalence of 2 to 8 per 100,000 ([12] among others), with a significant increase of prevalence after age 60. It is 20% to 60% more common in men than women ([12] among others). A recent meta-analysis suggests a rate of FALS of approximately 5%[13]; however, the prevalence varies from 17% to 23% in prospective studies including active investigations of relatives (reviewed in[14]).

There are several geographic clusters of ALS. Western Pacific ALS was described in Chamorro natives of Guam and the Mariana islands, where it had an incidence of 50 to 100 times greater than the rest of the world.[15] Other hotspots of Western Pacific ALS are the Kii Peninsula of Japan and a small area in western New Guinea.[16] During its peak incidence, the male/female ratio of Western Pacific ALS was 2:1, with a median age of onset of 44.[15,17] More recently, there has been a dramatic decrease in the prevalence of Western Pacific ALS[18] suggesting that there may have been exposure to an environmental toxin that is no longer present in a population with a genetic predisposition for the disease. Excessive consumption on Guam during World War II of the neurotoxin β-N-methylamino-l-alanine, which is present in seeds of the *Cycas circinalis*, has been proposed as a cause[19,20]; however, it is unlikely that a neurotoxic amount of β-N-methylamino-l-alanine could have been ingested from eating these seeds. More recently, it has been hypothesized that a sufficiently high concentration of β-N-methylamino-l-alanine was obtained by the Chamorros' ingestion of bats, a favorite food, because the bats feed on the cycads and can thereby concentrate it. Bats are no longer prevalent on Guam, a potential explanation for the decrease in the incidence of ALS.[19,21] This hypothesis needs to be proven, and the possibility that genetics explains the disease clusters remains (discussed later).

SMA is the most common autosomal-recessive neuromuscular disease and the most common cause of floppy infant syndrome. A recent study showed a carrier frequency of 1 in 54 and an incidence of 1 in 11,000 in the United States.[22] The incidence and prevalence of SBMA have been estimated at 3.3 per 100,000 for the male population.[23] Most of the cases of Hirayama disease are reported in Japan, where the peak age of onset ranges from 15 to 17 years.[24]

GENETICS OF SELECTED MNDS

Knowledge of the pathogenesis of ALS has significantly increased through the identification of mutations that cause FALS. The most common inheritance pattern of FALS is autosomal-dominant with complete penetrance; however, an autosomal-dominant pattern with incomplete penetrance, autosomal-recessive, and X-linked pattern have also been reported.[14]

Cu/Zn superoxide dismutase 1 (*SOD1*) was the first gene identified as a cause of FALS and the most extensively studied to date. SOD1 mutations account for approximately 20% of FALS cases[25] (reviewed in[14]). Some FALS cases were subsequently found to be caused by mutations in two RNA binding proteins, TAR DNA-binding protein-43 (TDP-43) and fused in sarcoma (FUS). More recently, expansions of a GGGGCC hexanucleotide repeat in a noncoding region of chromosome 9 open reading frame 72 (*C9ORF72*) has been identified as the most frequent cause of FALS.[26,27] The latter expansion is present in 37% to 46% of FALS and 6% to 20% of sporadic ALS of European descent.[26–28] Other causes of FALS include mutations in alsin, angiogenin, senataxin, optineurin, ubiquilin 2, VAMP-associated protein type B, polyphosphoinositide phosphatase, and valosin-containing protein. It should be noted that incomplete penetrance in many pedigrees has been associated with the previously mentioned genes.

There are more than 100 genes that have been reported to impact the risk of sporadic ALS or its course (http://alsod.iop.kcl.ac.uk/). For example, intermediate-length polyglutamine expansions in ATXN2 gene were detected in 4.7% of ALS cases unselected for family history versus 1.4% of normal control subjects.[29] Furthermore, it was shown that ATXN-2 can modify the MN toxicity of TDP-43.[29] An abnormally low number of copies of survival of motor neuron 1 (*SMN1*) gene has been associated with ALS.[30] *Epha4*, which encodes a receptor in the ephrin axonal repellent system, has been shown to affect the survival in MND and SMA.[31]

Mutations in transient receptor potential melastatin 2 (*TRPM2*) have been suggested to play a role in the pathogenesis of Western Pacific ALS.[32] TRPM2 encodes a calcium-permeable cation channel that is highly expressed in the brain. Inactivation of the channel by the mutation results in decreased intracellular Ca^{2+}, which is postulated to result in neurodegeneration through downstream signaling pathways.[32]

SMA is an autosomal-recessive disease that results from deletions of the telomeric *SMN1* gene in about 95% to 98% of patients. The remainder of SMA cases is caused by small intragenic mutations or mutations that convert SMN1 to SMN2 by disrupting exon 7.[33] The *SMN2* gene differs from *SMN1* by a single nucleotide, leading to alternative splicing, so that only 10% of *SMN2* transcripts code for full length functional SMN protein. The number of copies of *SMN2* per chromosome varies among normal individuals, from no copies in 10% to 15% of the population to five in most normal individuals.[33,34] The number of *SMN2* copies correlates with the severity of phenotype of patients with SMA. A total of 95% to 100% of the most severely affected patients with SMA with early onset (SMA 1 patients) have one or two copies of *SMN2*, whereas at least three copies of *SMN2* are present in SMA 3 patients.[35]

SBMA is an X-linked disease caused by an expansion of a trinucleotide CAG repeat, which encodes a polyglutamine tract in the first exon of the androgen receptor gene.[36]

CLINICAL MANIFESTATIONS OF SELECTED MNDS

ALS usually runs a relentlessly progressive course, resulting in death because of respiratory failure, typically 2 to 3 years after onset.[37] The onset of ALS peaks between the ages of 50 and 75, although the onset could be in the 20s (and rarely earlier) and in the 80s. The clinical manifestations of ALS are mainly secondary to dysfunction of UMNs and LMNs (**Table 1**). Muscle atrophy, fasciculations, hyperreflexia, and pathologic reflexes (including a hyperactive jaw jerk) are usually present, in the absence of ptosis, ocular motor abnormalities, and sensory impairment. In some cases, UMN signs may be lacking, even in the advanced stages of the disease.[38] In other cases, UMN involvement may be the most prominent feature of ALS, especially early in the course of the disease, making it difficult to differentiate from PLS.

The initial symptoms usually appear in a limb, and can progress in a segmental pattern. For example, if a lower limb is initially involved, the contralateral lower limb or ipsilateral upper limb is usually the next to be affected. It is speculated that UMN and LMN loss progresses along contiguous three-dimensional anatomic planes because of a self-propagated seeded aggregation reminiscent of a prion disease, in which spread occurs to neighboring neurons and glial cells.[39,40] A bulbar onset of symptoms occurs in 20% to 30% of the patients, usually in older women.[16,41] In a minority of cases ALS begins with progressive respiratory insufficiency secondary to involvement of LMNs that innervate the diaphragm and other respiratory muscles.[42,43] All cases of ALS that live long enough eventually develop involvement of the bulbar and respiratory muscles, resulting in death unless mechanical ventilation is used. At times, especially with an initial bulbar onset, the course of ALS may be rapid, with survival less than 1 year after the diagnosis. Bladder and bowel function is usually spared even in the advanced stages of ALS, presumably because the degree of neurodegeneration in the MNs of Onuf nucleus is less severe than in other MNs.[44] Similarly, extraocular muscle involvement is usually not clinically apparent except in patients on long term mechanical ventilation.[45]

Sporadic ALS and FALS can differ in some respects. The mean age of onset of high-penetrance *SOD1* mutations is 46 to 47 and the weakness more frequently starts in the lower limbs.[14] A4V, the most common *SOD1* mutation in the United States, is associated with an especially rapid course of progression.[46] However, some of the other mutations such as D90A, which is recessively inherited and the most common *SOD1* mutation in some European countries, are usually associated with a slower course and longer survival.[14,46] The age of onset is slightly younger in patients with high-penetrant *FUS* mutations and older with TDP-43 mutations than with *SOD1* mutations.[14,47,48] Bulbar-onset ALS and onset in upper limbs are more often encountered in patients with FUS and TDP-43 mutations respectively than in sporadic ALS. In addition, patients with *FUS* mutations tend to have a shorter survival.[47,48] ALS cases with an

Table 1	
Clinical features of UMN and LMN dysfunction	
UMN	**LMN**
Weakness	Weakness
Slowed rapid alternating movements	Muscle atrophy
Spasticity, clasp knife phenomenon	Fasciculations
Hyperreflexia	Cramps
Pathologic reflexes, including Babinski and Hoffmann	Attenuated or absent reflexes
Presence of reflexes in atrophic limbs	Bulbar palsy
Pseudobulbar palsy (labile affect, spastic speech, dysarthria, brisk jaw jerk, and gag reflex)	

expanded hexanucleotide repeat in *C9ORF72* have an earlier mean age of onset compared with those without the repeat (56–59 vs 61–62 years old); shorter survival (20 vs 26 months); and more frequent family history of dementia and parkinsonism.[28,49]

Although ALS is primarily a disease of MNs, other regions of the nervous system, such as the frontal and temporal cortex, autonomic system, sensory tracts, and basal ganglia, can be affected. This is evident in the case of ALS-frontotemporal dementia (ALS-FTD), in which there is significant impairment in cognitive functions and behavior because of degeneration of nonmotor cortex along with MN involvement. The finding that the same genes that cause FALS can lead to ALS and ALS-FTD and FTD in individuals within the same pedigree or in different pedigrees supports the close relationship of these disorders. Impairment of cognition, including apathy, irritability, disinhibition, and restlessness can occur in up to 50% of ALS-FTD cases with one of eight patients exhibiting clear FTD.[50,51] Impaired word finding consistent with FTD is found in one-third of patients with ALS.[52] Involvement of cortical and extrapyramidal systems is also seen in Western Pacific ALS leading to varied clinical syndromes: ALS, a combined parkinsonism-dementia complex, or a combination of ALS, Parkinsonism and dementia.[53]

SMA is categorized on the basis of the age of onset and the maximum motor function achieved: the onset of disease in SMA 0 is in utero; SMA 1 (Werdnig-Hoffmann disease) has onset from birth to 6 months; SMA 2 (Kugelberg-Welander syndrome), 3, and 4 have onset at 3 to 15 months, 15 months to the teenage years, and adult onset (mean age, 37 years), respectively (reviewed in[54]). SMA 0 and 1 present with hypotonia, problems with sucking and breathing, and inability to sit, with survival of less than 2 years when there is no mechanical ventilation. SMA 2 patients are not able to walk, whereas types 3 and 4 lose their ability to walk later in life. Other symptoms of SMA 2, 3, and 4 include proximal greater than distal muscle weakness, tremors, and fasciculations. Respiratory muscle weakness may occur in the later stages as a result of weakness of intercostal muscles, whereas diaphragm, facial, and bulbar muscles remain relatively spared. Reflexes are typically attenuated or absent.

SBMA has an onset between 30 and 60 years in males. The initial symptoms consist of postural tremors, fasciculations, muscle cramps, and weakness of facial and bulbar muscles, that is frequently manifest as a nasal voice and dysphagia. The disease course is slowly progressive with loss of ambulation usually 15 to 20 years after the onset.[55] Weakness is usually more severe in proximal than distal limb muscles. Respiratory tract infection secondary to aspiration is often the terminal event; however, patients can have a normal life expectancy.[55] Patients can have elevated creatine kinase (CK) and mild distal sensory loss. The extraocular and sphincter muscles are spared. Other symptoms that arise from androgen insensitivity include diabetes, glucose intolerance, gynecomastia, testicular atrophy, and erectile dysfunction.[56] Female carriers are usually asymptomatic, but may have high CK, hypertension, dyslipidemia, glucose intolerance, and bulbar muscle weakness (later in life).

Monomelic amyotrophy is a pure LMN syndrome, usually starting between age 15 and 25 with a progression that generally lasts less than 5 years.[53] The disorder can occur unilaterally or bilaterally. At times a similar process can affect the lower limbs.[53,57] Imaging studies including cervical spinal MRI with flexion and extension views are important to rule out structural lesions. The typically normal imaging studies in cases of monomelic amyotrophy suggest that it may represent a benign, focal form of MND.[58,59]

WORK-UP AND DIFFERENTIAL DIAGNOSIS OF MND

Several diagnostic criteria have been proposed for ALS, based on the presence of UMN signs and evidence for acute and chronic denervation in the electromyography

(EMG) (**Table 2**). EMG signs of denervation include fibrillations, positive sharp waves, fasciculations, neurogenic units, and a neurogenic pattern of recruitment. The EMG can also be helpful in differentiating ALS from mimics. Nerve conduction studies are usually normal or show diminished amplitude of compound motor action potentials.

Genetic testing can expedite the diagnosis in selected cases of familial or sporadic MND. Commercial testing is available for most of the genetic causes of FALS. Genetic testing for FALS should be considered in patients with a family history of ALS, cognitive and behavioral impairment, or unexplained neurodegenerative disease, but is generally not recommended for typical cases of sporadic ALS, at least partly because of the cost versus benefit. In cases with pure LMN involvement or phenotypic features of SMA or SBMA, genetic testing for SMN and androgen receptor mutations should be considered. In these cases, it is important to differentiate ALS from the less common MNDs (SMBA, SMA, and monomelic amyotrophy) because of the different prognoses and potential implication for family members.

ALS should be differentiated from other diseases that cause weakness, fasciculations, muscle atrophy, and UMN signs (**Tables 3** and **4**). The most common mimics of ALS are compressive myelopathy (especially myeloradiculopathy caused by

Table 2
Diagnostic criteria for ALS

Revised El Escorial Criteria[83]	Awaji Criteria[84] (Proposed to Increase the Sensitivity of Revised El Escorial Criteria for Early Diagnosis of ALS)
To make a diagnosis of ALS, there should be clinical or electrophysiologic evidence of progression within a region or to other regions as well as exclusion of ALS mimics by EMG, appropriate imaging, and laboratory studies Definite ALS • UMN and LMN signs* in three regions** Probable ALS • UMN and LMN signs in two regions with some UMN signs rostral to LMN signs Probable laboratory-supported ALS • UMN and LMN signs, or only UMN signs in one region with evidence by EMG of denervation in two regions Possible ALS • UMN and LMN signs in one region or UMN signs in at least two regions * LMN degeneration with muscle denervation is demonstrated by the finding on EMG of: fibrillations; positive waves; large, long duration polyphasic motor units; unstable and complex motor units; and reduced recruitment ** LMN degeneration in lumbar and cervical regions is defined by the presence of denervation in two muscles innervated by two different nerves and nerve roots. LMN degeneration is defined by the presence of denervation in only one muscle in the thoracic and cranial regions	Definite ALS • Clinical or electrophysiologic evidence of LMN *** and UMN signs in the bulbar region and at least two spinal regions or the presence of LMN and UMN signs in three spinal regions Probable ALS • Clinical or electrophysiologic evidence by LMN and UMN signs in at least two regions with some UMN signs necessarily rostral to (above) the LMN signs Possible ALS • Clinical or electrophysiologic signs of UMN and LMN dysfunction are in only one region, or UMN signs alone in two or more regions, or LMN signs rostral to UMN signs ALS mimics should be excluded by EMG, appropriate neuroimaging, and clinical laboratory studies *** EMG evidence for denervation has equal value to clinical LMN signs; when there is clinical suspicion for ALS, fasciculations have equivalent value to fibrillations and positive waves in determining denervation

Table 3
MND mimics with UMN signs

Disease	Distinguishing Features
• Spondylosis	Pain and sensory signs frequent; MRI abnormalities
• Multiple sclerosis	Sensory signs frequent; MRI lesions, CSF oligoclonal bands
• Sarcoidosis	Systemic involvement (eg, lung, lymph node, eye, skin)
• Vasculitis, collagen vascular disease	Serology (ANCA), imaging studies
• HTLV-1 and -2 myelopathy	Slowly progressive spastic paraparesis with sensory loss and sphincter symptoms. HTLV-1 and -2 antibody
• Adrenomyeloneuropathy[85]	Spastic paraparesis, sphincter impairment, polyneuropathy with slow tempo; high levels of VLCFA, *ABCD1* genotyping
• Prion diseases, especially the amyotrophic form of Creutzfeldt-Jakob disease[86–88]	Nonmotor signs, especially myoclonus and rapidly evolving dementia, are usually prominent; abnormal EEG
• Hereditary spastic paraparesis[89]	Pure UMN syndrome, positive family history, exclusion of other causes of myelopathy, genetic testing (can be AD, AR, and X linked); SPG4 is the most common subtype and accounts for 50% of AD cases; SPG 11 the most common AR type; SPG 11, 17, and 31 are associated with hand amyotrophy
• Neurolymphomatosis	CSF analysis, nerve root enhancement on the MRI, lymphomatous infiltration in nerve biopsy
• Radiation-induced radiculomyelopathy	History of radiation treatment, presence of myokymic discharges on EMG
• Lyme disease	Lyme antibody, CSF pleocytosis
• Polyglucosan body disease[90]	Polyglucosan bodies in nerve or muscle biopsy, GBE1 genotyping, sensory loss, ± neurogenic bladder, cognitive dysfunction, extrapyramidal disease

Abbreviations: AD, autosomal dominant; ANCA, antineutrophil cytoplasmic antibodies; AR, autosomal recessive; CSF, cerebrospinal fluid; GBE, glycogen brancher enzyme; HTLV, Human T-lymphotropic virus; VLCFA, very long chain fatty acids.

cervical spondylosis); motor neuropathy or neuronopathy (especially multifocal motor neuropathy or a paraneoplastic syndrome); polyradiculopathy (especially chronic inflammatory demyelinating polyradiculoneuropathy); diseases of the neuromuscular junction (myasthenia gravis and Eaton-Lambert syndrome); and myopathies (especially inclusion body myositis). Differentiation can usually be made because MND mimics are frequently associated with pain, sensory impairment, ocular motor abnormalities, or bladder or bowel involvement. It is essential to obtain imaging studies (preferably MRIs) of the highest level of involvement: brain for cases with bulbar involvement, and cervical spine for upper limb involvement. This is mainly to exclude the mimics rather than to provide confirmation of the diagnosis of ALS.

Viral infections that cause lower motor neuronopathy (West Nile virus, poliovirus, and nonpolio enteroviruses, such as enterovirus 71) are distinguished from LMN forms

Table 4
MND mimics with LMN but not UMN signs

Motor Neuronopathy	Neuropathy- Radiculopathy	Nerve Hyperexcitability	Neuromuscular Junction Diseases	Myopathy

• Acute viral diseases
  ○ Poliomyelitis
  ○ Enterovirus 71[91]
  ○ WNV
• Postpolio syndrome
• Hexosaminidase A deficiency (adult-onset Tay-Sachs)[92]
• Paraneoplastic motor neuronopathy[60,61]
	• Multifocal motor neuropathy
	• Guillain-Barré syndrome
	• CIDP and its variants
	• POEMS
	• Porphyria
	• Lead intoxication
	• Amyloidosis
	• Polyglucosan body disease (it can involve LMNs or present as a myopathy)
		• Benign fasciculations
		• Fasciculation cramp syndrome
		• Isaacs syndrome
		• Morvan syndrome
			• Myasthenia gravis (including muscle-specific kinase antibody related myasthenia)
			• LEMS
			• Botulism
			• Congenital myasthenia
				• Sporadic inclusion body myositis
				• Familial inclusion body myositis
				• Chronic polymyositis
				• Myofibrillar myopathy
				• Nemaline rod disease
				• Polyglucosan body disease
				• Amyloidosis
				• Congenital myopathies

Abbreviations: CIDP, chronic inflammatory demyelinating polyneuropathy; LEMS, Lambert-Eaton myasthenic syndrome; MG, myasthenia gravis; POEMS, polyneuropathy, organomegaly, endocrinopathy, monoclonal gammopathy, and skin changes; WNV, West Nile virus.

of MND because they have an acute onset. West Nile CNS infection has emerged as a not infrequent cause of LMN dysfunction in the United States. Cerebrospinal fluid studies including serologic tests (specially spinal fluid IgM antibody against the virus), and polymerase chain reaction testing are used to diagnose the latter conditions. Postpolio syndrome, especially postpolio syndrome, is a pure LMN neuronopathy characterized by late-onset weakness with progressive atrophy of limbs that were affected by prior poliomyelitis. In contrast to ALS, postpolio syndrome has no UMN signs, is slowly progressive, and tends to have a relatively benign course. Adult-onset hexosaminidase A deficiency can present with proximal weakness, however, some cases may have spasticity, hyperreflexia, cognitive, psychiatric, cerebellar, and extrapyramidal features. Diagnosis is made by hexosaminidase A enzymatic assay. A self-limited, subacute motor neuronopathy has been reported in association with an underlying lymphoma.[60] These paraneoplastic motor neuronopathies can be associated with antibodies to Hu and Yo.[61,62] As a result of these associations, serum protein immunoelectrophoresis/immunofixation and a paraneoplastic antibody profile are not infrequently part of the work-up of patients with MND. Imaging studies (including positron emission tomography) to detect an underlying lymphoma or carcinoma should be considered in selected cases, including those with seropositivity to paraneoplastic autoantibodies.

Other categories of MND mimics include polyradiculopathies and neuropathies. Similar to ALS multifocal motor neuropathy usually presents with asymmetric limb onset weakness and fasciculations without sensory impairment. Multifocal motor neuropathy usually targets hand muscles. Muscle atrophy can be rather mild even when severe weakness is present, and UMN signs are usually not present. Multifocal motor neuropathy can be differentiated from ALS based on of the presence of conduction blocks on nerve conduction study and, in some cases, antibodies to GM1. Other neuropathies that may mimic ALS include chronic inflammatory demyelinating polyradiculoneuropathy and POEMS syndrome (polyneuropathy, organomegaly, endocrinopathy, monoclonal gammopathy, and skin changes); however, in contrast to ALS, these condition have a demyelinating range of slowing on nerve conduction studies. A nerve biopsy is often necessary to diagnose polyglucosan body disease or amyloidosis. Repetitive nerve stimulation and measurement of acetylcholine receptor binding antibodies, muscle-specific kinase antibodies, and P/Q calcium channel antibodies help differentiate a neuromuscular junction disease from MND. Measurement of CK may help differentiate a myopathy from ALS; however, an elevation of CK three to four times normal is frequently reported in ALS cases, with occasional elevations more than 1000 U/L. Higher levels of CK (up to eight times normal) can be seen in SBMA.[63] CK is often normal in patients with inclusion body myositis, one of the most common ALS mimics. A muscle biopsy should be considered if the CK is markedly elevated or if myopathic motor units are present on needle EMG. A nerve hyperexcitability syndrome is differentiated from MND based on the lack of significant muscle weakness, the presence of neuromyotonic and myokymic discharges on needle EMG, and seropositivity to antibodies to voltage-gated potassium channel in some cases.

PATHOLOGY AND PATHOGENESIS OF MND

Autopsy tissue from ALS demonstrates: a loss of MNs; astrocytosis of the motor cortex, brainstem, and spinal cord; secondary degeneration and atrophy of the pyramidal tracts and anterior roots; secondary neurogenic atrophy of skeletal muscles.[64,65] Although the pathology predominantly affects the motor system, it often involves other systems, such as frontal and temporal cortex. Evidence of degeneration of long tracts of the spinal cord besides the lateral and anterior pyramidal tracts has been reported in some cases of FALS.[66] As in the case with other neurodegenerative diseases, MNs of patients with ALS can display intracellular aggregates that form inclusion bodies (**Table 5**).

Table 6 summarizes the proposed pathogenicity of some of the more common genetic causes of MND. Wild-type SOD1 is an intracellular antioxidant involved in the clearance of toxic superoxide free radicals. More than 100 different mutations in *SOD1* account for about 20% of the familial cases (http://alsod.iop.kcl.ac.uk/misc/FAQs.aspx). Several transgenic mice have been produced that express different FALS-associated mutant SOD1s and develop ALS. Studies of these transgenic mice have shown that MND in these mice is primarily caused by a toxic gain of function of the mutant SOD1, rather than reduced enzymatic activity. Several pathogenic features seem to be at play resulting in MN degeneration including oxidative damage; glutamate excitotoxicity; intracellular aggregates of misfolded proteins; mitochondrial dysfunction; and abnormalities in axonal transport, neurotrophic factors, and RNA processing (reviewed in[67]). Although the toxicity of mutant SOD1 is not fully understood, misfolding and aggregation is generally thought to underlie the basis for MN degeneration. Aggregates of mutant SOD1 could cause toxicity by sequestering SOD1-binding proteins that are critical for viability of the MN or by exposing a toxic domain of SOD1. The expression of mutant SOD1 in non-MN cells, such as astrocytes, microglia, and oligodendrocytes, as well as MNs have an influence on the onset and progression of the

Table 5 Inclusion bodies in MND		
Type of Inclusion	**Cellular Location**	**Characteristics**
Ubiquinated inclusions[93,94]	Cell bodies or dendrites of LMNs Also in hippocampus and cerebral cortex in ALS-FTD	Contains ubiquitin and may contain dorfin, TDP-43, ubiquilin 2, FUS, optineurin, (contains SOD1 in *SOD1* mutations) Intracytoplasmic, fibrillary (skein-like) inclusions, compact inclusions, and Lewy body–like inclusions Highly sensitive and specific for ALS
Bunina bodies[95]	LMNs, other neurons (eg, STN, RF)	Eosinophilic, possible lysosomal origin
Hyaline conglomerates	LMNs, rarely Betz cells	NF proteins and SOD1 Pale, hyaline appearance, argyrophilic Only seen in cases of mutant SOD1-induced FALS
Basophilic inclusions	MNs, basal ganglia, thalamus, cerebellum	± ubiquitin Frequent in some cases of juvenile-onset ALS
Spheroids	Large inclusions in proximal part of axons of the LMNs	Phosphorylated heavy, light, and medium NFs; negative or subtle staining for ubiquitin Not specific for ALS

Abbreviations: NF, neurofilament; RF, reticular formation; STN, sub-thalamic nucleus.

Table 6
Mutated genes that cause MNDs

Gene (Encoded Protein)	Phenotype, (Target Cells)	Suggested Mechanism
SOD1 (Cu/Zn superoxide dismutase)	ALS (LMN, UMN, can be LMN predominant)	Mitochondrial toxicity of misfolded mutant SOD1 in MNs and astrocytes,[67,96,97] abnormalities of axonal transport,[98] malfunction of the astrocytic EAAT2 transporter resulting in impaired reuptake of glutamate with resultant excitotoxicity,[67] endoplasmic reticulum dysfunction in responding to misfolded proteins (endoplasmic reticulum stress),[99,100] paradoxical increase of extracellular superoxide radicals, resulting in oxidative stress, through the activation of NADPH oxidase (Nox) pathway.[101]
C9ORF72 (unknown)[26,102,103]	ALS, ALS-FTD, FTD (LMN, UMN)	Abnormal RNA produced as a result of pathogenic expanded repeat could cause neurotoxicity because of a loss in function or because of disruption of transcription or splicing/processing of mRNAs (due to sequestration of RNA-binding proteins).
TARDBP (TDP-43)[71,104]	ALS, ALS-FTD, FTD	Abnormal cytoplasmic accumulation and loss of normal nuclear localization of TDP-43 in neurons and glia of UMNs and LMNs, neocortex, and hippocampus. MN toxicity could be caused by a loss of function of nuclear TDP-43 causing abnormalities in RNA splicing and messenger RNA processing or a gain of function caused by cytoplasmic aggregation, or a combination of both.

(continued on next page)

Table 6
(continued)

Gene (Encoded Protein)	Phenotype, (Target Cells)	Suggested Mechanism
FUS (FUS/TLS)[104]	ALS (LMN, UMN), ALS-FTD	Inclusions immunoreactive for FUS in neuronal and glial cells. Neurotoxicity could be the result of a toxic gain-of-function, a loss-of-function mechanism by depletion of physiologic FUS, or a combination of both.
SMN gene[72] (SMN)	SMA (LMN)	SMN is involved in the formation of snRNP complexes, which are important for pre-mRNA splicing. Lack of SMN function results in altered snRNP structures and abnormal splicing of RNA with resultant MN toxicity. SMN's interaction with RNA binding proteins is important in localization and transport of mRNA in MNs. Lack of function of SMN results in disturbance of protein synthesis in MN axons and synapses.
Androgen receptor (androgen receptor)[103,105]	SBMA, Kennedy disease (LMN, DRG)	Abnormal polyglutamate aggregates could cause altered function through aberrant protein interactions, transcriptional dysregulation, mitochondrial dysfunction, RNA toxicity, impaired axonal transport, and excitotoxicity.

Abbreviation: snRNP, small nuclear ribonucleoproteins.

disease in mutant SOD1 mice. Of note, abnormalities of the structure and function of wild-type SOD1 have been described in sporadic ALS suggesting that abnormalities in SOD1 may be a final common pathway in the sporadic and familial disease.[68]

TDP-43 is a nuclear factor that functions in regulating transcription and alternative splicing of RNA.[69,70] The importance of TDP-43 in ALS was brought home by studies that showed that all cases of sporadic ALS have TDP-43 cytoplasmic inclusions.[71] In contrast, ALS cases secondary to mutant SOD1 have cytoplasmic aggregates of ubiquitinated SOD1 in neural cells without TDP-43, suggesting that mutant SOD1-induced FALS ALS has a different pathophysiology than sporadic ALS, and that the response of mutant SOD1 FALS transgenic mouse to treatment may not predict the response in sporadic ALS. It may be that the displacement of TDP-43 from the nucleus of neural cells in patients with ALS triggers a loss in function with respect to its interactions with RNA (eg, splicing) as well as a toxic gain in function. The hexanucleotide expanded repeat found in the noncoding region of C9ORF72 may induce FALS because of "toxicity" of RNA or because of a loss in function. The toxicity of this expanded region of the RNA may at least partly be related to sequestration of RNA-binding proteins, as seems to be the case in myotonic dystrophy. The importance of TDP-43, FUS, and the expanded hexanucleotide repeat of *C9ORF72* in FALS (and SMN in SMA) has focused investigators on the role of RNA in MND pathogenesis. SMA is caused by loss of function of SMN, which is present in the cytoplasm and nucleus of all cells and plays a critical role in pre-mRNA splicing (see **Table 6**).[72] SBMA is caused by an expansion of a trinucleotide CAG repeat, which encodes a polyglutamine tract in the first exon of the androgen receptor gene located on chromosome Xq12–21.[36] The normal CAG repeat number is 17 to 26, whereas the disease is associated with 40 to 52 repeats. An increasing number of repeats is associated with earlier onset and more severe disease.[36,73] Inclusions containing the amino-terminal of the polyglutamine-expanded androgen receptor accumulate in the nucleus of LMNs and dorsal root ganglia, resulting in neuronal death.[74]

TREATMENT

Riluzole is the only medication that has been shown to be effective in ALS; however, its effect is relatively small. Administration of riluzole, 50 mg twice a day, improves 1-year survival by about 15% and prolongs overall survival by 2 to 3 months (reviewed in[75,76]). The prolongation of survival may be more significant if riluzole is started early in the course of the disease. Although some patients with PMA and PLS may benefit from riluzole, the efficacy of riluzole in these conditions has not been proven.[75]

The cornerstones of symptomatic treatment of ALS include walking assists, management of respiratory impairment, nutritional support, treatment of sialorrhea, and palliative care. Although FVC is the most commonly used respiratory parameter, maximal inspiratory pressure, sniff nasal pressure, supine FVC, and nocturnal oximetry are more sensitive than FVC in detecting early respiratory impairment in ALS.[77] Elevated serum bicarbonate and low serum chloride in the setting of respiratory symptoms may predict the occurrence of respiratory failure.[76] Early institution of noninvasive positive pressure ventilation probably improves survival and slows the rate of decline of the FVC.[78] **Box 1** summarizes the indications of noninvasive positive

---

Box 1
Indications for starting noninvasive positive pressure ventilation in ALS[75,76]

Any of the following symptoms or signs of respiratory muscle weakness:

- Shortness of breath (dyspnea, tachypnea, orthopnea, use of accessory respiratory muscles at rest)
- Nocturnal arousals
- Excessive daytime drowsiness and fatigue
- Morning headache
- Paradoxic respiration

AND

Any of the following abnormalities on respiratory function tests:

- FVC <80% of predicted value
- Sniff nasal pressure <40 cm H_2O
- Maximal inspiratory pressure <60 mm H_2O
- Nocturnal desaturation <90% for more than 1 cumulative minute on overnight oximetry
- Morning blood gas P_{CO_2} >45 mm Hg

pressure ventilation in ALS.[75,76] More recently, diaphragm pacing has been used in selected patients with ALS with moderately impaired respiratory function and viable phrenic nerves and diaphragm as determined by nerve conduction study, fluoroscopy, or ultrasonography (reviewed in[79]). Ongoing studies are being conducted to assess the efficacy of diaphragm pacing in improving quality of life and survival in patients with ALS. Another measure that is thought to improve survival and quality of life in patients with ALS is percutaneous endoscopic gastrostomy. Because the percutaneous endoscopic gastrostomy procedure has a higher complication rate when significant respiratory impairment is present, it should preferably be done when the FVC is greater than 50% predicted.[75–77] Other parameters that determine the timing of percutaneous endoscopic gastrostomy include the presence of bulbar symptoms, weight loss of more than 10%, and the patient's general condition.

Some of the promising treatment approaches to MND include stem cell transplantation and methods to lower the level of pathogenic RNAs. MN cell transplantation faces the difficulty of making appropriate and functional connections to target muscles. Therefore, transplantation of precursor neural cells seems to be a more realistic approach to prevent surviving MNs from degeneration because of their supportive and trophic effect (reviewed in[80]). Antisense oligonucleotides and RNA interference have been proposed or are being used to knock down SOD1 or

---

Case study

A 46 year old developed weakness of the right hand with difficulty buttoning 6 years after a cervical spinal fusion. She had no sensory symptoms or pain. The family history was significant for dementia in a grandmother. An MRI of the cervical spine showed postoperative changes, but no nerve root compression or central spinal stenosis. She initially underwent carpal and cubital tunnel release 8 months later with no improvement. She then developed progressive weakness in the left hand, weakness of the right arm, difficulty rising from a chair, and muscle twitching and occasional cramping in the extremities and trunk. On examination, the cranial nerves were normal, except for a brisk jaw jerk. Moderate weakness, muscle atrophy, and frequent fasciculations were noted in multiple muscle groups of both arms. No significant weakness was present in the lower limbs but the muscle tone was increased. Reflexes were diffusely brisk and the Hoffmann reflex was present bilaterally. Nerve conduction study showed normal sensory nerve action potentials. The amplitudes of the right median and ulnar motor nerve action potentials were reduced with mildly slowed conduction velocities, and slight prolongation of distal and F wave latencies. Needle EMG demonstrated widespread denervation and fasciculations in all muscles tested in the upper and lower limbs and thoracic paraspinal muscles. Serum protein immunoelectrophoresis and serologic testing for Lyme disease, collagen vascular disease, vasculitis, and paraneoplastic antibody panel antibodies were negative.

A diagnosis of ALS was made based on the history of progressive weakness and clinical evidence of UMN involvement and LMN signs, with fasciculations in the upper limbs and EMG demonstration of widespread denervation involving three myotomes. ALS mimics (specially cervical radiculomyelopathy) were excluded with appropriate imaging and laboratory tests. A genetic test was not performed, but could have been considered because the age of onset was earlier than typical ALS and there was a family history of dementia.

Riluzole was started after the diagnosis of ALS was made. During the next 2 years, the patient developed progressive dysphagia, dysarthria, and deteriorating respiratory muscle weakness. A percutaneous endoscopic gastrostomy was placed, and she was started on noninvasive positive pressure ventilation. Diaphragm pacing was started about 3 years after the onset of symptoms. One year later palliative care was instituted. The patient died of complications of progressive respiratory insufficiency 5 years after the onset of symptoms and 2 years after diaphragm pacing had been started.

C9ORF72 expression or alter the splicing of SMN2 (reviewed in[81]). Other treatment approaches for SMA include strategies to activate *SMN2* gene expression or stabilize SMN protein (reviewed in[82]).

REFERENCES

1. Parent A, Carpenter MB. Carpenter's human neuroanatomy. 9th edition. Baltimore (MD): Williams & Wilkins; 1996.
2. Tomlinson BE, Irving D. The numbers of limb motor neurons in the human lumbosacral cord throughout life. J Neurol Sci 1977;34(2):213–9.
3. Strick PL, Burke RE, Kanda K, et al. Differences between alpha and gamma motoneurons labeled with horseradish peroxidase by retrograde transport. Brain Res 1976;113(3):582–8.
4. Willis WD. The case for the Renshaw cell. Brain Behav Evol 1971;4(1):5–52.
5. Alvarez FJ, Fyffe RE. The continuing case for the Renshaw cell. J Physiol 2007; 584(Pt 1):31–45.
6. Baldissera F, Hultborn H, Illert M. Integration in spinal neuronal systems. In: Handbook of Physiology, vol 2. The Nervous System: Motor Control American Physiological Society. Bethesda: V.B. Brooks; 1981. p. 509–95.
7. Kandel ER, Schwartz JH, Jassell TM. Principles of neural science. 4th edition. New York: McGraw-Hill, Health Professions Division; 2000.
8. Phani S, Re DB, Przedborski S. The role of the innate immune system in ALS. Front Pharmacol 2012;3:150.
9. Lee Y, Morrison BM, Li Y, et al. Oligodendroglia metabolically support axons and contribute to neurodegeneration. Nature 2012;487(7408):443–8.
10. Sasaki S, Iwata M. Immunocytochemical and ultrastructural study of the motor cortex in patients with lower motor neuron disease. Neurosci Lett 2000;281(1): 45–8.
11. Ince PG, Evans J, Knopp M, et al. Corticospinal tract degeneration in the progressive muscular atrophy variant of ALS. Neurology 2003;60(8): 1252–8.
12. Yoshida S, Mulder DW, Kurland LT, et al. Follow-up study on amyotrophic lateral sclerosis in Rochester, Minn., 1925 through 1984. Neuroepidemiology 1986; 5(2):61–70.
13. Byrne S, Walsh C, Lynch C, et al. Rate of familial amyotrophic lateral sclerosis: a systematic review and meta-analysis. J Neurol Neurosurg Psychiatry 2011; 82(6):623–7.
14. Andersen PM, Al-Chalabi A. Clinical genetics of amyotrophic lateral sclerosis: what do we really know? Nat Rev Neurol 2011;7(11):603–15.
15. Kurland LT, Mulder DW. Epidemiologic investigations of amyotrophic lateral sclerosis. I. Preliminary report on geographic distribution and special reference to the Mariana Islands, including clinical and pathologic observations. Neurology 1954;4(6):438–48.
16. Mitsumoto H, Przedborski S, Gordon PH. Amyotrophic lateral sclerosis. New York: Taylor & Francis; 2006.
17. Kurland LT, Mulder DW. Epidemiologic investigations of amyotrophic lateral sclerosis. I. Preliminary report on geographic distribution, with special reference to the Mariana Islands, including clinical and pathologic observations. Neurology 1954;4(5):355–78.
18. Plato CC, Galasko D, Garruto RM, et al. ALS and PDC of Guam: forty-year follow-up. Neurology 2002;58(5):765–73.

19. Spencer PS, Nunn PB, Hugon J, et al. Motorneurone disease on Guam: possible role of a food neurotoxin. Lancet 1986;1(8487):965.
20. Armon C. Western Pacific ALS/PDC and flying foxes: what's next? Neurology 2003;61(3):291–2.
21. Cox PA, Sacks OW. Cycad neurotoxins, consumption of flying foxes, and ALS-PDC disease in Guam. Neurology 2002;58(6):956–9.
22. Sugarman EA, Nagan N, Zhu H, et al. Pan-ethnic carrier screening and prenatal diagnosis for spinal muscular atrophy: clinical laboratory analysis of >72,400 specimens. Eur J Hum Genet 2012;20(1):27–32.
23. Guidetti D, Sabadini R, Ferlini A, et al. Epidemiological survey of X-linked bulbar and spinal muscular atrophy, or Kennedy disease, in the province of Reggio Emilia, Italy. Eur J Epidemiol 2001;17(6):587–91.
24. Hosokawa T, Fujieda M, Wakiguchi H, et al. Pediatric Hirayama disease. Pediatr Neurol 2010;43(2):151–3.
25. Rosen DR. Mutations in Cu/Zn superoxide dismutase gene are associated with familial amyotrophic lateral sclerosis. Nature 1993;364(6435):362.
26. Renton AE, Majounie E, Waite A, et al. A hexanucleotide repeat expansion in C9ORF72 is the cause of chromosome 9p21-linked ALS-FTD. Neuron 2011; 72(2):257–68.
27. DeJesus-Hernandez M, Mackenzie IR, Boeve BF, et al. Expanded GGGGCC hexanucleotide repeat in noncoding region of C9ORF72 causes chromosome 9p-linked FTD and ALS. Neuron 2011;72(2):245–56.
28. van Rheenen W, van Blitterswijk M, Huisman MH, et al. Hexanucleotide repeat expansions in C9ORF72 in the spectrum of motor neuron diseases. Neurology 2012;79(9):878–82.
29. Elden AC, Kim HJ, Hart MP, et al. Ataxin-2 intermediate-length polyglutamine expansions are associated with increased risk for ALS. Nature 2010; 466(7310):1069–75.
30. Corcia P, Camu W, Halimi JM, et al. SMN1 gene, but not SMN2, is a risk factor for sporadic ALS. Neurology 2006;67(7):1147–50.
31. Van Hoecke A, Schoonaert L, Lemmens R, et al. EPHA4 is a disease modifier of amyotrophic lateral sclerosis in animal models and in humans. Nat Med 2012. [Epub ahead of print].
32. Hermosura MC, Cui AM, Go RC, et al. Altered functional properties of a TRPM2 variant in Guamanian ALS and PD. Proc Natl Acad Sci U S A 2008;105(46): 18029–34.
33. Ogino S, Wilson RB, Gold B. New insights on the evolution of the SMN1 and SMN2 region: simulation and meta-analysis for allele and haplotype frequency calculations. Eur J Hum Genet 2004;12(12):1015–23.
34. Markowitz JA, Singh P, Darras BT. Spinal muscular atrophy: a clinical and research update. Pediatr Neurol 2012;46(1):1–12.
35. Mailman MD, Heinz JW, Papp AC, et al. Molecular analysis of spinal muscular atrophy and modification of the phenotype by SMN2. Genet Med 2002;4(1):20–6.
36. La Spada AR, Wilson EM, Lubahn DB, et al. Androgen receptor gene mutations in X-linked spinal and bulbar muscular atrophy. Nature 1991;352(6330):77–9.
37. Rowland LP, Shneider NA. Amyotrophic lateral sclerosis. N Engl J Med 2001; 344(22):1688–700.
38. Kim WK, Liu X, Sandner J, et al. Study of 962 patients indicates progressive muscular atrophy is a form of ALS. Neurology 2009;73(20):1686–92.
39. Polymenidou M, Cleveland DW. The seeds of neurodegeneration: prion-like spreading in ALS. Cell 2011;147(3):498–508.

40. Ravits JM, La Spada AR. ALS motor phenotype heterogeneity, focality, and spread: deconstructing motor neuron degeneration. Neurology 2009;73(10): 805–11.
41. Hardiman O, van den Berg LH, Kiernan MC. Clinical diagnosis and management of amyotrophic lateral sclerosis. Nat Rev Neurol 2011;7(11):639–49.
42. Fromm GB, Wisdom PJ, Block AJ. Amyotrophic lateral sclerosis presenting with respiratory failure. Diaphragmatic paralysis and dependence on mechanical ventilation in two patients. Chest 1977;71(5):612–4.
43. Scelsa SN, Yakubov B, Salzman SH. Dyspnea-fasciculation syndrome: early respiratory failure in ALS with minimal motor signs. Amyotroph Lateral Scler Other Motor Neuron Disord 2002;3(4):239–43.
44. Kihira T, Yoshida S, Yoshimasu F, et al. Involvement of Onuf's nucleus in amyotrophic lateral sclerosis. J Neurol Sci 1997;147(1):81–8.
45. Mizutani T, Aki M, Shiozawa R, et al. Development of ophthalmoplegia in amyotrophic lateral sclerosis during long-term use of respirators. J Neurol Sci 1990; 99(2–3):311–9.
46. Cudkowicz ME, McKenna-Yasek D, Sapp PE, et al. Epidemiology of mutations in superoxide dismutase in amyotrophic lateral sclerosis. Ann Neurol 1997;41(2): 210–21.
47. Millecamps S, Salachas F, Cazeneuve C, et al. SOD1, ANG, VAPB, TARDBP, and FUS mutations in familial amyotrophic lateral sclerosis: genotype-phenotype correlations. J Med Genet 2010;47(8):554–60.
48. Kirby J, Goodall EF, Smith W, et al. Broad clinical phenotypes associated with TAR-DNA binding protein (TARDBP) mutations in amyotrophic lateral sclerosis. Neurogenetics 2010;11(2):217–25.
49. Byrne S, Elamin M, Bede P, et al. Cognitive and clinical characteristics of patients with amyotrophic lateral sclerosis carrying a C9orf72 repeat expansion: a population-based cohort study. Lancet Neurol 2012;11(3):232–40.
50. Phukan J, Elamin M, Bede P, et al. The syndrome of cognitive impairment in amyotrophic lateral sclerosis: a population-based study. J Neurol Neurosurg Psychiatry 2012;83(1):102–8.
51. Grossman AB, Woolley-Levine S, Bradley WG, et al. Detecting neurobehavioral changes in amyotrophic lateral sclerosis. Amyotroph Lateral Scler 2007;8(1): 56–61.
52. Lomen-Hoerth C, Murphy J, Langmore S, et al. Are amyotrophic lateral sclerosis patients cognitively normal? Neurology 2003;60(7):1094–7.
53. Brown RH, Swash M, Pasinelli P. Amyotrophic lateral sclerosis. 2nd edition. Abingdon (England) and Boca Raton (FL): Informa Healthcare; Distributed in North America by Taylor & Francis; 2006.
54. Mercuri E, Bertini E, Iannaccone ST. Childhood spinal muscular atrophy: controversies and challenges. Lancet Neurol 2012;11(5):443–52.
55. Atsuta N, Watanabe H, Ito M, et al. Natural history of spinal and bulbar muscular atrophy (SBMA): a study of 223 Japanese patients. Brain 2006;129(Pt 6):1446–55.
56. Sinnreich M, Sorenson EJ, Klein CJ. Neurologic course, endocrine dysfunction and triplet repeat size in spinal bulbar muscular atrophy. Can J Neurol Sci 2004; 31(3):378–82.
57. Hamano T, Mutoh T, Hirayama M, et al. MRI findings of benign monomelic amyotrophy of lower limb. J Neurol Sci 1999;165(2):184–7.
58. Willeit J, Kiechl S, Kiechl-Kohlendorfer U, et al. Juvenile asymmetric segmental spinal muscular atrophy (Hirayama's disease): three cases without evidence of "flexion myelopathy." Acta Neurol Scand 2001;104(5):320–2.

59. Ammendola A, Gallo A, Iannaccone T, et al. Hirayama disease: three cases assessed by F wave, somatosensory and motor evoked potentials and magnetic resonance imaging not supporting flexion myelopathy. Neurol Sci 2008;29(5):303–11.

60. Schold SC, Cho ES, Somasundaram M, et al. Subacute motor neuronopathy: a remote effect of lymphoma. Ann Neurol 1979;5(3):271–87.

61. Verma A, Berger JR, Snodgrass S, et al. Motor neuron disease: a paraneoplastic process associated with anti-hu antibody and small-cell lung carcinoma. Ann Neurol 1996;40(1):112–6.

62. Khwaja S, Sripathi N, Ahmad BK, et al. Paraneoplastic motor neuron disease with type 1 Purkinje cell antibodies. Muscle Nerve 1998;21(7):943–5.

63. Chahin N, Sorenson EJ. Serum creatine kinase levels in spinobulbar muscular atrophy and amyotrophic lateral sclerosis. Muscle Nerve 2009;40(1):126–9.

64. Charcot JM, Joffroy A. Deux cas d'atrophy musculaire progressive avec lesions de la substance grise et des faisceaux antero-lateraux de la moelle epiniere. Arch Physiol Neurol Pathol 1869;2:744–60.

65. Hirano A, Arumugasamy N, Zimmerman HM. Amyotrophic lateral sclerosis. A comparison of Guam and classical cases. Arch Neurol 1967;16(4):357–63.

66. Hirano A, Nakano I, Kurland LT, et al. Fine structural study of neurofibrillary changes in a family with amyotrophic lateral sclerosis. J Neuropathol Exp Neurol 1984;43(5):471–80.

67. Rothstein JD. Current hypotheses for the underlying biology of amyotrophic lateral sclerosis. Ann Neurol 2009;65(Suppl 1):S3–9.

68. Bosco DA, Morfini G, Karabacak NM, et al. Wild-type and mutant SOD1 share an aberrant conformation and a common pathogenic pathway in ALS. Nat Neurosci 2010;13(11):1396–403.

69. Kabashi E, Valdmanis PN, Dion P, et al. TARDBP mutations in individuals with sporadic and familial amyotrophic lateral sclerosis. Nat Genet 2008;40(5):572–4.

70. Neumann M, Sampathu DM, Kwong LK, et al. Ubiquitinated TDP-43 in frontotemporal lobar degeneration and amyotrophic lateral sclerosis. Science 2006;314(5796):130–3.

71. Mackenzie IR, Bigio EH, Ince PG, et al. Pathological TDP-43 distinguishes sporadic amyotrophic lateral sclerosis from amyotrophic lateral sclerosis with SOD1 mutations. Ann Neurol 2007;61(5):427–34.

72. Burghes AH, Beattie CE. Spinal muscular atrophy: why do low levels of survival motor neuron protein make motor neurons sick? Nature reviews. Neuroscience 2009;10(8):597–609.

73. Doyu M, Sobue G, Mukai E, et al. Severity of X-linked recessive bulbospinal neuronopathy correlates with size of the tandem CAG repeat in androgen receptor gene. Ann Neurol 1992;32(5):707–10.

74. Li M, Miwa S, Kobayashi Y, et al. Nuclear inclusions of the androgen receptor protein in spinal and bulbar muscular atrophy. Ann Neurol 1998;44(2):249–54.

75. Andersen PM, Abrahams S, Borasio GD, et al. EFNS guidelines on the clinical management of amyotrophic lateral sclerosis (MALS)–revised report of an EFNS task force. Eur J Neurol 2012;19(3):360–75.

76. Miller RG, Jackson CE, Kasarskis EJ, et al. Practice parameter update: the care of the patient with amyotrophic lateral sclerosis: drug, nutritional, and respiratory therapies (an evidence-based review): report of the quality standards subcommittee of the American Academy of Neurology. Neurology 2009;73(15):1218–26.

77. Rezania K, Goldenberg FD, White S. Neuromuscular disorders and acute respiratory failure: diagnosis and management. Neurol Clin 2012;30(1):161–85, viii.

78. Miller RG, Jackson CE, Kasarskis EJ, et al. Practice parameter update: the care of the patient with amyotrophic lateral sclerosis: multidisciplinary care, symptom management, and cognitive/behavioral impairment (an evidence-based review): report of the Quality Standards Subcommittee of the American Academy of Neurology. Neurology 2009;73(15):1227–33.

79. Scherer K, Bedlack RS. Diaphragm pacing in amyotrophic lateral sclerosis: a literature review. Muscle Nerve 2012;46(1):1–8.

80. Gowing G, Svendsen CN. Stem cell transplantation for motor neuron disease: current approaches and future perspectives. Neurotherapeutics 2011;8(4): 591–606.

81. Muntoni F, Wood MJ. Targeting RNA to treat neuromuscular disease. Nat Rev Drug Discov 2011;10(8):621–37.

82. Van Meerbeke JP, Sumner CJ. Progress and promise: the current status of spinal muscular atrophy therapeutics. Discov Med 2011;12(65):291–305.

83. Brooks BR, Miller RG, Swash M, et al. El Escorial revisited: revised criteria for the diagnosis of amyotrophic lateral sclerosis. Amyotroph Lateral Scler Other Motor Neuron Disord 2000;1(5):293–9.

84. de Carvalho M, Dengler R, Eisen A, et al. Electrodiagnostic criteria for diagnosis of ALS. Clin Neurophysiol 2008;119(3):497–503.

85. Poll-The BT, Engelen M. Peroxisomal leukoencephalopathy. Semin Neurol 2012; 32(1):42–50.

86. Roos R, Gajdusek DC, Gibbs CJ Jr. The clinical characteristics of transmissible Creutzfeldt-Jakob disease. Brain 1973;96(1):1–20.

87. Kovanen J. Clinical characteristics of familial and sporadic Creutzfeldt-Jakob disease in Finland. Acta Neurol Scand 1993;87(6):469–74.

88. Worrall BB, Rowland LP, Chin SS, et al. Amyotrophy in prion diseases. Arch Neurol 2000;57(1):33–8.

89. Schule R, Schols L. Genetics of hereditary spastic paraplegias. Semin Neurol 2011;31(5):484–93.

90. Moses SW, Parvari R. The variable presentations of glycogen storage disease type IV: a review of clinical, enzymatic and molecular studies. Curr Mol Med 2002;2(2):177–88.

91. Ooi MH, Wong SC, Lewthwaite P, et al. Clinical features, diagnosis, and management of enterovirus 71. Lancet Neurol 2010;9(11):1097–105.

92. Mitsumoto H, Sliman RJ, Schafer IA, et al. Motor neuron disease and adult hexosaminidase A deficiency in two families: evidence for multisystem degeneration. Ann Neurol 1985;17(4):378–85.

93. Neumann M, Kwong LK, Sampathu DM, et al. TDP-43 proteinopathy in frontotemporal lobar degeneration and amyotrophic lateral sclerosis: protein misfolding diseases without amyloidosis. Arch Neurol 2007;64(10):1388–94.

94. Deng HX, Chen W, Hong ST, et al. Mutations in UBQLN2 cause dominant X-linked juvenile and adult-onset ALS and ALS/dementia. Nature 2011; 477(7363):211–5.

95. Tomonaga M, Saito M, Yoshimura M, et al. Ultrastructure of the Bunina bodies in anterior horn cells of amyotrophic lateral sclerosis. Acta Neuropathol 1978; 42(2):81–6.

96. Vande Velde C, Miller TM, Cashman NR, et al. Selective association of misfolded ALS-linked mutant SOD1 with the cytoplasmic face of mitochondria. Proc Natl Acad Sci U S A 2008;105(10):4022–7.

97. Cassina P, Cassina A, Pehar M, et al. Mitochondrial dysfunction in SOD1G93A-bearing astrocytes promotes motor neuron degeneration: prevention by mitochondrial-targeted antioxidants. J Neurosci 2008;28(16):4115–22.
98. Borchelt DR, Wong PC, Becher MW, et al. Axonal transport of mutant superoxide dismutase 1 and focal axonal abnormalities in the proximal axons of transgenic mice. Neurobiol Dis 1998;5(1):27–35.
99. Kikuchi H, Almer G, Yamashita S, et al. Spinal cord endoplasmic reticulum stress associated with a microsomal accumulation of mutant superoxide dismutase-1 in an ALS model. Proc Natl Acad Sci U S A 2006;103(15):6025–30.
100. Nishitoh H, Kadowaki H, Nagai A, et al. ALS-linked mutant SOD1 induces ER stress- and ASK1-dependent motor neuron death by targeting Derlin-1. Genes Dev 2008;22(11):1451–64.
101. Harraz MM, Marden JJ, Zhou W, et al. SOD1 mutations disrupt redox-sensitive Rac regulation of NADPH oxidase in a familial ALS model. J Clin Invest 2008; 118(2):659–70.
102. Wojciechowska M, Krzyzosiak WJ. Cellular toxicity of expanded RNA repeats: focus on RNA foci. Hum Mol Genet 2011;20(19):3811–21.
103. Todd PK, Paulson HL. RNA-mediated neurodegeneration in repeat expansion disorders. Ann Neurol 2010;67(3):291–300.
104. Mackenzie IR, Rademakers R, Neumann M. TDP-43 and FUS in amyotrophic lateral sclerosis and frontotemporal dementia. Lancet Neurol 2010;9(10): 995–1007.
105. Banno H, Adachi H, Katsuno M, et al. Mutant androgen receptor accumulation in spinal and bulbar muscular atrophy scrotal skin: a pathogenic marker. Ann Neurol 2006;59(3):520–6.

Spinal Cord Tumors
New Views and Future Directions

Laszlo L. Mechtler, MD[a,b,c],*, Kaveer Nandigam, MD[d]

KEYWORDS

- Intramedullary spinal tumors • Ependymoma • Hemangioblastoma • Astrocytoma
- Ganglioglioma • Spine cysts • MRI • DTI

KEY POINTS

- About 90% of spinal intramedullary tumors are ependymomas or astrocytomas.
- Ependymomas commonly cause central cord syndrome because of their location.
- Myxopapillary ependymomas compose 90% of filum terminale tumors.
- Astrocytomas compose 90% of all primary spinal cord tumors in those less than 10 years of age and up to 60% of primary spinal cord tumors in adolescents.
- Astrocytomas typically present in an asymmetric eccentric location within the cord.
- Contrary to intracranial astrocytomas, low-grade spinal astrocytomas enhance commonly.
- Spinal cord hemangioblastomas are associated with Von Hippel-Lindau disease in 25% and typically show flow voids in the periphery of the tumor.

INTRODUCTION

Spinal cord tumors are uncommon neoplasms that, without treatment, can cause significant neurologic morbidity and mortality. The historic classification of spine tumors is based on the use of myelography with 3 main groups as schematically depicted in **Fig. 1**: (1) extramedullary extradural, (2) intradural extramedullary, and (3) intradural intramedullary. Using this scheme, spinal tumors are characterized as either arising inside the dura mater (intradural) or outside (extradural). This article focuses on *intramedullary spinal cord tumors*, with an emphasis on new diagnostic modalities[1] and treatment options. Because of the rarity of these lesions, the

[a] Dent Imaging and Neuro-Oncology Center, Dent Neurologic Institute, 3980 Sheridan Drive, Buffalo, NY 14226, USA; [b] Roswell Park Cancer Institute, Buffalo, NY, USA; [c] American Society of Neuro-Imaging, Minneapolis, MN, USA; [d] Dent Neurologic Institute, 3980 Sheridan Drive, Buffalo, NY 14226, USA
* Corresponding author. Dent Imaging and Neuro-Oncology Center, Dent Neurologic Institute, 3980 Sheridan Drive, Buffalo, NY 14226.
E-mail address: lmechtler@dentinstitute.com

Neurol Clin 31 (2013) 241–268
http://dx.doi.org/10.1016/j.ncl.2012.09.011
0733-8619/13/$ – see front matter © 2013 Elsevier Inc. All rights reserved.

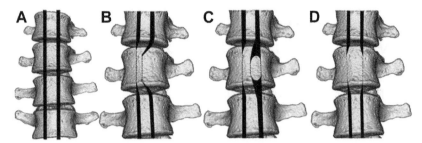

Fig. 1. Historic classification of spine tumors based on myelography. Myelographic spine tumor classification. (*A*) Normal, (*B*) extradural extramedullary, (*C*) intradural extramedullary, and (*D*) intradural intramedullary.

heterogeneous clinical presentation, and varied treatment strategies, it is not feasible to perform a prospective randomized study; a multicenter prospective case series or cohort study would require the standardization of treatment and outcomes.[2] Data from national registries and improved imaging capabilities have allowed spine tumor specialists the opportunity to study and treat these unusual and rare tumors with more confidence and better results.

EPIDEMIOLOGY OF INTRAMEDULLARY SPINE TUMORS

Intramedullary spinal tumors account for 5% to 10% of all spinal tumors in adults and approximately 35% in children. About 90% of the tumors of the spinal cord are glial tumors, of which most of these neoplasms are ependymomas and astrocytomas. Ependymomas represent about 60% and astrocytomas 30%.[3] Of the remaining 10%, hemangioblastomas account for 2% to 8%[4] and 2% are intramedullary metastases.[5] Intramedullary tumors are more common in children, with extramedullary tumors being more common in adults.

The rarity of these tumors has significant ramifications on potential outcomes because it impacts research allocation and treatment decisions. Most descriptive epidemiologic studies in primary spinal cord tumors include intradural extramedullary tumors, such as meningiomas, and nerve sheath tumors. Some recent studies have focused on the actual frequency of intramedullary tumors. Data from the central registries in the National Program of Cancer Registration and Surveillance, Epidemiology, and End results programs for 2004 to 2007 and 1999 to 2007 were analyzed.[1] This study provided the first comprehensive population-based incidence of primary spinal cord tumors, covering approximately 99.2% of the US population from 2004 to 2007.

Men had higher rates than women for ependymomas, lymphomas, and nerve sheath tumors but lower rates than women for meningiomas. The most common intradural spinal tumors histologically are meningiomas (33%), nerve sheath tumors (27%), and ependymomas (21%).[1] The overall incidence of spinal tumors, malignant and nonmalignant combined, was 0.97 per 100 000.[3] Seventy-eight percent of the primary spinal tumors were nonmalignant, accounting for most incident cases diagnosed between 2004 and 2007. As a result of mandating the collection of nonmalignant primary spinal tumors in conjunction with malignant primary spinal tumors in a 2004 population-based surveillance of cancers, the authors were able to capture the burden of the disease more completely in the US population.[1,2]

Tumors of the spinal cord are much less frequent than intracranial tumors. Overall prevalence is about 4 intracranial lesions for every 1 spinal tumor, which varies based on tumor histology. The intracranial-to-spine ratio for astrocytomas is approximately 10:1, whereas that for ependymomas can range from 2:1 to 3:1, depending on the specific histologic variant. The anatomic distribution of intramedullary spinal cord tumors is proportional to the length of the cord, with thoracic segment having the most (50%–55%), lumbosacral the second most (25%–30%), and the cervical segment the least (15%–25%).[6,7]

CLINICAL SYMPTOMS

In general, a spinal cord lesion may be suspected when there are bilateral motor and sensory signs or symptoms that do not involve the head and face. Several distinct spinal cord syndromes are recognized. These syndromes are used in a clinical evaluation because they often result from distinct pathologic conditions, such as stroke, infectious, demyelinating, trauma, or neoplasms. These spinal cord syndromes are summarized in **Table 1**.

Segmental Syndrome

Segmental syndrome or total cord transection syndrome can result from acute trauma as well as subacute/chronic processes, such as transverse myelitis, multiple sclerosis, or neoplasms. Tumors that cause segmental syndrome are usually epidural metastases with compression fractures and are associated with a relatively subacute onset of complete paralysis. The loss of function occurs in all ascending and descending spinal cord pathways and, thus, results in the loss of all types of sensation and loss of movement below the level of the lesion.[8]

Brown-Séquard Syndrome

This syndrome occurs when a lesion is on one side of the spinal cord (lateral cord syndrome) affecting contralateral pain and thermal sensation and ipsilateral proprioception and vibratory sensation. The loss of pain and temperature sensation begins 1 or 2 segments below the lesion. Associated motor paralysis on the side of the lesion completes the syndrome. The unilateral involvement of the descending autonomic fibers does not produce bladder symptoms. The most common causes are trauma, demyelination, and rarely disk herniation and infarctions. Extramedullary tumors are

Table 1
Cord syndromes caused by spine tumors

Syndrome	Cause
Complete cord transection	• Metastatic epidural disease, pathologic fractures, intramedullary cord metastasis/hemorrhage (ie, melanoma)
Brown-Séquard syndrome	• Astrocytoma, ganglioglioma, meningiomas, nerve sheath tumor, and hemangioblastoma
Ventral cord syndrome	• Usually vascular but also anterior epidural metastatic disease, radiation myelopathy, astrocytoma
Central cord syndrome	• Ependymoma, syringomyelia, lipoma, metastases
Posterior cord syndrome (Lhermitte sign)	• Epidural metastases, astrocytoma, hemangioblastoma
Conus medullaris syndrome	• Ependymoma, syringomyelia, lymphoma, astrocytoma
Cauda equina syndrome	• Epidural metastasis, myxopapillary ependymoma, meningioma, nerve sheath tumor, leptomeningeal disease, paraganglioma

the more common neoplastic cause of this syndrome; but intramedullary astrocytomas, gangliogliomas, hemangioblastomas, and metastases[9] may cause similar findings.

Ventral Cord Syndrome

The clinical presentation of *ventral spinal cord syndrome* includes complete motor paralysis below the level of the lesion caused by the interruption of the corticospinal tracts, with a loss of pain and temperature sensation below the level of the lesion caused by the interruption of the spinothalamic tract. There is sparing of proprioception and vibratory sensation caused by intact dorsal columns. Flaccid anal sphincter, urinary retention, and intestinal obstruction may be associated with anterior cord syndrome. The most common causes of anterior spinal cord syndrome include occlusion or dissection of the anterior spinal artery. An acute disk herniation, cervical spondylosis, vasculitis, and sickle cell disease are also associated with this syndrome. Anterior epidural metastatic disease is the most common neoplastic cause. Rare neuro-oncological causes include radiation myelopathy, and astrocytoma is also in the differential diagnosis.[10]

Central Cord Syndrome

Central cord syndrome occurs when a lesion affects the center of the spinal canal, mainly the central gray matter and adjacent crossing spinothalamic tracts, causing paresis in the upper extremities more than the lower extremities. There is a loss of pain and temperature sensation in a shawl-like distribution over the upper neck, shoulders, and upper trunk, with light touch, position, and vibratory sensation relatively preserved (disassociated sensory loss). There are usually no bladder symptoms. The classic causes of central cord syndrome are slow-growing lesions, such as syringomyelia, or intramedullary tumors, such as ependymomas. However, central cord syndrome is also seen in patients with hyperextension injury and longstanding cervical spondylosis.[11]

Dorsal Cord Syndrome

Dorsal cord syndrome results from bilateral involvement of the dorsal columns, the corticospinal tracts, and descending central autonomic tracts. The main symptoms of dorsal column syndrome include gait ataxia, paresthesias, weakness, and bladder control symptoms. Lhermitte sign often occurs in patients with posterior column involvement, especially in the cervical spine,[12,13] which is characterized by a sensation of electrical shocks running down the spine and into the limbs, occurring with bending the head forward or backward. The causes of dorsal cord syndrome include multiple sclerosis, tabes dorsalis, subacute combined degeneration, compressive myelopathy caused by cervical spondylitic disease, as well as epidural and intradural extramedullary tumors, and radiation myelopathy.[10]

Conus Medullaris Syndrome

Conus medullaris syndrome in its pure form presents with sphincter disturbances, saddle anesthesia (S3–S5), impotence, and the absence of lower extremity abnormalities. Lower extremity weakness tends to be mild, and spontaneous pain tends to be bilateral and symmetric. The causes of conus medullaris syndrome include disk herniation as well as the following neoplasms: myxopapillary ependymomas, lymphomas, and astrocytomas.

Cauda Equina Syndrome

This syndrome is caused by a loss of function in 2 or more of the 18 nerve roots consti-tuting the cauda equina. Deficits usually affect both legs but are often asymmetric. Low back pain tends to be radicular in nature. Weakness also seems to be associated with the loss of reflexes and is more unilateral compared with the conus medullaris syndrome whereby weakness occurs late and is usually bilateral. The rectal sphincter paralysis usually occurs later, and sensory loss usually occurs in a dermatomal distri-bution. The multiple causes of cauda equina syndrome include epidural metastases, myxopapillary ependymoma, paraganglioma, leptomeningeal disease, nerve sheath tumors, and meningiomas.[14,15]

COMMON SPINAL INTRAMEDULLARY TUMORS
Ependymoma

Half of all ependymomas are located below the foramen magnum and involve either the spinal cord (55%) or the cauda equina region (45%). The mean age of presentation is around 40 years, and there is a slight male predominance. Intramedullary ependy-momas have a predilection for the cervical spinal cord such that 67% percent of tumors arise from or extend into this region.[16,17] Ependymomas of the cord are typi-cally solitary tumors that arise from the ependymal lining of the central canal causing a diffuse enlargement of the cord over several levels and associated with syrinx in about 50% of the cases. Spinal cord ependymomas have only a slight tendency to infiltrate the adjacent neural tissue and have a delicate capsule forming a plane of cleavage to separate the tumor from the spinal cord. The World Health Organization (WHO) recognizes 5 histologic variants of ependymoma, which include cellular, papil-lary, epithelial, tanycytic, and myxopapillary subtypes. Ependymomas are also commonly divided into typical, WHO grade II, or anaplastic WHO grade III varieties. In addition, 2 low-grade (WHO grade I) forms, myxopapillary ependymoma and sub-ependymoma, have also been recognized. Anaplastic ependymomas (WHO grade III) are less common in the spinal cord and have additional pathologic features, such are increased cellularity, mitotic activity, pleomorphic nuclei, vascular hyper-plasia, nuclear atypia, and necrosis.[18] Anaplastic ependymomas (WHO grade III) have a malignant behavior and have a tendency for progression. Myxopapillary epen-dymomas of the filum terminale are a histologic variant accounting for about 13% of all ependymomas but more than 80% of all ependymomas that are located in the conus medullaris and filum terminale. Cellular ependymomas occur in the spinal cord more often.[18]

Magnetic resonance imaging (MRI) of the spine has reduced the average duration from symptom onset to diagnosis from 24 to 36 months to 14 months; as a conse-quence, the incidences of weakness and sphincter involvement has decreased. The most common complaint (95%) at the time of diagnosis is back pain. Most patients have dysesthesias without sensory loss, which is attributed to the location of the spinal ependymomas around the central canal; the symmetric expansion of the central canal causes an interruption of the crossing spinalthalamic tracts (central cord syndrome). When pain and numbness are in a radicular pattern involving the legs, the underlying tumors are usually myxopapillary ependymomas predominantly involving the cauda equina. Spinal ependymomas also have a tendency of causing microhemorrhages, and delayed diagnosis may lead to superficial hemosiderosis with involvement of the caudal cranial nerves. Unexplained superficial hemosiderosis seen on a cranial MRI should prompt a spinal investigation with MRI for the exclusion of spinal ependymoma.

The association between neurofibromatosis type II (NF2) and spinal ependymoma is well known.[19,20] This disease is autosomal dominant caused by mutation of the merlin or schwannomin gene on chromosome 22 (this is a member of the protein 401 family). NF2 has been described as multiple inherited schwannomas, meningiomas, and ependymomas. The frequency of polar tumoral cysts that are seen rostral or caudal to the tumor is about 50% to 90%.[11] On T1-weight images, cellular ependymomas tend to be isointense to slightly hyperintense to the spinal cord. On T2-weighted images, they appear hyperintense. Hemosiderin is commonly seen as an area of hypointensity, showing a so-called cap sign, which occurs in about 20% to 64% of cord ependymomas. Short-tau inversion-recovery (STIR) sequences show hyperintensity, although 80% of these cases on postcontrast T1-weight images enhance homogeneously. Minimal or no enhancement is actually relatively rare. Diffusion tensor imaging (DTI) may show the tumor displacing the fiber tracts rather than interrupting them, as shown in **Fig. 2**.[16,17,21–24]

Myxopapillary ependymoma of the conus medullaris and filum terminale are relatively common spinal intradural neoplasms, predominantly seen in children and young adults, although they may be observed at an older age. There is a slight male predominance. This tumor is a WHO grade I with low mitotic activity and glial fibrillary acidic protein (glial fibrillary acidic protein [GFAP])/S100 positivity. They make up about one-third of all ependymomas and 90% of filum terminale tumors. They appear as

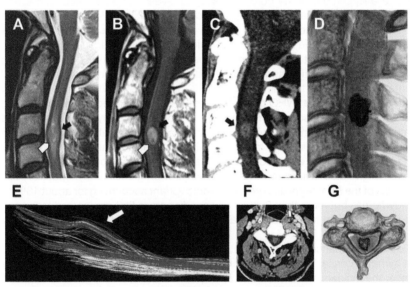

Fig. 2. MRI and computed tomography (CT) images of a spinal intramedullary ependymoma. Patient is a 55-year-old man who presented with progressive 1-year history of shawl-like dissociated sensory loss in the upper extremities as well as weakness typical of a central cord syndrome. Multiple sclerosis workup was negative. (A) T2-weighted (W) sagittal image shows a central cord mass (*black arrow*) with mild edema, with a rostral and a caudal (*white arrowhead*) small polar cysts. On T1W sagittal with contrast (B), there is diffuse tumor enhancement. The polar cyst (*white arrowhead*) does not enhance with contrast. Diffusion tensor imaging/tractography (E) confirms the noninfiltrative nature of this mass with fibers being displaced (*white arrow*). Postcontrast images obtained on a 320-slice CT (C, F) and 3-dimensional reconstruction in the sagittal (D) and axial (G) planes elaborates the bony structures surrounding this well-demarcated enhancing ovoid (*blue*) spinal cord mass that was consistent with a cellular ependymoma.

isointense to hypointense masses on T1-weighted images and as isointense to hypo-intense masses on T2-weighted images. They tend to be extramedullary and present as a cauda equina syndrome. They usually span 2 to 4 vertebral segments as seen in **Fig. 3**, and they usually fill the lumbo-sacral thecal sac. There may be posterior verte-bral scalloping as well as intravertebral foraminal widening. At times on T1- and T2-weighted images, they may be hyperintense because of the accumulation of mucin. On T2-weighted images, they may also be hypointense because the tumor margin is consistent with hemosiderin. STIR sequences tend to be hyperintense and the contrast enhancement is usually avid. Myxopapillary ependymomas are the most common subtype of ependymomas that are associated with hemorrhage. They may have local seeding or even subarachnoid dissemination.[16,18,25,26]

Astrocytoma

Intramedullary spinal astrocytomas account for 3% to 4% of all central nervous system (CNS) astrocytomas. In adults, they compose about 30% to 35% of all intramedullary spinal cord tumors. They are more common in children, composing 90% of all primary spinal cord tumors in those less than 10 years of age and up to 60% of primary spinal cord tumors in adolescents. Gender distribution between male and female patients is fairly even. In adults, the average age of onset is 29 years, a presentation that is earlier than that of ependymomas. The tumor arises in the cervical spinal cord in approxi-mately 60% of patients. Tumors spanning the entire cord from the cervico-medullary junction to the conus medullaris, called holocord tumors, can occur but are very rare. Histologically, gliomas can be differentiated as pilocytic (WHO grade I), fibrillary (WHO grade II), anaplastic (WHO grade III), and glioblastoma multiforme (WHO grade IV) (**Box 1**).[27] Fibrillary astrocytomas show widespread parenchymal infiltration and

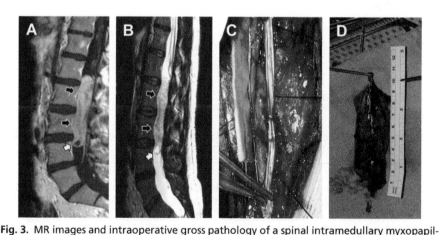

Fig. 3. MR images and intraoperative gross pathology of a spinal intramedullary myxopapil-lary ependymoma. A 38-year-old man who presented with radicular pain as well as sexual dysfunction. A large sausagelike mass with scalloping fills the intraspinal canal at L2–L5 (*black arrows*). On T1-weighted (W) sagittal contrast images (*A*), it is strongly enhancing with a caudal tumor cyst (*white arrow*). T2W images (*B*) confirm a relative hypointense mass that is probably caused by its myxoid pathology (micropapillae of hyalinized blood vessels surrounded by mucinous matrix) or blood products (hemosiderin). Intraoperatively (*C*), the tumor was found to be gelatinous and originating from the filum terminale. The tumor was completely excised with relative ease (*D*). Pathology was consistent with a myxo-papillary ependymoma. No treatment was recommended. Patient is disease free and asymp-tomatic since his diagnosis 10 years ago.

Box 1
Classification of intramedullary tumors

Neuroepithelial tumors (90%)

- Ependymal cell tumors (60%)
  - Ependymoma (WHO grade II)
  - Anaplastic ependymoma (WHO grade III)
  - Subependymoma (WHO grade I)
  - Myxopapillary ependymoma (WHO grade I)
- Astrocytic tumors (30%)
  - Pilocytic astrocytoma (WHO grade I)
  - Fibrillary astrocytoma (WHO grade II)
  - Anaplastic astrocytoma (WHO grade III)
  - Glioblastoma multiforme (WHO grade IV)
- Oligodendroglioma tumors
  - Oligodendroglioma (WHO grade II)
  - Anaplastic oligodendroglioma (WHO grade III)

Mixed neuronal/glial tumors (<1%)

- Ganglioglioma (WHO grade I)
- Gangliocytoma (WHO grade I)

Mesenchymal tumors (<8%)

- Hemangioblastoma (2%–8%) (WHO grade I)
- Lipoma
- Melanocytoma

Metastatic tumors (2%)

Hematopoietic tumors

- Primary CNS lymphoma
- Leukemia

Data from Louis DN, Ohgaki H, Wiestler OD, et al. The 2007 WHO classification of tumors of the central nervous system. Acta Neuropathol 2007;114:97–109.

---

variable degrees of nuclear atypia and increased cellularity. The presence of mitoses warrants an anaplastic designation. Pilocytic astrocytomas tend to displace rather than infiltrate the cord. Statistically, about 85% to 90% of astrocytomas are low grade (either fibrillary or pilocytic), whereas 10% to 15% are high grade (mostly anaplastic). Glioblastoma multiforme occurs in 0.2% to 1.5% of all cord astrocytomas.[28,29] In general, astrocytomas cause asymmetric enlargement of the cord. The incidence of primary spinal cord astrocytomas is reported to be at 2.5 per 100 000 per year, which is tenfold less frequent than primary astrocytomas.

The initial clinical presentation of spinal cord astrocytomas is often back pain and progressive weakness. Astrocytomas have an affinity to white matter tracts, which topographically are peripheral in the spinal cord. *Hence, the asymmetric presentation is characteristic of these tumors.* Unlike ependymomas, paresthesias are more common than dysesthesias. The average duration of symptoms before diagnosis is about 3.5 years for low-grade astrocytomas and about 6 months for malignant astrocytomas. On T1-weighted images, there is cord expansion, usually less than 4 segments. Holocord presentation is exceedingly rare but is histologically most consistent with pilocytic astrocytoma.[30]

In general, astrocytomas are T1 hypointense to isointense. On T2-weighted images, they are hyperintense. Blood products occur in a minority of cases. *Unlike most intracranial low-grade astrocytomas, spinal astrocytomas enhance with gadolinium.* The enhancement pattern is usually mild to moderate and patchy. Contrast enhancement does not predict tumor grade or behavior, especially in pilocytic astrocytomas.[31] Axial MRI images show an asymmetric expansion of the cord. In fact, the frequency of nonenhancing spinal cord astrocytoma is 18%.[16,17] The MRI appearance of an intramedullary astrocytoma with diffusion tractography is shown in **Fig. 4.**

Spinal astrocytomas and ependymomas often demonstrate associated cysts. There are 3 distinct types of cysts associated with these intramedullary spine tumors:

1. Tumoral cyst
2. Rostral or caudal cysts (polar cysts)[32]
3. Reactive dilatation of the central canal (syringomyelia)

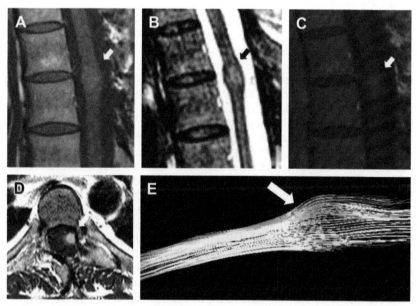

Fig. 4. MRI appearance of an intramedullary astrocytoma with diffusion tractography. A 48-year-old man with vague back pain and normal examination was operated on 9 years ago for an intramedullary mass (*arrows*). Laminectomy without biopsy was performed. T1-weighted (W) noncontrast (*A*) and T2W sagittal images (*B*) show a focal asymmetric enlargement of the left cord that enhances homogenously on T1W sagittal (*C*) and axial (*D*) contrast images. The images and clinical history are consistent with a pilocytic astrocytoma. 3 T MRI diffusion tractography (*E*) confirms typical findings in a noninfiltrative astrocytoma with fanning of the fibers around the tumor. Fluorodeoxyglucose positron emission tomography (not shown) showed hypermetabolism of the tumor, which is also characteristic of pilocytic astrocytomas, despite being WHO grade I. Patient continues to be neurologically intact and asymptomatic and has not had any adjuvant treatment.

The cysts located rostral or caudal to the tumor are typically non-neoplastic with gliotic linings and filled with fluid similar to cerebral spinal fluid. By contrast, those within neoplastic masses are lined by abnormal glial cells and are xanthochromic or blood filled. The polar cysts have also been described as satellite or reactive cysts. They usually do not enhance with T1-weighted postcontrast MRI and, in fact, are a form of a syringohydromyelia. In comparison, tumoral cysts are associated with a variable surrounding solid component and enhance in most cases. Characterization of the nature of the cysts is important because reactive cysts simply collapse after excision of the solid component, whereas tumoral cysts have to be surgically removed. The third type of cyst seen in association with spinal tumors is secondary reactive dilatation of the central canal most likely related to the partial obstruction of the central canal by the tumor mass. Distinction between rostral/caudal cysts and reactive dilatation of the central canal might be difficult. It is important to differentiate tumoral cysts from the other two types of cysts because intratumoral cysts should be surgically excised along with the tumor given their potential to cause tumor recurrence when not excised. In the surgical series of 100 intramedullary tumors, 45% were associated with a syrinx.[33] A syrinx was more likely to be found above the tumor level than below it. Hemangioblastomas were the most common tumor type to be associated with syrinx. The higher the spinal level, the more likely a syrinx was encountered.[34,35]

Hemangioblastoma

Hemangioblastomas are benign WHO grade I tumors. Their annual incidence is about 0.02 per 100 000 people. They compose about 2% to 8% of all intramedullary spinal cord tumors.[4] The cell of origin is uncertain but likely vascular endothelial growth factor (VEGF)–secreting cells[36] of undifferentiated mesenchymal origin.[37] They occur sporadically in about 75% and are associated with von Hippel-Lindau disease in the remaining 25%.[38] Mutations on the short arm of chromosome 3p25 are seen in patients with von Hippel-Lindau disease (VHL) with hemagioblastomas.[39] Cervical and thoracic segments are commonly involved, with a predilection for dorsolateral cord surface. The tumors can be single or multiple and tend to be smaller than 10 mm in diameter in patients with VHL.[40] With sporadic spinal hemangioblastomas, the tumors can get bigger, up to 6 cm in diameter.[40] Grossly, they are well demarcated with a capsule and have characteristic abnormally dilated tortuous vessels on the surface.[41] Microscopic pathology shows gliosis and Rosenthal fibers, with prominent small capillaries and venous vessels.[42] The tumor's mitotic activity, measured as KI-67 activity, is less than 1% for intramedullary tumors compared with up to 25% for tumors that extend into both intramedullary and extramedullary space.[43] These tumors are isointense on T1-weighted images and hyperintense on T2 weighted images.[40] They may have mixed heterogeneity if intralesional hemorrhage is present. Contrast enhancement is usually homogenous and well demarcated, with superficial heterogeneous enhancement within the flow voids, as seen in **Fig. 5**. The surrounding vasogenic edema is usually mild. Flow voids are more common in tumors greater than 15 mm in size.[40] Because of the presence of dilated vessels, these tumors are often mistaken for a vascular malformation. The presence of a syrinx, which is uncommon with vascular malformations but seen in 30% to 60%[40,41,44] of patients with hemangioblastoma, may help differentiate the two. A spinal cyst with an enhancing mural nodule and a nonenhancing cyst rim is another characteristic feature of a hemangioblastoma. Spinal angiography may demonstrate enlarged feeding arteries, intense nodular stains, and early draining veins.[45] In terms of natural history, the cysts associated with the tumors tend to grow faster than the tumor itself. The symptomatic mass effect is predominantly caused by the cysts. The tumor alternates between a growth phase

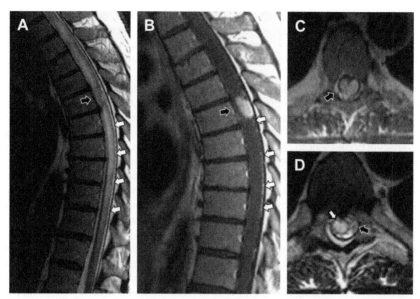

Fig. 5. MR images of intramedullary hemangioblastoma. A 58-year-old man with human immunodeficiency virus and diabetes presents with left-sided numbness, left partial foot drop, and left upper abdominal pain progressing over a period of 6 months. A T2-weighted (W) sagittal image (*A*) shows a heterogeneous mass at T-6 (*black arrow*) associated with extensive cord edema. White arrows show a hypointense linear structure consistent with a vessel posterior to the cord. On the contrast sagittal T1W image (*B*), an enhancing intramedullary bilobulated mass is seen (*black arrow*). Furthermore, an enhancing engorged vessel is seen posterior and caudal to tumor (*white arrows*). Axial T1W contrast (*C*) shows an interesting bilobulated intramedullary and extramedullary snowman appearance (*black arrow*). T2W axial (*D*) hyperintensity (*white arrow*) is consistent with extensive holocord edema that resolved after surgery. The black arrow is a signal void from an abnormal vessel. Pathology was consistent with a hemangioblastoma.

and a quiescent phase with no growth. Hence, the tumor may remain of the same size for several years in a quiescent phase.[38] For this reason, follow-up monitoring with serial imaging at regular intervals is recommended. The first-line treatment is micro-surgical resection using feeder vessels coagulation[44] or temporary arterial occlusion.[46] A cerebrospinal fluid (CSF) fistula is a complication of surgery in less than 5% patients.[44] The presence of multiple tumors may necessitate a more aggressive approach with stereotactic radiosurgery.[47] There has been growing interest in the use of the VEGF inhibitor, bevacizumab, which has shown to cause tumor regression in a single case study.[48] The prognosis in usually excellent,[49] although the tumor recurrence is common in patients with von Hippel-Lindau disease.

RARE SPINAL INTRAMEDULLARY TUMORS
Ganglioglioma

Gangliogliomas are mostly benign WHO grade I tumors. Rarely, they can transform into more aggressive anaplastic gangliogliomas, which are WHO grade III tumors. Only about 15 cases of anaplastic ganglioglioma are reported in the literature.[50] These tumors are comprised of ganglion cells as well as neoplastic glial elements. They constitute roughly about 1% of intramedullary spinal cord tumors.[51] They predominantly occur in the pediatric age group, with three-fourths of the patient's being younger than 16 years of age at diagnosis.[52] There is a male preponderance, with a sex ratio of 1.7:1.[52] There are case reports of these tumors being found in patients with NF1,[53] NF2,[54] Floating-Harbor syndrome,[55] and Peutz-Jeghers syndrome.[56] There are no known definite genetic associations.

In a large case series,[52] the cervicothoracic segment was most commonly involved in about 37.5%, thoracic in 28.5%, cervicomedullary in 14.0%, cervical in 12.5%, and conus in 7.0% of patients with intramedullary spinal ganglioglioma. These tumors favor eccentric locations.[57] They are elongated tumors that extend over an average of 8 vertebral bodies length compared with about 4 vertebral bodies length in intramedullary astrocytomas and ependymomas.[57] Microscopically, they consist of clusters of large ganglion cells, fibrosis, desmoplasia, and calcifications.[58] Antisynaptophysin antibody marker for neoplastic neurons is helpful in confirming pathologic diagnosis.[58]

On a computed tomography (CT) scan, gangliogliomas appear hypodense or CSF dense with patchy contrast enhancement despite their solid nature. About 85% of these tumors show mixed signal intensity on the T1-weighted images.[57] They tend to be hyperintense on T2-weighted images,[59] although roughly about 40% appear heterogeneous on T2 as well as on contrast-enhanced images.[57] The enhancement pattern is mostly patchy, along with pial surface enhancement. About 20% of these tumors show focal enhancement, and 15% of them are nonenhancing.[57] Surrounding vasogenic edema is uncommon and seen in less than 10% of tumors.[57] To differentiate a high-grade anaplastic ganglioglioma from a benign tumor, a preoperative fluorodeoxyglucose positron emission tomography (FDG-PET) or a thallium-201 single-photon emission CT (^{201}TI-SPECT) scan can be helpful.[60] Tumoral cysts are seen in about 40% of patients. These tumors are commonly associated with bony erosions and vertebral column deformities, such as scoliosis. The first-line treatment is gross total resection with laminectomy. Adjuvant radiotherapy and chemotherapy with temozolomide is usually reserved for anaplastic high-grade tumors.[50] The 5-year survival rates are close to 90%, whereas the 10-year survival rates are about 80%.[52,61] Tumor recurrence following surgery occur in about 30% of patients[52] and, hence, require close follow-up with serial imaging.

Oligodendroglioma

Primary spinal oligodendroglioma constitutes 2% of spinal cord tumors. Fewer than 50 cases have been reported in the literature. According to the WHO grading, oligodendrogliomas are WHO grade II, whereas anaplastic oligodendroglioma are WHO grade III.[27] Sixty percent of patients are older than 18 years, with a slight male predominance. The most common site of involvement is the thoracic cord.[24] On MRI, oligodendrogliomas are isointense to the spinal cord on T1-weighted images, hyperintense on T2-weighted images, and show heterogeneous contrast enhancement. As in the brain, hemorrhages and calcifications are relatively common findings.[24,62]

Paraganglioma

Paraganglioma are extra-adrenal pheochromocytomas originating from the chromaffin cells of the autonomic nervous system. They have also been called chemodectomas and glomus tumors, which is terminology based on the anatomic site. Spinal paragangliomas are almost always located in the intradural extramedullary compartment, predominantly within the cauda equina and filum terminale. Paraganglioma are slightly more common in male patients, with a mean age at presentation of about 46 years. Spinal paragangliomas have little or no secretory activity, and the most common symptom is low back pain and radiculopathy. Paragangliomas present with hypointense or isointense signal on T1-weighted images, which are relatively well delineated round, ovoid or lobulated masses with prominent flow voids. On T2-weighted images, there is isointensity to hyperintensity with a possible hemosiderin rim as well as tumoral cyst formation.[63] Angiography may be indicated for preoperative embolization. Surgical excision is usually curative.[24]

Melanocytoma

Melanocytoma are benign, although at times locally aggressive tumors arising from melanocytes within the leptomeninges along the neural axis. Most of these leptomeningeal tumors are extramedullary, with only about 18 cases of intramedullary melanocytomas reported in the literature. On T1-weighted images, they seem to be isointense to hypointense. The degree of melanization affects signal intensities on MRI, which creates variability in their appearance on neuroimaging.[64] On T2-weighted images, they are hypointense to the normal cord. On gradient echo images, there is a blooming effect caused by melanin susceptibility artifact. Heterogeneous enhancement is noted on contrast studies. The cervical/thoracic region is the most common location. Complete cervical resection is usually curative. Subtotal resection is usually followed by external beam radiation therapy.[65]

Lipoma

Lipomas are benign intramedullary tumors. They are thought to arise from premature disjunction of the neural ectoderm from the cutaneous ectoderm during embryonic neurulation before neural tube closure, which allows mesenchymal access to the neural groove, and subsequent development into fat that is indistinguishable from normal body fat.[66] They are commonly seen in the pediatric age group, and occasionally in young adults. Although no syndromic association is known, a single case study reported intramedullary spinal lipoma in a patient with multifocal dysembryoplastic neuroepithelial tumors.[66] They are slow-growing tumors and become symptomatic because of the mass effect from their size. They can occur as a solitary cord lesion or multiple mass lesions. The common initial presentations include pain, dysesthetic sensory changes, gait difficulties, weakness, and incontinence.[67] They tend to favor the cervical segment over the thoracolumbar cord and have a predilection for dorsal location.[68] On gross and microscopic pathology, the tumor resembles normal adipose tissue as found elsewhere in the body.[42] On a CT scan, they have the appearance of a hypodense mass lesion. On MRI, they are hyperintense on T1- and T2-weighted images and show signal cancellation on fat-suppressed or STIR images. They are nonenhancing on postcontrast MRI. Occasional calcifications may show susceptibility signal change on susceptibility-weighted imaging (SWI). MR images of an intramedullary spinal lipoma are shown in **Fig. 6**.

The natural history is usually of a slow-growing mass lesion with progressive myelopathic symptoms. Surgical resection is the first line of treatment. Carbon dioxide lasers are occasionally used for debulking procedures. The timing or the need for surgery is controversial. Lack of cleavage plane and the intermingling of neural and fibrofatty tissue at the periphery of the tumor makes total tumor removal extremely difficult.[69] Based on limited published data, improvement of neurologic symptoms postoperatively is not universal. Total or near-total resection has been shown to produce about 90% of long-term progression-free survival at 16 years compared with only 35% at 10 years for partial resection and debulking procedures.[70] Other than the immediate postoperative morbidity, the long-term survival is usually excellent.

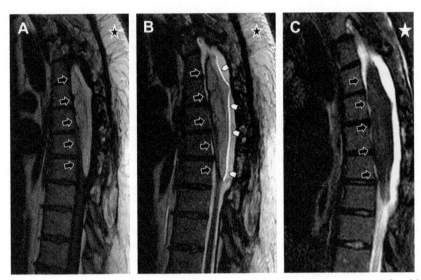

Fig. 6. MR images of intramedullary spinal lipoma. A T3–T8 mass is seen on T1-weighted (W) sagittal (*A*) noncontrast study, consistent with intramedullary mass (*black arrows*) that is hyperintense (short T1). Multilevel laminectomy defect is seen posterior to this. Pathology was consistent with a lipoma. On the T2W (*B*) images there is chemical shift artifact (*white arrowheads*). Chemical shift is caused by the differences between resonance frequencies between fat and water. Fat suppression is the process of using specific MRI parameters to remove the deleterious effects of fat from the resulting images, which is well seen on the STIR sagittal (*C*) where the signal within the lipoma as well as the subcutaneous fat (*star*) is hypointense (suppressed).

Primary CNS Lymphoma

Intramedullary lymphomas are highly aggressive tumors with a poor prognosis. About 90% of the spinal lymphomas arise from large B cells, whereas the rest are T-cell lymphomas.[71] These tumors are considered extremely rare, with a published case series reporting an annual incidence of roughly 1 case diagnosed per year at a large academic hospital.[72] They compose only 1% to 2% of patients with primary CNS lymphoma. Patients who are immunocompetent tend to be middle-aged or older, with a median age of 62.5 years,[72] whereas patients who are immunocompromised are usually younger, in their 30s to 40s. A slight male preponderance is seen. The most commonly known risk factor is immunosuppression, either caused by human immunodeficiency virus or postorgan transplant treatment. A rare case of CNS Epstein-Barr virus infection causing spinal lymphoma has been reported in the literature.[72] The most common initial presentations include back pain as the presenting complain in about 30% of the newly diagnosed patients,[72] progressive myelopathy, and radiculopathy. Occasionally, symptoms may precede the MR appearance.[73] Spine lymphoma favors cervical segment over the thoracolumbar segments.[74] The tumor tends to contact the subarachnoid space.[75] The tumor size is usually greater than 15 mm in diameter.[75] Multifocality is a characteristic of intramedullary spinal lymphoma. More than 50% of spinal lymphomas are multifocal, including intracranial lesions.[72]

On gross pathology, it has indistinct margins, with the cut surfaces being gray or brown. The tumor is usually soft to firm, friable, and granular and may contain hemorrhages and necrosis.[42] The tumor diffusely spreads and extends beyond its macroscopic borders, with cells arranged around blood vessels and encircled by reticulin fibers. Immunohistochemical staining with B- and T-cell markers is helpful in the iden-tification of the cells of origin. One of the major pitfalls with establishing the diagnosis is that the tumor may shrink or vanish following steroid administration, compromising the ability to obtain a histologic diagnosis.

The tumor shows high attenuation on a CT scan with homogeneous contrast enhancement. On MRI, it is usually isointense to hypointense on T1-weighted images[76] and hypointense on T2-weighted images with surrounding hyperintense signal from vasogenic edema.[77] It is homogeneously enhancing on the postcontrast images,[76] with restricted diffusion caused by hypercellularity, diffusion-weighted imaging (DWI). The MRI appearance of an intramedullary spinal lymphoma is shown in **Fig. 7**. Multi-focal persistently enhancing lesions in contact with the subarachnoid space with conus medullaris or cauda equina involvement are characteristic of an intramedullary spinal lymphoma. There may be foci of susceptibility signal changes caused by hemorrhage or calcifications. About 10% of tumors show leptomeningeal involvement.[74] FDG-PET is further helpful in establishing the diagnosis and may show lesion hypermetabolism. The major differential includes multiple sclerosis, neuromyelitis optica, neurosarcoido-sis, transverse myelitis, and immune-mediated paraneoplastic myelopathy syndromes.

Survival typically is less than 1 year without chemotherapy and less than 6 months in patients who are immunocompromised. Treatment is initiated at diagnosis because of the aggressive nature of the tumor. Corticosteroids and methotrexate-based chemo-therapy with or without radiation are the first line of treatment. Systemic side effects are common. Surgery is not helpful. KI-67 expression is shown to be inversely related to survival[78] and may help with prognostication. The prognosis is generally poor, with a 2-year survival of about 36%.[72]

TREATMENT OF PRIMARY INTRAMEDULLARY SPINAL CORD TUMORS

The most important factor in determining long-term neurologic and functional outcome after surgery for patients with intramedullary spinal cord tumors is patients'

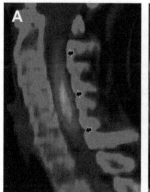
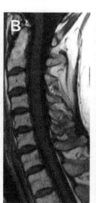
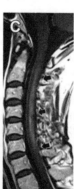
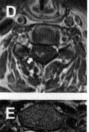
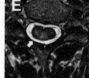

Fig. 7. MR images of spinal intramedullary lymphoma. A 65-year-old woman with a history of non-Hodgkin B-cell lymphoma diagnosed 6 years ago status-post chemotherapy who underwent a PET scan (*A*) for restaging and was found to have a FDG hypermetabolic spinal cord mass from C-2 to C-7 (*black arrows*). T1-weighted (*W*) noncontrast (*B*) sagittal and contrast sagittal (*C*) and axial (*D*) imaging confirms a diffusely enhancing mass with a minimal edema (*white arrow*). This mass is best seen on T2W axial (*E*) images (*white arrow*). Despite being asymptomatic, patient underwent external beam radiation with significant MR response. Unfortunately, patient was also found to have periventricular and corpus callosum enhancement consistent with recurrent lymphoma in the brain.

preoperative neurologic status.[2,79] The second most important factor is the tumor histopathology and grading. Furthermore, the presence of syringomyelia or a cystic component seems to be associated with poor neurologic outcome. Advances in microsurgical techniques and intraoperative electrophysiologic monitoring have significantly reduced operative morbidity. The guiding principle of tumor resectability has been the ability to identify a tumor–spinal cord plane of dissection on neuroimaging. Tumors, such as ependymomas and hemangioblastomas, often exhibit a plane of dissection that facilitates the resection. The absence of a tumor-normal spinal cord interface in infiltrative tumors, such as astrocytomas, permits only subtotal resection or biopsy in hopes of preventing neurologic decline. The exception to this rule is pilocytic astrocytomas (WHO grade I).

In a surgical center experience of 102 patients, gross total resection was achieved in 91.0% of ependymomas, 14.3% of astrocytomas, and 92.0% of hemangioblastomas.[79] When analyzed by tumor location, there was no difference in neurologic outcomes at a mean follow-up of 41.8 months. The incidence of recurrence was 7.3% for ependymoma and 47.6% for astrocytomas. No recurrence was noted in hemangioblastomas. A conclusion drawn from the study was that tumor histology is the most important predictor of neurologic outcome following surgical resection because it predicts resectability and recurrence. The treatment of recurrent tumors is largely based on tumor histology and remains controversial. Incompletely resected low-grade astrocytomas are routinely followed by serial MRI for evidence of tumor progression, and radiation therapy is offered to patients with enlarging tumors or recurrence. Secondary resection is offered to patients with recurring ependymomas. Ependymomas are very amenable to safe, complete removal with a low recurrence rate. Radiation may be indicated in the setting of malignant astrocytoma, recurrent ependymoma, or when a significant portion of the tumor cannot be resected.[80,81]

Intramedullary astrocytomas are typically low-grade tumors treated by surgical resection and monitored for recurrence by clinical and radiographic follow-up. In cases of subtotal resection, some advocate the use of radiation to the residual tumor; this is especially true for fibrillary astrocytomas. At the time of recurrence, radiation therapy should be considered for those tumors not amenable to further surgical intervention.[81] Pilocytic astrocytomas are more amenable to aggressive surgery. Radiation is not usually recommended for pilocytic astrocytomas and hemangioblastomas.[32] Malignant astrocytomas of the spinal cord, however, have a poor prognosis; and radical resection results in high morbidity. Therefore, conservative tumor removal or tissue diagnosis followed by radiation therapy is common practice. In historical studies, the recommended dose of radiation therapy for spinal cord gliomas has been reported to be between 45 Gy and 50 Gy in 25 to 30 fractions given over a course of 5 weeks.[82] Particle beam therapies, such as protons, have been investigated as a means to improve the therapeutic gain of radiotherapy by reducing the integral dose to surrounding normal tissue. Patients with spinal cord gliomas treated with proton beam radiation seem to do significantly worse than their photon-treated counterparts. Stereotactic radiosurgery for intramedullary tumors has been described in small studies with a brief follow-up. A new technique being applied to selected primary spinal cord tumors is an image-guided radiosurgery performed with computer-controlled linear accelerator (linac) based techniques. In the future, this treatment strategy may prove useful in select cases in which complete surgical excision is not possible or after multiple recurrences.[83] The spinal cord is sensitive to the effects of radiation. Overdoses must be avoided to reduce the risk of radiation-induced myelopathy, which is reversible to some extent. The accepted spinal cord tolerance level is 5000 to 5500 cGy administered over 5 to 6 weeks using 180 to 200 cGy daily fractions.

Because of the rarity of spinal cord malignant gliomas, there are only a few cases of chemotherapy-treated tumors. Temozolomide may be a viable option as a concurrent treatment with radiotherapy or an adjuvant regimen for malignant intramedullary spinal cord tumors. Based on activity in intracranial glioblastoma multiforme, the antiangiogenic drug bevacizumab, a humanized monoclonal antibody that inhibits VEGF-A, has been used for the treatment of recurrent high-grade intramedullary gliomas.[84–87] Radiation-induced myelopathy and vascular tumors (hemangioblastomas) may respond to antiangiogenic agents, such as bevacizumab.[88] Improved imaging capabilities as discussed in this article and data from national registries will allow neuro-oncologists the opportunity to study and treat these unusual and rare tumors with more confidence and improved outcomes.

Intramedullary Spinal Metastatic Disease

Intramedullary spinal cord metastasis (ISCM) is a relatively rare sequela of systemic cancer with arguably the worst prognosis of all intramedullary spinal cord tumors. It is diagnosed in less than 1% of systemic patients with cancer.[5] Lung and breast cancers are the most frequent source,[89] although a multitude of different systemic cancers have been associated, including malignant melanoma,[90] renal cell carcinoma,[91] colon carcinoma,[5] papillary thyroid carcinoma,[92,93] cystic adenocarcinoma,[83] epithelioid hemangioepithelioma,[83] prostate adenocarcinoma,[94] choriocarcinoma,[95] gastric adenocarcinoma,[96] ovarian carcinoma,[97] urothelial carcinoma,[98] squamous cell cervical carcinoma,[99] mesothelioma,[100] acute lymphoblastic leukemia,[101] and gliosarcoma.[102] Intracranial cancers, such as pituitary carcinoma,[103] pituitary stalk and hypothalamus germinoma,[104] and supratentorial glioblastoma,[105] are also reported to metastasize to the spinal cord. Location of a supratentorial glioblastoma adjacent to CSF space is thought to be a risk factor for leptomeningeal seeding and subsequent cord invasion.[105]

Motor weakness is the most common presenting symptom, followed by pain and sensory disturbances.[89] Rarely, they may present with a Brown-Séquard syndrome.[9] At the time of diagnosis, most patients with ISCM have a known primary cancer often associated with cerebral and other systemic metastases.[89] In about 3% of patients, the spinal intramedullary lesion is the initial manifestation of the malignant disease.[106] About 90% of patients with ISCM have intracranial metastases, which is 6 times more frequent than those with vertebral metastases.[107] Cervical, thoracic, and lumbar spinal segments are equally effected.[89] Size of the tumors range, on average, from 5 mm up to 6 cm.[83] MRI would typically show an isointense lesion on T1-weighted images and a hyperintense lesion with extensive surrounding edema on a T2-weighted sequence. Postcontrast images would show either a ring-enhancing or a homogenously enhancing lesion. The presence of hemorrhage may produce heterogeneous enhancement. Metastatic tumors that are most likely to present with an intramedullary hemorrhage are choriocarcinoma,[95] papillary thyroid carcinoma,[92] and malignant melanomas.[108] In these cases, the SWI or gradient echo images show hypointense hemorrhagic lesions. MR images of a spinal intramedullary metastatic lesion from a breast cancer are shown in **Fig. 8**.

There are 3 principal treatment modalities available for ISCM, including radiotherapy, chemotherapy, and microsurgical resection of a focal intramedullary mass. The optimal modality and survival benefit with each modality is unclear at this time. Nevertheless, the prognosis remains poor, with a median survival of 4 to 6 months from the time of diagnosis.[89] The 6-month survival rate after radiotherapy was reported to be about 36%.[107] In a retrospective review, a modest survival benefit with improvement in quality of life was noted following surgery.[109] A small series of

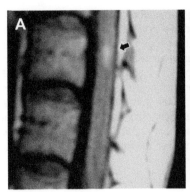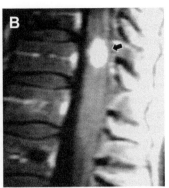

Fig. 8. MR images of spinal metastatic lesion from a breast cancer. A 50-year-old patient with breast cancer with known history of metastatic disease. Intramedullary hemorrhagic hyperintense thoracic cord lesion at T11 lesion (*arrow*) is seen on the noncontrast sagittal T1-weighted (W) images (*A*) that avidly enhances with contrast (*B*). This lesion responded to radiation therapy and the patient's conus medullaris syndrome improved.

9 patients showed an improved survival of about 20 months in patients with metastatic intramedullary melanoma compared with less than 3 months for patients with nonmelanoma metastases.[90] In addition, patients in this series who were ambulatory preoperatively remained ambulatory postoperatively. Hence, surgical resection was thought to help in preserving ambulatory status in symptomatic patients, although its benefit in extending survival is not convincing.[90] Linac-based stereotactic radiosurgery for spinal intramedullary metastatic disease is emerging as a safer alternative[83] and is likely most appropriate for palliative treatment in symptomatic patients. Although several small case series reported different treatment options, a lack of controlled clinical trials, mainly caused by the rarity of these tumors coupled with poor survival from systemic disease burden, makes it difficult to draw reliable conclusions on optimal therapy or prognostic factors.

NOVEL NEUROIMAGING IN INTRAMEDULLARY SPINE TUMORS

The introduction of MRI to clinical practice has been one of the most important advances in the care of patients with spine tumors. The characterization of spine tumors by MRI involves determining, in the context of patient's age and sex, the location of the lesion and whether or not it enhances after gadolinium injection. The fundamental question is whether the mass is intra-axial (intramedullary) or extra-axial (extramedullary). With the exception of MRI, most imaging modalities play a limited role in imaging the spinal cord. Radiographs fail to provide visualization of the cord, although scalloping of the posterior aspect of the vertebral body that occurs in some cases of long-standing intramedullary lesions with substantive cord expansion may be detected. CT and/or CT myelography allows for the visualization of the cord and the identification of areas of gross enlargement but does not provide good resolution of internal structures.[110,111] High-resolution PET is also capable of allowing clinicians to evaluate spinal cord lesions and tumors anatomically as well as metabolically.[112]

The advantages of the MRI are its multiplane capabilities, superior contrast agent resolution, and flexible protocols that play an important role in assessing tumor location and extent, in directing biopsy, in planning appropriate therapy, and in evaluating therapeutic results. The mainstay of spinal cord imaging is the T2-weighted axial and sagittal sequences using fast spin echo, which produces highly detailed T2-weighted sequences in only a few minutes. T1-weighted images should be performed in the axial and sagittal planes with and without gadolinium contrast. Fat suppression studies (STIR) are also particularly sensitive to spinal cord abnormalities as well as to the involvement of adjacent bone marrow. Gradient-echo or susceptibility-weighted sequences are most sensitive to detecting hemorrhage, calcification, and flow voids. MR myelography can generate images that are compatible with those obtained by conventional myelography. Conventional CT myelography is being largely replaced by MR and should be reserved for patients who are not MRI candidates. The role of angiography is mainly limited to diagnose and preoperative embolization of spinal vascular malformation and hypervascular spinal tumors. The MRI appearance of different intramedullary spinal tumors is summarized as a schematic diagram in **Fig. 9.**

The 3-T MR scanner is currently considered the state-of-the-art imaging modality for spinal cord disease. Signal-to-noise ratio increases approximately by twofold compared with MRI using 1.5 T. Using advanced parallel acquisition techniques which combine the signals of several coil elements to reconstruct the image, the signal-to-noise ratio is improved along with accelerated acquisition to reduce scan time. Parallel reconstruction algorithms that reconstruct either the global image from the images produced by each coil or fourier plane of the image from the frequency signals of each coil, are used to further improve image quality with better spatial resolution, and reduced artifacts. The major advantage of the 3-T MRI is improved quality of high-end imaging, such as DWI, diffuse-tensor tractography, SWI, perfusion-weighted imaging (PWI), and MR spectroscopy (MRS).[1] Visualization of the angio architecture of vascular malformations and cord tumors has been aided by the addition of 3-dimensional contrast-enhanced MR angiography, which is a natural extension of standard MRI and should be used in all cases of suspected vascular-related myelopathy. This point is especially true in patients who have hemangioblastomas, paragangliomas, and vascular malformations.[113]

Molecular mobility is an essential contrast mechanism exploited in DWI, reflecting in a measurement of the apparent diffusion coefficient (ADC). The greater the density of structures impeding water mobility, the lower the ADC. Therefore, ADC is considered a noninvasive indicator of cellularity or cell density. DWI is an excellent sequence in the study of acute ischemic infarctions. There have been publications of spinal cord infarctions with restricted diffusion. In addition, DWI and ADC may be markers for hypercellularity, especially in tumors of the spinal cord that include lymphoma and primitive neuroectodermal tumors.[1] In these so-called blue cell tumors, the ADC is lower than in other tumors because of its hypercellularity, which may help in the differential diagnosis of enhancing spinal cord masses (**Box 2**).[114] DWI sequences have been adapted to perform DTI by acquiring data in 6 or more directions. A tensor is used to describe diffusion in an anisotropic system. DTI allows us to visualize the location, orientation, and anisotropy of the white matter tracts in the brain and spine. DTI can be used to provide maps of white matter fiber tracts (tractography) adjacent to spinal cord tumors.[57] *DTI tractography* maps of desired white matter tracts (ie, corticospinal tract) can be overlaid onto high-resolution anatomic images. DTI has the potential to help differentiate destructive intramedullary tumors from tumors that displace normal tissue, which can, in turn, decrease surgical morbidity.[21,115]

SWI is a relatively novel technique that helps in the detection of calcification, iron content, and deoxygenated hemoglobin with higher sensitivity than other MR techniques. SWI can increase the visibility of hemorrhagic, calcified, and vascular tumors and may reflect the tumor grade and improve the differential diagnosis. Iron and

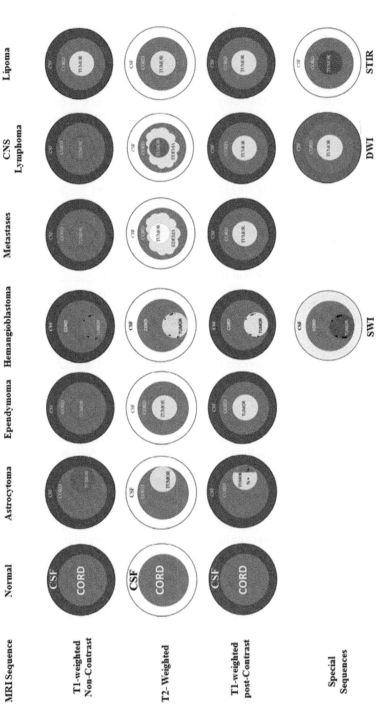

Fig. 9. MRI appearance of different intramedullary spinal tumors. Schematic summary of various tumor-related MR imaging findings in intramedullary tumors. Astrocytomas are commonly found in eccentric location within the cord, and about two-thirds of the spinal astrocytomas enhance. Ependymomas are commonly located centrally. Hemangioblastomas show flow voids in the periphery of the tumor and are hypointense on SWI sequence. Lipomas have similar hyperintense appearance on T1-weighted and T2-weighted images and show hypointense signal suppression on STIR images.

Box 2
Differential diagnosis of spinal cord enlargement

- Intramedullary tumor
  - Ependymoma
  - Astrocytoma
  - Hemangioblastoma
- Demyelinating disease
  - Multiple sclerosis
  - Devic disease
  - Transverse myelitis
  - Acute disseminated encephalomyelitis
- Granulomatosis disease
  - Sarcoid
- Vascular lesions
  - Acute infarction
  - Arteriovenous malformation
  - Cavernous malformation
  - Hemorrhage, posttraumatic
  - Venous hypertension
- Infection
  - Tuberculosis
  - Toxoplasmosis
  - Syphilis
  - Cytomegalic virus infection

---

calcium can be discriminated by their paramagnetic versus diamagnetic behaviors on SWI, which may help identify tumors that are more prone to calcify, such as oligodendroglioma. Aggressive tumors tend to have rapidly growing vasculature and many microhemorrhages. Hence, the ability to detect these changes in the tumor could lead to better determination of the tumor's biologic behavior. SWI imaging of the spinal cord can potentially help in confirming hemosiderin that is often seen with ependymomas and in the evaluation of hemangioblastomas of the spinal cord.[1,116] MRS is a noninvasive imaging technique that offers metabolic information on spine tumor biology that is not available from anatomic imaging. However, because of technical challenges, MRS has been rarely applied to spinal cord tumors. MRS may be used preoperatively, to differentiate between neoplastic from non-neoplastic disease, and expand the differential diagnosis. Elevation of choline indicates increased cellular turnover and, therefore, can serve as a marker of neoplastic disease.[117] MR PWI has enjoyed great clinical and research success in the assessment of cerebrovascular reserve and as an adjunct for assessing biologic behavior of cerebral neoplasms. PWI uses rapid data acquisition techniques to generate temporal data series that capture first-pass kinetics of a contrast agent as it passes through a tissue matrix. PWI can measure the degree of tumor angiogenesis and capillary permeability, both of which are important biologic markers of malignancy, grading, and prognosis, particularly in gliomas.[118] Intraoperative MRI surgical suites have been in operation for more than 15 years. Field strength for these intraoperative MRI systems ranges from 0.1 to 3 T. The main advantages of intraoperative MRI are its excellent soft tissue discrimination and 3-dimensional visualization of the operative site and its near real-time imaging to evaluate the extent of tumor or hemorrhage. The use of intraoperative MRI has led to advances in the extent of tumor resection.[119]

Neuroimaging is entering an exciting new era in which we can ask and expect to answer sophisticated questions concerning intramedullary spine tumors. The shift to high-end imaging incorporating DWI, DTI, MRS, PWI, SWI, PET, and intraoperative MRI as part of the mainstream clinical imaging protocol has provided neurologists, neuro-oncologists, and neurosurgeons a window of opportunity to assess the biologic behavior of intramedullary spine neoplasms. These novel approaches may, in the future, be routinely used preoperatively, intraoperatively, and in therapeutic monitoring. The ultimate success of spine surgery will depend on the incorporation of anatomic and functional imaging with high-field MRI to diagnose patients sooner and more accurately, when patients' performance status is minimally affected. Postoperative prognosis depends on preoperative neurologic morbidity, tumor histology, and post-operative residual disease. Most intramedullary tumors are potentially resectable (ependymoma, pilocytic astrocytoma, and hemangioblastoma) and curable without adjuvant treatment. Tumors that are more infiltrative (astrocytoma, ganglioglioma, oligodendroglioma) or malignant (anaplastic ependymoma or astrocytoma, glioblastoma, metastases, lymphoma) need to be treated with the input of a multidisciplinary team consisting of neurosurgeons, neuro-oncologists, neuroimagers, and radiation oncologists; patients should be followed closely with the same imaging modalities that were instrumental in the initial diagnosis.

ACKNOWLEDGMENTS

The authors would like to thank Drs Vernice Bates, Joe Fritz, and Kalyan Shastri for their help with the article.

REFERENCES

1. Mechtler L. Neuroimaging in neuro-oncology. Neurol Clin 2009;27:171–201, ix.
2. Harrop JS, Ganju A, Groff M, et al. Primary intramedullary tumors of the spinal cord. Spine 2009;34:S69–77.
3. Duong LM, McCarthy BJ, McLendon RE, et al. Descriptive epidemiology of malignant and nonmalignant primary spinal cord, spinal meninges, and cauda equina tumors, United States, 2004-2007. Cancer 2012;118:4220–7.
4. Lonser RR, Weil RJ, Wanebo JE, et al. Surgical management of spinal cord hemangioblastomas in patients with von Hippel-Lindau disease. J Neurosurg 2003;98:106–16.
5. Vassiliou V, Papamichael D, Polyviou P, et al. Intramedullary spinal cord metastasis in a patient with colon cancer: a case report. J Gastrointest Cancer 2012; 43:370–2.
6. Tihan T, Chi JH, McCormick PC, et al. Pathologic and epidemiologic findings of intramedullary spinal cord tumors. Neurosurg Clin N Am 2006;17:7–11.
7. Newton HB, Newton CL, Gatens C, et al. Spinal cord tumors: review of etiology, diagnosis, and multidisciplinary approach to treatment. Cancer Pract 1995;3: 207–18.
8. Miller DH, McDonald WI, Blumhardt LD, et al. Magnetic resonance imaging in isolated noncompressive spinal cord syndromes. Ann Neurol 1987;22:714–23.

9. Kaballo MA, Brennan DD, El Bassiouni M, et al. Intramedullary spinal cord metastasis from colonic carcinoma presenting as Brown-Sequard syndrome: a case report. J Med Case Rep 2011;5:342.

10. Novy J. Spinal cord syndromes. Front Neurol Neurosci 2012;30:195–8.

11. Harrop JS, Sharan A, Ratliff J. Central cord injury: pathophysiology, management, and outcomes. Spine J 2006;6:198S–206S.

12. Lim DC, Gagnon PJ, Meranvil S, et al. Lhermitte's Sign developing after IMRT for head and neck cancer. Int J Otolaryngol 2010;2010:907960.

13. Newton HB, Rea GL. Lhermitte's sign as a presenting symptom of primary spinal cord tumor. J Neurooncol 1996;29:183–8.

14. Fraser S, Roberts L, Murphy E. Cauda equina syndrome: a literature review of its definition and clinical presentation. Arch Phys Med Rehabil 2009;90:1964–8.

15. Gardner A, Gardner E, Morley T. Cauda equina syndrome: a review of the current clinical and medico-legal position. Eur Spine J 2011;20:690–7.

16. Koeller KK, Rosenblum RS, Morrison AL. Neoplasms of the spinal cord and filum terminale: radiologic-pathologic correlation. Radiographics 2000;20:1721–49.

17. Smith AB, Soderlund KA, Rushing EJ, et al. Radiologic-pathologic correlation of pediatric and adolescent spinal neoplasms: part 1, Intramedullary spinal neoplasms. AJR Am J Roentgenol 2012;198:34–43.

18. Kahan H, Sklar EM, Post MJ, et al. MR characteristics of histopathologic subtypes of spinal ependymoma. AJNR Am J Neuroradiol 1996;17:143–50.

19. Plotkin SR, O'Donnell CC, Curry WT, et al. Spinal ependymomas in neurofibromatosis type 2: a retrospective analysis of 55 patients. J Neurosurg Spine 2011;14:543–7.

20. Aguilera DG, Mazewski C, Schniederjan MJ, et al. Neurofibromatosis-2 and spinal cord ependymomas: report of two cases and review of the literature. Childs Nerv Syst 2011;27:757–64.

21. Ducreux D, Fillard P, Facon D, et al. Diffusion tensor magnetic resonance imaging and fiber tracking in spinal cord lesions: current and future indications. Neuroimaging Clin N Am 2007;17:137–47.

22. Smith JK, Lury K, Castillo M. Imaging of spinal and spinal cord tumors. Semin Roentgenol 2006;41:274–93.

23. Waldron JS, Cha S. Radiographic features of intramedullary spinal cord tumors. Neurosurg Clin N Am 2006;17:13–9.

24. Traul DE, Shaffrey ME, Schiff D. Part I: spinal-cord neoplasms-intradural neoplasms. Lancet Oncol 2007;8:35–45.

25. Schwartz TH, McCormick PC. Intramedullary ependymomas: clinical presentation, surgical treatment strategies and prognosis. J Neurooncol 2000;47:211–8.

26. Stephen JH, Sievert AJ, Madsen PJ, et al. Spinal cord ependymomas and myxopapillary ependymomas in the first 2 decades of life: a clinicopathological and immunohistochemical characterization of 19 cases. J Neurosurg Pediatr 2012;9:646–53.

27. Louis DN, Ohgaki H, Wiestler OD, et al. The 2007 WHO classification of tumours of the central nervous system. Acta Neuropathol 2007;114:97–109.

28. Tinchon A, Oberndorfer S, Marosi C, et al. Malignant spinal cord compression in cerebral glioblastoma multiforme: a multicenter case series and review of the literature. J Neurooncol 2012. [Epub ahead of print].

29. Santi M, Mena H, Wong K, et al. Spinal cord malignant astrocytomas. Clinicopathologic features in 36 cases. Cancer 2003;98:554–61.

30. Wilson PE, Oleszek JL, Clayton GH. Pediatric spinal cord tumors and masses. J Spinal Cord Med 2007;30(Suppl 1):S15–20.

31. Koeller KK, Rushing EJ. From the archives of the AFIP: pilocytic astrocytoma: radiologic-pathologic correlation. Radiographics 2004;24:1693–708.
32. Horger M, Ritz R, Beschorner R, et al. Spinal pilocytic astrocytoma: MR imaging findings at first presentation and following surgery. Eur J Radiol 2011;79: 389–99.
33. Samii M, Klekamp J. Surgical results of 100 intramedullary tumors in relation to accompanying syringomyelia. Neurosurgery 1994;35:865–73 [discussion: 73].
34. Houten JK, Cooper PR. Spinal cord astrocytomas: presentation, management and outcome. J Neurooncol 2000;47:219–24.
35. Henson JW. Spinal cord gliomas. Curr Opin Neurol 2001;14:679–82.
36. Morii K, Tanaka R, Washiyama K, et al. Expression of vascular endothelial growth factor in capillary hemangioblastoma. Biochem Biophys Res Commun 1993;194:749–55.
37. Frank TS, Trojanowski JQ, Roberts SA, et al. A detailed immunohistochemical analysis of cerebellar hemangioblastoma: an undifferentiated mesenchymal tumor. Mod Pathol 1989;2:638–51.
38. Wanebo JE, Lonser RR, Glenn GM, et al. The natural history of hemangioblastomas of the central nervous system in patients with von Hippel-Lindau disease. J Neurosurg 2003;98:82–94.
39. Latif F, Tory K, Gnarra J, et al. Identification of the von Hippel-Lindau disease tumor suppressor gene. Science 1993;260:1317–20.
40. Chu BC, Terae S, Hida K, et al. MR findings in spinal hemangioblastoma: correlation with symptoms and with angiographic and surgical findings. AJNR Am J Neuroradiol 2001;22:206–17.
41. Na JH, Kim HS, Eoh W, et al. Spinal cord hemangioblastoma: diagnosis and clinical outcome after surgical treatment. J Korean Neurosurg Soc 2007;42: 436–40.
42. Haberland C. Clinical neuropathology: text and color atlas. New York: Demos; 2007.
43. Imagama S, Ito Z, Wakao N, et al. Differentiation of localization of spinal hemangioblastomas based on imaging and pathological findings. Eur Spine J 2011;20: 1377–84.
44. Bostrom A, Hans FJ, Reinacher PC, et al. Intramedullary hemangioblastomas: timing of surgery, microsurgical technique and follow-up in 23 patients. Eur Spine J 2008;17:882–6.
45. Abul-Kasim K, Thurnher MM, McKeever P, et al. Intradural spinal tumors: current classification and MRI features. Neuroradiology 2008;50:301–14.
46. Clark AJ, Lu DC, Richardson RM, et al. Surgical technique of temporary arterial occlusion in the operative management of spinal hemangioblastomas. World Neurosurg 2010;74:200–5.
47. Daly ME, Choi CY, Gibbs IC, et al. Tolerance of the spinal cord to stereotactic radiosurgery: insights from hemangioblastomas. Int J Radiat Oncol Biol Phys 2011;80:213–20.
48. Omar AI. Bevacizumab for the treatment of surgically unresectable cervical cord hemangioblastoma: a case report. J Med Case Rep 2012;6:238.
49. Garces-Ambrossi GL, McGirt MJ, Mehta VA, et al. Factors associated with progression-free survival and long-term neurological outcome after resection of intramedullary spinal cord tumors: analysis of 101 consecutive cases. J Neurosurg Spine 2009;11:591–9.
50. Schneider C, Vosbeck J, Grotzer MA, et al. Anaplastic ganglioglioma: a very rare intramedullary spinal cord tumor. Pediatr Neurosurg 2012. [Epub ahead of print].

51. Lee JC, Glasauer FE. Ganglioglioma: light and electron microscopic study. Neurochirurgia 1968;11:160–70.
52. Jallo GI, Freed D, Epstein FJ. Spinal cord gangliogliomas: a review of 56 patients. J Neurooncol 2004;68:71–7.
53. Hayashi Y, Nakada M, Mohri M, et al. Ganglioglioma of the thoracolumbar spinal cord in a patient with neurofibromatosis type 1: a case report and literature review. Pediatr Neurosurg 2011;47:210–3.
54. Sawin PD, Theodore N, Rekate HL. Spinal cord ganglioglioma in a child with neurofibromatosis type 2. Case report and literature review. J Neurosurg 1999;90:231–3.
55. Nelson RA, McNamara M, Ellis W, et al. Floating-Harbor syndrome and intramedullary spinal cord ganglioglioma: case report and observations from the literature. Am J Med Genet A 2009;149A:2265–9.
56. De Tommasi A, Luzzi S, D'Urso PI, et al. Molecular genetic analysis in a case of ganglioglioma: identification of a new mutation. Neurosurgery 2008;63:976–80 [discussion: 80].
57. Patel U, Pinto RS, Miller DC, et al. MR of spinal cord ganglioglioma. AJNR Am J Neuroradiol 1998;19:879–87.
58. Miller DC, Lang FF, Epstein FJ. Central nervous system gangliogliomas. Part 1: pathology. J Neurosurg 1993;79:859–66.
59. Cheung YK, Fung CF, Chan FL, et al. MRI features of spinal ganglioglioma. Clin Imaging 1991;15:109–12.
60. Kincaid PK, El-Saden SM, Park SH, et al. Cerebral gangliogliomas: preoperative grading using FDG-PET and 201Tl-SPECT. AJNR Am J Neuroradiol 1998;19: 801–6.
61. Hamburger C, Buttner A, Weis S. Ganglioglioma of the spinal cord: report of two rare cases and review of the literature. Neurosurgery 1997;41:1410–5 [discussion: 5–6].
62. Fountas KN, Karampelas I, Nikolakakos LG, et al. Primary spinal cord oligodendroglioma: case report and review of the literature. Childs Nerv Syst 2005;21: 171–5.
63. Faro SH, Turtz AR, Koenigsberg RA, et al. Paraganglioma of the cauda equina with associated intramedullary cyst: MR findings. AJNR Am J Neuroradiol 1997; 18:1588–90.
64. Demirci A, Kawamura Y, Sze G, et al. MR of parenchymal neurocutaneous melanosis. AJNR Am J Neuroradiol 1995;16:603–6.
65. Eskandari R, Schmidt MH. Intramedullary spinal melanocytoma. Rare Tumors 2010;2:e24.
66. White RD, Kanodia AK, Sammler EM, et al. Multifocal dysembryoplastic neuroepithelial tumour with intradural spinal cord lipomas: report of a case. Case Rep Radiol 2011;2011:734171.
67. Lee M, Rezai AR, Abbott R, et al. Intramedullary spinal cord lipomas. J Neurosurg 1995;82:394–400.
68. Bhatoe HS, Singh P, Chaturvedi A, et al. Nondysraphic intramedullary spinal cord lipomas: a review. Neurosurg Focus 2005;18:ECP1.
69. Naim Ur R, Salih MA, Jamjoom AH, et al. Congenital intramedullary lipoma of the dorsocervical spinal cord with intracranial extension: case report. Neurosurgery 1994;34:1081–3 [discussion: 4].
70. Pang D, Zovickian J, Oviedo A. Long-term outcome of total and near-total resection of spinal cord lipomas and radical reconstruction of the neural placode, part II: outcome analysis and preoperative profiling. Neurosurgery 2010;66:253–72 [discussion: 72–3].

71. Lee DK, Chung CK, Kim HJ, et al. Multifocal primary CNS T cell lymphoma of the spinal cord. Clin Neuropathol 2002;21:149–55.
72. Flanagan EP, O'Neill BP, Porter AB, et al. Primary intramedullary spinal cord lymphoma. Neurology 2011;77:784–91.
73. Herrlinger U, Weller M, Kuker W. Primary CNS lymphoma in the spinal cord: clinical manifestations may precede MRI detectability. Neuroradiology 2002;44:239–44.
74. Koeller KK, Smirniotopoulos JG, Jones RV. Primary central nervous system lymphoma: radiologic-pathologic correlation. Radiographics 1997;17:1497–526.
75. Kuker W, Nagele T, Korfel A, et al. Primary central nervous system lymphomas (PCNSL): MRI features at presentation in 100 patients. J Neurooncol 2005;72:169–77.
76. Slone HW, Blake JJ, Shah R, et al. CT and MRI findings of intracranial lymphoma. AJR Am J Roentgenol 2005;184:1679–85.
77. Coulon A, Lafitte F, Hoang-Xuan K, et al. Radiographic findings in 37 cases of primary CNS lymphoma in immunocompetent patients. Eur Radiol 2002;12:329–40.
78. Szczuraszek K, Mazur G, Jelen M, et al. Prognostic significance of Ki-67 antigen expression in non-Hodgkin's lymphomas. Anticancer Res 2008;28:1113–8.
79. Karikari IO, Nimjee SM, Hodges TR, et al. Impact of tumor histology on resectability and neurological outcome in primary intramedullary spinal cord tumors: a single-center experience with 102 patients. Neurosurgery 2011;68:188–97 [discussion: 97].
80. Armstrong TS, Vera-Bolanos E, Gilbert MR. Clinical course of adult patients with ependymoma: results of the Adult Ependymoma Outcomes Project. Cancer 2011;117:5133–41.
81. Isaacson SR. Radiation therapy and the management of intramedullary spinal cord tumors. J Neurooncol 2000;47:231–8.
82. Kahn J, Loeffler JS, Niemierko A, et al. Long-term outcomes of patients with spinal cord gliomas treated by modern conformal radiation techniques. Int J Radiat Oncol Biol Phys 2011;81:232–8.
83. Veeravagu A, Lieberson RE, Mener A, et al. CyberKnife stereotactic radiosurgery for the treatment of intramedullary spinal cord metastases. J Clin Neurosci 2012;19:1273–7.
84. Kim WH, Yoon SH, Kim CY, et al. Temozolomide for malignant primary spinal cord glioma: an experience of six cases and a literature review. J Neurooncol 2011;101:247–54.
85. Chamberlain MC, Johnston SK. Recurrent spinal cord glioblastoma: salvage therapy with bevacizumab. J Neurooncol 2011;102:427–32.
86. Raco A, Esposito V, Lenzi J, et al. Long-term follow-up of intramedullary spinal cord tumors: a series of 202 cases. Neurosurgery 2005;56:972–81 [discussion: 81].
87. Kaley TJ, Mondesire-Crump I, Gavrilovic IT. Temozolomide or bevacizumab for spinal cord high-grade gliomas. J Neurooncol 2012;109:385–9.
88. Chamberlain MC, Eaton KD, Fink J. Radiation-induced myelopathy: treatment with bevacizumab. Arch Neurol 2011;68:1608–9.
89. Sung WS, Sung MJ, Chan JH, et al. Intramedullary spinal cord metastases: a 20-year institutional experience with a comprehensive literature review. World Neurosurg 2012. [Epub ahead of print].
90. Wilson DA, Fusco DJ, Uschold TD, et al. Survival and functional outcome after surgical resection of intramedullary spinal cord metastases. World Neurosurg 2012;77:370–4.

91. Kaya RA, Dalkilic T, Ozer F, et al. Intramedullary spinal cord metastasis: a rare and devastating complication of cancer–two case reports. Neurol Med Chir 2003;43:612–5.

92. Choi IJ, Chang JC, Kim DW, et al. A case report of "spinal cord apoplexy" elicited by metastatic intramedullary thyroid carcinoma. J Korean Neurosurg Soc 2012;51:230–2.

93. Jeon MJ, Kim TY, Han JM, et al. Intramedullary spinal cord metastasis from papillary thyroid carcinoma. Thyroid 2011;21:1269–71.

94. Lieberson RE, Veeravagu A, Eckermann JM, et al. Intramedullary spinal cord metastasis from prostate carcinoma: a case report. J Med Case Rep 2012;6:139.

95. Ko JK, Cha SH, Lee JH, et al. Intramedullary spinal cord metastasis of choriocarcinoma. J Korean Neurosurg Soc 2012;51:141–3.

96. Cemil B, Gokce EC, Kirar F, et al. Intramedullary spinal cord involvement from metastatic gastric carcinoma: a case report. Turk Neurosurg 2012;22:496–8.

97. Miranpuri AS, Rajpal S, Salamat MS, et al. Upper cervical intramedullary spinal metastasis of ovarian carcinoma: a case report and review of the literature. J Med Case Rep 2011;5:311.

98. Abdulazim A, Backhaus M, Stienen MN, et al. Intramedullary spinal cord metastasis and multiple brain metastases from urothelial carcinoma. J Clin Neurosci 2011;18:1405–7.

99. Ding DC, Chu TY. Brain and intramedullary spinal cord metastasis from squamous cell cervical carcinoma. Taiwan J Obstet Gynecol 2010;49:525–7.

100. Chamberlain MC, Eaton KD, Fink JR, et al. Intradural intramedullary spinal cord metastasis due to mesothelioma. J Neurooncol 2010;97:133–6.

101. Kim W, Min CK, Shim YS, et al. Intramedullary spinal cord metastasis of acute lymphoblastic leukemia as the initial manifestation of relapse. Leuk Lymphoma 2008;49:1214–6.

102. Fischer S, Lee W, Aulisi E, et al. Gliosarcoma with intramedullary spinal metastases: a case report and review of the literature. J Clin Oncol 2007;25:447–9.

103. Sivan M, Nandi D, Cudlip S. Intramedullary spinal metastasis (ISCM) from pituitary carcinoma. J Neurooncol 2006;80:19–20.

104. Shah KC, Chacko G, John S, et al. Spinal intramedullary metastasis from intracranial germinoma. Neurol India 2005;53:374–5.

105. Tantongtip D, Rukkul P. Symptomatic leptomeningeal and entirely intramedullary spinal cord metastasis from supratentorial glioblastoma: a case report. J Med Assoc Thai 2011;94(Suppl 7):S194–7.

106. Gasser T, Sandalcioglu IE, El Hamalawi B, et al. Surgical treatment of intramedullary spinal cord metastases of systemic cancer: functional outcome and prognosis. J Neurooncol 2005;73:163–8.

107. Hashii H, Mizumoto M, Kanemoto A, et al. Radiotherapy for patients with symptomatic intramedullary spinal cord metastasis. J Radiat Res 2011;52:641–5.

108. Ishii T, Terao T, Komine K, et al. Intramedullary spinal cord metastases of malignant melanoma: an autopsy case report and review of the literature. Clin Neuropathol 2010;29:334–40.

109. Kalayci M, Cagavi F, Gul S, et al. Intramedullary spinal cord metastases: diagnosis and treatment - an illustrated review. Acta Neurochir 2004;146:1347–54 [discussion: 54].

110. Seidenwurm DJ, Wippold FJ 2nd, Cornelius RS, et al. ACR Appropriateness Criteria (R) myelopathy. J Am Coll Radiol 2012;9:315–24.

111. Lane B. Practical imaging of the spine and spinal cord. Top Magn Reson Imaging 2003;14:438–43.

112. Sandu N, Popperl G, Toubert ME, et al. Current molecular imaging of spinal tumors in clinical practice. Mol Med 2011;17:308–16.
113. Pattany PM, Saraf-Lavi E, Bowen BC. MR angiography of the spine and spinal cord. Top Magn Reson Imaging 2003;14:444–60.
114. Andre JB, Bammer R. Advanced diffusion-weighted magnetic resonance imaging techniques of the human spinal cord. Top Magn Reson Imaging 2010;21:367–78.
115. Vertinsky AT, Krasnokutsky MV, Augustin M, et al. Cutting-edge imaging of the spine. Neuroimaging Clin N Am 2007;17:117–36.
116. Wang M, Dai Y, Han Y, et al. Susceptibility weighted imaging in detecting hemorrhage in acute cervical spinal cord injury. Magn Reson Imaging 2011;29:365–73.
117. Marliani AF, Clementi V, Albini-Riccioli L, et al. Quantitative proton magnetic resonance spectroscopy of the human cervical spinal cord at 3 Tesla. Magn Reson Med 2007;57:160–3.
118. Liu X, Germin BI, Ekholm S. A case of cervical spinal cord glioblastoma diagnosed with MR diffusion tensor and perfusion imaging. J Neuroimaging 2011;21:292–6.
119. Duprez TP, Jankovski A, Grandin C, et al. Intraoperative 3T MR imaging for spinal cord tumor resection: feasibility, timing, and image quality using a "twin" MR-operating room suite. AJNR Am J Neuroradiol 2008;29:1991–4.

Management of Spasticity from Spinal Cord Dysfunction

Jeffrey A. Strommen, MD

KEYWORDS

- Spasticity • Upper motor neuron syndrome • Chemodenervation
- Intrathecal baclofen • Benzodiazepines • Clonodine • Tizanidine

KEY POINTS

- Management of spasticity must be individualized based on specific patient goals.
- Begin with a foundation of conservative management and build upon this depending on the defined goals.
- Understand that some degree of spasticity may provide functional benefit and treatment may lead to functional decline.
- Involvement of the rehabilitation team in these treatment decisions is important to assure that the goals of treatment are being met.

INTRODUCTION

Spasticity is a common but not inevitable sequelae associated with damage or dysfunction of the upper motor neuron pathway within the central nervous system. Classically, as defined by Lance, spasticity is a motor disorder characterized by a velocity-dependent increase in tonic stretch reflexes (muscle tone) with exaggerated tendon jerks, resulting from hyperexcitability of the stretch reflex, as one component of the upper motor neuron syndrome.[1] This is somewhat simplified, however, because in the clinical setting, spasticity may also be characterized by spasms, stiffness, clonus, and pain, all of which have functional consequences. Because it has become more clear that spasticity has many potential pathophysiological mechanisms and is clearly influenced by multiple afferent (cutaneous and proprioceptive) pathways, a more appropriate definition with clinical relevance may be "disordered sensory-motor control, resulting from an upper motor neuron lesion, presenting as intermittent or sustained involuntary activation of muscles."[2,3] It is important to understand that spasticity is just one component of the upper motor neuron syndrome, which may have deleterious functional consequences. In addition to the positive symptom of spasticity, negative symptoms such as weakness and lack of coordination may equal or exceed the impairment, leading to functional decline (**Table 1**).

Department of Physical Medicine and Rehabilitation, Mayo Clinic, Rochester, MN, USA
E-mail address: strommen.jeffrey@mayo.edu

Neurol Clin 31 (2013) 269–286
http://dx.doi.org/10.1016/j.ncl.2012.09.013
0733-8619/13/$ – see front matter © 2013 Elsevier Inc. All rights reserved.

neurologic.theclinics.com

Case study

JB is a 40-year-old man who had a spinal cord injury at the age of 34 years related to a motor vehicle accident. His injury is classified at C7 ASIA A, and he functions from a power wheelchair base with caregiver assistance. He was initially flaccid, but after the spinal shock cleared, 4 weeks after the injury, his tone began to increase. This situation was managed well with stretching and wheelchair positioning initially, but during rehabilitation, spasticity increased, with JB requiring more assistance with transfers and experienced significant sleep disruption because of flexor spasms. Baclofen was initiated with at a dose of 10 mg twice a day and gradually increased to 10 mg 4 times a day, which significantly improved the tone during the day, but he still had frequent flexor spasms at night. Valium was initiated at 5 mg at bedtime with marked improvement. JB was dismissed home but returned 4 months later with reports of significant clonus of his feet that caused distress and early heel cord contractures. Attempts to increase the dose of baclofen led to unacceptable sedation. Local chemodenevation was performed with botulinum toxin injections into the gastrocnemius and soleus muscles, which improved the clonus and allowed improved stretching. Intermittently, the spasticity would increase in a relatively acute manner and he would experience associated headache and flushing. In general, these episodes of increased spasticity and autonomic dysreflexia were related to urinary tract infections, which resolved with appropriate antibiotic treatment, but occasionally were also caused by constipation. JB presents now with 6 months of gradually worsening spasticity with abdominal spasm, flexor spasms of the lower extremities, and increased care needs. Extensive evaluation including abdominal imaging, laboratory, urologic evaluation, and magnetic resonance imaging to exclude syringomyelia were all unremarkable. Given the previous sedating effects of escalating the dose of baclofen, the patient chose not to increase or add oral medication. A 50-μg intrathecal test dose was performed. Baseline tone was Ashworth 3 bilaterally, which reduced to 1 after injection. His pain and caregiver burden improved. The patient elected to undergo implantation of an intrathecal baclofen pump with excellent spasticity control and discontinuation of all oral spasticity medication.

The literature has reported that up to 80% of patients with spinal cord injury have spasticity[4–6] and that of these patients, 41% listed this as a major obstacle to reintegration and nearly 50% as requiring pharmacologic treatment. Similarly, spasticity is reported in 60% to 80% of those with multiple sclerosis with the quality of life inversely related to the degree of spasticity.[7]

The rationale for treatment of spasticity is individualized in that spasticity may not always have a negative impact on function; rather in some cases, it may provide some benefit. In this situation, treatment of spasticity has the potential to lead to further functional decline. **Boxes 1** and **2** and list the negative and potentially beneficial effects of spasticity.

PATHOPHYSIOLOGY

The exact pathophysiology of spasticity is uncertain but is clearly very complex. Motor control requires a feedback loop that integrates information regarding position,

Table 1
Upper motor neuron syndrome

Positive Symptoms	Negative Symptoms
Spasticity	Paralysis
Hyperreflexia	Weakness
Release of primitive reflexes (Babinski)	Loss of dexterity
Dystonia	Fatigue
Athetosis	—

Box 1
Potential positive benefits of spasticity
Standing
Transfers
Gait
Bone density
Possibly improved circulation
Muscle mass

muscle activity, and velocity. This regulation is provided through muscle spindle and Golgi tendon organs as well as multiple spinal interneurons and supraspinal influences. In practical terms, spasticity is related to an imbalance of inhibition and excitation. A recent comprehensive review of the potential mechanisms by Elbasiouny and colleagues[8] has attempted to evaluate several potential mechanisms and assess the likelihood of involvement and relative significance in the pathophysiology of spasticity. The most likely mechanisms are thought to be related to the enhancement of excitability of motor neurons through activation of persistent inward currents due to loss of descending control and enhanced excitability of interneurons. In addition, the mechanism of axonal sprouting playing a role with local Ia afferents sprouting after injury forming new synapses on the motor neurons and contributing to several spinal mechanisms underling spasticity is likely. Fusimotor hyperexcitability may also play a role, with hyperactivity of gamma motor neurons and Golgi tendon organs leading

Box 2
Negative effects of spasticity
Impairment
Pain
Fatigue
Sleep difficulties
Joint contractures
Bowel/bladder dysfunction
Pressure ulcers
Activity and Participation
Decreased mobility
Inadequate seating
Difficulty with activities of daily living
Falls
Sexual dysfunction
Vocational disability
Social isolation
Impaired self esteem
Increased caregiver burden

to exaggerated stretch reflexes and impaired control of the muscle spindles and stretch reflex gain.[9] Finally, alteration in other spinal mechanisms such as reduction of postactivation depression, uncontrolled activation of persistent inward currents, reduction of presynaptic inhibition, and reduction in Ia reciprocal inhibition clearly play a role. The role and degree of each of these mechanisms in the development of spasticity is uncertain, but they provide multiple potential targets for intervention.

CLINICAL MEASUREMENTS

The most commonly used measures of spasticity with high reliability are the Ashworth and modified Ashworth scales (**Table 2**).[10,11] These are clinically useful and reliable measurements that can be used as an ordinal value, but by themselves, they poorly define the potential of impact of spasticity. These measures are performed in a supine relaxed position and thus are inadequate to assess the effect of activity on spasticity. It is not uncommon in clinical practice to find minimal spasticity on supine clinical examination and then note a marked increased, and functionally limiting, tone with activities such as transfers, gait, or bowel/bladder management. Although these measures serve as a clinical and research measure, the clinician must observe the patient during activities to determine the true impact of spasticity. Additional clinical measures include the Penn spasm frequency scale and the spasm frequency score, both of which can be used to monitor treatment efficacy (**Table 3**). Multiple other potential measures incorporating electrophysiological, neurophysiologic, and biomechanical measures are also available, but in the author's experience, they are useful only in the research realm. A more comprehensive review of these techniques is found in a review by Biering-Sorensen.[12,13]

TREATMENT
Introduction

The degree and impact of spasticity varies based on the injury and also individually as to how this impairs or enhances function. Assessment and treatment goals thus must

Table 2
Spasticity scales

	Grade	Criteria
Ashworth Scale	0	No increase in tone
	1	Slight increase in tone, giving a "catch" when the limb is moved in flexion or extension
	2	More marked increase in tone, but limb easily flexed
	3	Considerable increase in tone; passive movement difficult
	4	Limb rigid in flexion or extension
Modified Ashworth Scale	0	No increase in muscle tone
	1	Slight increase in muscle tone, manifested by a catch and release or by minimal resistance at the end of the ROM when the affected part is moved in flexion or extension
	1+	Slight increase in muscle tone, manifested by a catch, followed by minimal resistance throughout the remainder (less than half) of the ROM
	2	More marked increase in muscle tone through most of the ROM, but affected part easily moved
	3	Considerable increase in muscle tone; passive movement difficult
	4	Affected part rigid in flexion or extension

Abbreviation: ROM, range of motion.

Table 3
Spasm scales

Penn Spasm Frequency Scale	0	No spasms
	1	Mild spasms at stimulation
	2	Irregular strong spasms, less than once per hour
	3	Spasms more often than once per hour
	4	Spasms more than 10 times/h
Spasm Frequency Score	1	No spasms
	2	One or fewer spasms per day
	3	Between 1 and 5 spasms/d
	4	5 to <10 spasms/d
	5	10 or more spasms/d, or continuous contraction

be determined on an individual case basis. As previously noted, spasticity may enhance activities such as transfers, whereby, for example, the patient uses the extensor spasticity to rise to a standing position and pivot to the wheelchair. Similarly, the ambulatory patient may find that the extensor spasm helps to control the knee flexion moment, thus preventing knee collapse because of the underlying weakness. Treatment of spasticity in this setting may lead to increased dependence on mobility and activities of daily living. Spasticity that negatively affects function, leading to pain or secondary complications such as contracture and pressure wounds, or that increases caregiver burden is likely to require treatment. Treatment goals may include *improved* range of motion, mobility, gait, orthotic fit, positioning, ease of hygiene, and cosmesis. Treatment goals may also include *reduced* pain, energy expenditure, and pain and caregiver burden. Any treatment should be expected to affect these treatment goals and if not, should be reassessed.

Multiple considerations should be taken into account when developing an individualized treatment plan. The *chronicity* as well as the *severity* play a role in choosing the appropriate treatment options. During early stages after spinal cord injury, delaying pharmacologic interventions may be appropriate in that these may lead to secondary issues such as difficulty with blood pressure management, bowel management, or worsening of fatigue. Early tone may also enhance respiratory function and mobility. Once these secondary conditions stabilize, pharmacologic intervention may be more warranted. The *distribution* of spasticity will also affect the treatment recommendations. In general, those with diffuse spasticity will require a more systemic treatment such as with oral pharmacologic agents, whereas those with more focal functional limiting spasticity such as excessive finger flexor tone or lower extremity adductor tone may benefit from local treatment such as use of botulinum toxin or phenol injections. The locus of injury or dysfunction, whether cerebral or spinal, will affect treatment both in relation to the effectiveness of various agents as well as the potentials side effects such as lowered seizure threshold with Lioresal, which may need to be avoided in a patient with a traumatic brain injury. Those with cerebral cause of spasticity may also have significant cognitive and behavioral issues that could be negatively affected by some of these agents. Availability of care, support, and cost will certainly affect treatment choices as well. Effective treatment requires an individualized combination treatment regimen necessitating a broad knowledge of various treatment options. In general, no single treatment option will manage spasticity in all individuals. A treatment paradigm characterized by a foundation of the most conservative measures, which will be used for most patients, followed by progression to physical modalities, pharmacologic intervention, local chemodenervation, intrathecal delivery systems, and finally, surgery may be part of the treatment plan. Such a pyramid system was described by

Merritt,[14] which has been subsequently modified given the advances in treatment. The foundation of treatment is based on a daily stretching program as well as avoidance and identification of potentials noxious stimuli that exacerbate the spasticity. On this are built the treatments as described above (**Fig. 1**).

Prevention of Noxious Nociceptive Input

Spasticity is a dynamic process, not only in that it classically varies depending on factors such as position or velocity but also in that it varies day to day, which seems to be at least partly due to other external factors. A significant change in spasticity should alert the patient and physician to potentials systemic or local triggers. Worsening spasticity may be the initial symptom of a urinary tract infection, often in conjunction with urinary urgency, frequency, and incontinence. Typical features of fever and dysuria may be absent. Similarly, disruption of the bowel management program with constipation may also lead to a significant increase in tone and spasms. Other medical triggers could include deep venous thrombosis (DVT), decubitus ulcers, urinary tract stones, ingrown toenails, fractures, or even more serious causes such as an acute abdomen. Simple noxious external stimuli such as pinching of skin though improper position, zippers, tight stockings, and catheter straps will lead to an abrupt change in tone. Patient education is paramount so they and their caregivers can identify the potential cause and correct the problem before it escalates. The physician needs to be aware of these potential triggers and also understand that the general medical examination may be quite different in those with spinal cord dysfunction. The patient will not be able to localize the area of pain, and typical findings such as abdominal rebound and rigidity may be absent. These noxious stimuli are also those that may lead to autonomic dysreflexia, characterized by elevated blood pressure, headaches, facial flushing, and bradycardia in those with spinal cord lesion above T6.[13] Recognition of this by the patient is critical as determining the noxious stimulation is the only way to resolve the hypertension emergency, which may precipitate sudden cerebrovascular or cardiac events.

Physical Modalities

Stretching

Stretching remains the essential principle of management of all patients and should form the base from which further treatments are added. Stretching not only may briefly reduce the spasticity[15] but also, equally important, reduce the chronic rheologic changes such as stiffness, contractures, fibrosis, and atrophy. These rheologic issues may result from spastic muscles that remained shortened for long durations. This in turn leads to significant functional impairment because of reduced control of residual voluntary movements, impaired ability of weight bearing or position, and increased risk of secondary complications such as pressure sores. Stretching should be steady, continuous, and directional.[14] These passive stretching activities are initially provided by a physical therapist, but the ultimate goal is education to the patient and caregivers so that these can be performed on a daily basis. Prolonged passive standing though the use of a tilt table, standing frame, or standing wheelchair may also be used to provide stretch and has been shown to at least temporarily reduce tone.[16–19]

Splinting and positioning

Although splinting with devices such as an ankle-foot orthosis (AFO) is most commonly used to improve function by preventing excessive plantar flexion, either passive due to weakness or active due to tone, during the gait cycle, they may also improve spasticity and certainly reduce the risk of contracture. Proper positioning in bed and in the wheelchair not only can reduce the risk of contracture but also may

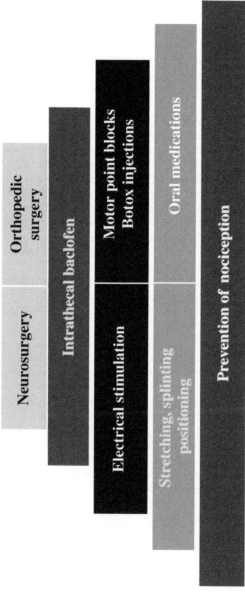

Fig. 1. Spasticity management options. (*Data from* Merritt JL. Management of spasticity in spinal cord injury. Mayo Clin Proc 1981;56(10):616.)

influence the degree of spasticity. Postures that should be avoided include a leg scissoring posture (bilateral hip extension, adduction, and internal rotation), the windswept position (hip flexion, abduction, and external rotation on one side and relative hip extension, adduction, and internal rotation on the other), and the fort-leg position, which can exacerbate the spasticity.[20] The affected joint can also be placed in a prolonged stretch position though serial casting, which involves placing the joint at the stretch through casting and changing this every 5 to 7 days with further stretch. Although there is some evidence for lower reflex activation with serial casting, this technique is mostly used for reduction of existing contractures because there is also a component of improved soft tissue extensibility with the prolonged stretch.[21] Serial casting to provide prolonged stretch in conjunction with botulinum toxin injection to reduce the tone is commonly used in combination.

Electrical Stimulation

A variety of electrical stimulation techniques may be used to reduce spasticity, with the most commonly used being muscle or peripheral nerve stimulation. Functional electrical stimulation (FES) is designed to provide coordinated contraction of muscle groups to produce a purposeful movement. This may involve activities such as walking, usually with bracing, riding an exercise bicycle, or performing upper extremity activities such as grasp. Although passive movements and stretching reduce spasticity as discussed, the addition of FES has been shown to be significantly more effective in those with complete[22–24] or incomplete[25] spinal cord injuries. Direct muscle stimulation to simulate isometric exercise of the quadriceps has also been shown to reduced spasticity but will little carry over 24 hours later.[26] Electrical stimulation has the disadvantage of being costly, often requiring skilled physical therapy intervention and with short-lived effect. The technique does, however, seem to have a more prominent role with neuromuscular reeducation techniques such as locomotor retraining.

Oral Pharmacologic Treatment

A variety of medication can be utilized to modulate spasticity but these effects need to be balanced against the potential for functional decline, reduced strength, and potentials side effects. General "muscle relaxants" such as carisoprodol and cyclobenzaprine seem to have little role in managing spasticity. Given the complex physiologic mechanisms, various other medications are available, and others are being developed, that can target these pathways and hopefully minimize the potential side effects. The list of proven medication is relatively limited at this time, but with either single or multiple agent combination, an individualized regimen can usually be developed under close supervision. **Table 4** lists the most common oral agents available. In general, the available medication can be grouped into agents that use (1) γ-aminobutyric acid (GABA) in the interneurons (diazepam, Lioresal0), (2) alpha-2 adrenergic agents acting in the central nervous system (tizanidine, clonidine), and (3) peripheral inhibition at muscle or neuromuscular level (dantrolene).

Lioresal (baclofen)

Baclofen is a structural analog of GABA with specific affinity for $GABA_B$ receptors. It is thought to reduce spasticity by enhancing inhibitory influences by increasing presynaptic inhibition through hyperpolarization, preventing the influx of calcium required for the release of neurotransmitters. Postsynaptically it likely acts by hyperpolarizing Ia afferents. The net effect is inhibition of monosynaptic and polysynaptic spinal reflexes.[27] With oral dosing, metabolism is 15% hepatic, with elimination primarily through the kidneys and a half-life of approximately 3.5 hours.[28] There are a variety of potential

Table 4
Common oral spasticity agents

Drug	MOA (Mechanism of Action)	Metabolism Elimination	Starting Dose	Range and Titration	Precautions
Lioresal (Baclofen)	Presynaptic inhibition of GABA$_B$ receptors, active both presynaptically and postsynaptically	Hepatic 15% Renal excretion 85% Half-life 2–4 h	5–10 mg bid	10 mg every 5–7 d, goal of tid, qid dosing Maximum 80 mg	Adjust with renal disease, avoid abrupt discontinuation
Diazepam (Valium)	Presynaptic inhibition by facilitating postsynaptic effects of GABA$_A$	Hepatic Renal excretion inactive Half-life 20–80 h	2.5 mg	As tolerated	Liver dosing Caution in elderly
Tizanidine (Xanaflex)	α_2 agonist, Presynaptic inhibition at α_2 receptors, blocks release of excitatory neurotransmitters, facilitated inhibitory neurotransmitter	Hepatic 95% Excretion: renal 60%, fecal 20% Half-life 2.5 h	2–4 mg	Increase by 2- to 4-mg increments every 5–7 d to tid dosing, maximum 36 mg	Sedation Possible hypotension
Clonidine	α_2 agonist, enhanced presynaptic inhibition	Hepatic 40%–60% Renal excretion 40%–60% unchanged Half-life 12–14 h	0.1 mg daily	Up to 0.4 mg/d	Hypotension Bradycardia
Dantrolene sodium (Dantrium)	Interferes with calcium release at sarcoplasmic reticulum	Hepatic metabolism Renal excretion	25 mg daily	25- to 50-mg increments every 5–7 d, goal qid dosing, maximum 400 mg	LFT monitoring

Abbreviation: LFT, liver function test.

side effects including sedation, drowsiness, and fatigue, which are generally the primary reason for discontinuation. Given these side effects, tolerance in those with cerebral-related spasticity may be more limiting. Another reason for discontinuation may be the precipitation of weakness. This can generally be explained by the effect of reducing clinical spasticity, which may have been functionally beneficial to the patient. By reducing the spasticity, the underlying volitional muscle weakness may be unmasked. This unmasking generally presents with increased difficulties with transfers and ambulation. Baclofen does have the potential to lower seizure threshold and can lead to seizures with abrupt discontinuation. Cautious use is recommended in those with a pre-existing seizure disorder, and a taper is always recommended when the drug is discontinued. Although there is no clear consensus on the taper speed, the author tapers approximately 10 mg/wk in the outpatient setting. When initiating treatment, 5 to 10 mg twice per day is generally recommended to assess tolerance. This dose is then increased to 3 or 4 times per day dosing, given the relatively short half-life, followed by 5 to 10 mg weekly titrations with a maximum recommended dose of 80 mg/d. Dosing up to 160 mg has been effective in some patients, given that there are no significant adverse effects related to sedation or weakness. Dosing may need to be adjusted in kidney disease given the fact that the drug undergoes primarily renal clearance.

There has been extensive clinical experience and use of baclofen, which is often the initial drug of choice for many clinicians. Despite the general acceptance, there is a relative paucity of scientific evidence for efficacy. In a recent study by Aydin[29] there was a clear improvement in spasticity with dosing up to 80 mg per day as measured by the Ashworth score as well as in measures of disability. This dosage also seems to be especially effective with flexor spasms.[27]

Benzodiazepines

Diazepam is likely the oldest antispasticity agent still in use. The mechanism of action is central, acting on the brainstem reticular formation and spinal polysynaptic pathways through $GABA_A$ receptors.[30] It binds postsynaptically, effectively increasing presynaptic inhibition or monosynaptic and polysynaptic pathways. Adverse effects have been a limiting factor in its use. Diazepam undergoes hepatic metabolism and is renally excreted as metabolites with a variable half-life ranging from 20 to 80 hours. Primary side effects are related to central nervous system depression, leading to sedation and impaired cognition, attention, and coordination. Additional effects include intoxication and withdrawal, which may lead to symptoms ranging from anxiety to seizures and coma.[27] This drug has somewhat fallen out of favor given these adverse effects and the very long half-life, particularly in the elderly. In the appropriate clinical setting it can be an effective and appropriate second agent. Diazepam is particularly useful as an adjunctive agent for nocturnal spasticity. Nocturnal dosing can generally begin at 5 mg and be increased to 10 mg if necessary. Daytime dosing is generally lower and must be slowly titrated as tolerated.

Clonazepam is a medication similar to diazepam but has a shorter time of activity and is more easily discontinued. It may be used for suppression of myotonia and dystonia and has shown some benefit in dystonia. Half-life is also relatively long at 18 to 28 hours but not as prolonged as that of diazepam, giving it some advantage with regard to the degree of central depression. It again seems to be most beneficial for nocturnal spasms that disrupt sleep. Doses range from 0.5 to 2 mg.

Tizanidine

Tizanidine is an imidazoline derivative that acts centrally at the alpha-adrenergic receptor, both at the supratentorial and spinal levels. The primary mechanism of action is blocking the release of excitatory amino acids, glutamate and aspartate, in addition to facilitating glycine, which is an inhibitory neurotransmitter.[27] Half-life is approximately 2.5 hours, and the drug is hepatically metabolized to an inactive compound, which is subsequently cleared by renal mechanisms. Given these facts, dosing needs to be adjusted in those with hepatic failure, and this drug is a better choice in those with renal compromise, in contrast to Lioresal. The most common side effects reported in clinical trials include drowsiness, sedation, and dizziness. As this drug acts at the α_2 receptors, hypotension is possible, especially when used in combination with other antihypertensive agents. This medication has been most studied in multiple sclerosis trials but is commonly used for spasticity of both spinal and cerebral causes. Tizanidine has been compared with Lioresal with regard to efficacy and side effects. Two studies have revealed that the 2 agents are equally effective but that tizanidine is better tolerated with regard to sedation and weakness.[31,32] No direct comparison of tizanidine with other agents in traumatic spinal cord injury have been completed, but a randomized controlled trial of tizanidine compared with placebo in traumatic spinal cord injury has shown a significant improvement in both the Ashworth and a biomechanical pendulum measure.[33] Adverse effects were, however, common in this group, leading to a discontinuation rate of 34%. This has certainly been this clinician's experience where significant sedation is a limiting factor. The author generally begins with Lioresal as the initial agent and if ineffective, then trial tizanidine. The starting dose is generally 2 to 4 mg at bedtime, increasing 2 to 4 mg every 5 to 7 days to 3 times a day dosing with a maximum daily dose of 36 mg/d. This can be used in combination with other agents, but the sedative effects are additive, requiring cautious adjustments.

Clonidine

Clonidine can be provided in either oral or transdermal form. It acts primarily as an α_2 agonist at both supraspinal and spinal sites. Half-life is approximately 15 to 19 hours, with the drug metabolized primarily by hepatic mechanisms but with a portion excreted renally in an active form. Dosing may thus need to be adjusted especially in renal disease. The primary side effects are hypotension and bradycardia, both of which are especially sensitive in spinal cord injury given the autonomic instability. Clonidine is generally used in conjunction with either Lioresal or tizanidine.[34] The starting dose is 0.1 mg daily with cautious and gradual increase as blood pressure tolerates. A transdermal formulation provides more uniform drug levels and needs to be applied only every 7 days. A small case series has revealed significant improvement, particularly with flexor spasms.[35] In those with hypertension and intermittent functionally impairing or painful flexor spasms, this is an excellent choice, beginning with Catapres TTS 1 (0.1 mg) and increasing to TTS 3 (0.3 mg) as tolerated.

Dantrolene sodium

Dantrolene is unique among other antispastic agents in that the mechanism of action is at the peripheral level, where it induces skeletal muscle relaxation by directly affecting the contractile response. It is suggested that its interference with the release of calcium ions from the sarcoplasmic reticulum results in the dissociation of the excitation–contraction coupling in skeletal muscle. The benefit of this dissociation is the lack of central nervous system effects such as sedation or confusion. The major drawback of the medication is the potential for serious hepatotoxity, with overall incidence reported at 1.8%, 0.3%, which were fatal. This effect was more likely in women older than 30 years and taking more than 300 mg for over 60 days.[36] Half-life is approximately 15 hours, and the drug is metabolized in the liver and eliminated in urine and bile. Dosing in initiated at 25 mg/d and slowly titrated by 25- to 50-mg increments every 5–7 days up to 100 mg 4 times per day. At the start of dantrolene sodium therapy, it is desirable to perform liver function studies (aspartate aminotransferase, alanine aminotransferase, alkaline phosphatase, total bilirubin) for a baseline or to establish whether there is preexisting liver disease. If baseline liver abnormalities exist and are confirmed, there is a clear possibility that the potential for dantrolene sodium hepatotoxicity could be enhanced. Appropriate interval monitoring needs to be performed, initially at least biweekly and then monthly for at least the first 6 months followed by every 3 months. If there is no significant response after 60 days, the medication should be discontinued. Dantrolene is generally recommended for spasticity of cerebral origin such as stroke or traumatic brain injury given the relative lack of central depressant effects; however, it must be used with caution and only with frequent liver function test monitoring.

Other medications

Gabapentin, developed primarily as an anticonvulsant and commonly used as a neuromodulatory agent for neuropathic pain may have some benefit in spasticity, but evidence is limited. Gruenthal and colleagues[37] reported an 11% reduction in the median Ashworth scale without other significant functional or treatment effects. This, however, may be a reasonable medication to test in the situation in which both neuropathic pain and spasticity are limiting or when it is suspected that the neuropathic pain is the primary noxious stimulus leading to increased spasticity.

The cannabinoids have been shown to improve spasticity in the population with multiple sclerosis.[38] There is a paucity of evidence for use in spinal cord injury. A single double-blind placebo-controlled study of 11 males with traumatic and nontraumatic injuries revealed a significant reduction of spasticity, as measures by the Ashworth scale, in patients receiving nabilone, but other outcome measures gave negative results.[39]

4-Aminopyridine has been shown to improve walking ability in persons with multiple sclerosis[40] but has little effect on spinal cord injury.

Local Treatments

Local treatment with focal neurolysis or chemodenervation has been used as a spasticity management tool in a variety of upper motor neuron disorders. The agents generally used are phenol or more commonly botulinum toxin A or B. Chemodenervation has the advantage of providing local muscle relaxation without the systemic or central side effects. Botulinum toxin, in particular, is easy to administer, titratable, and reversible. Phenol injections may be used for motor nerve blocks or motor point blocks. Phenol has the advantage of a longer effect, lasting up to 1 year, lesser cost, and better drug stability but has potential side effects of residual causalgia, edema, and skin sloughing. Botulinum toxin is also effective in reducing tone with selected graded weakness and can be used in conjunction with the previously discussed systemic treatments. The disadvantages of botulinum toxin are few but include cost and a relatively short-lived effect of 3 to 6 months. Selection of patients for chemodenervation include (1) clearly defined goals, (2) spasticity limited to a functional unit usually consisting of 4 to 6 upper extremity muscles or 2 to 4 lower limb muscles, and (3) determining that weakening the limb will not further compromise function. Relative contraindications to botulinum toxin include fixed contractures, coexisting neuromuscular disorders, use of aminoglycosides, pregnancy, or bleeding disorders. Botulinum toxin A varieties include onabotulinumtoxinA (Botox) and abobotulinumtoxin A (Dysport). Botulinum toxin B is available as Myobloc. Botox dosing in individual muscles vary from as little as 10 units in small hand muscles to 200 units in large lower limb muscles. The general upper limit dosing has gradually increased over the years; at present it should not generally exceed a total of 600 units. OnabotulinumtoxinA has been FDA approved for upper extremity spasticity but is used off-label for lower limb spasticity. Dysport dosing is not equivalent to Botox with regard to unit dosing, the generally accepted ratio is 4 to 5 units of Dysport for every unit of Botox.[41] Dysport or Myobloc does not have FDA approval for use in spasticity despite evidence that favors efficacy. Dosing can be repeated at 3-month intervals if necessary. Most research on the use of botulinum toxin for spasticity has been performed in spasticity of cerebral origin, as seen in cerebral palsy, stroke, and traumatic brain injuries. Given the relative diffuse nature of spasticity in spinal cord injury, its use is more limited, but it may serve as an additional tool for very specific goals such as reduced adductor tone to improve hygiene, gastrocnemius–soleus complex to reduce risk of contracture and finger flexors to improve hygiene, improve cosmesis, and reduce pain. Functional gains in activities such as gait are limited, but reduction of lower extremity tone, particularly of hamstrings and ankle plantar flexors, may help improve stance, transfers, and gait.

Intrathecal baclofen

Intrathecal baclofen in indicated in spasticity of either cerebral or spinal origin. Intrathecal baclofen in indicated in patients with severe spasticity who are unresponsive to oral baclofen and have failed other conservative and pharmacologic management, and/or experience unacceptable side effects at effective doses of oral medications. In general, it is recommended to wait 1 year postinjury to determine the natural history of the spasticity. The system is being implanted more frequently at earlier times in patients with severe pain, severe functional limitations, or impairment of rehabilitation because of severe spasticity that has failed other pharmacologic management. Realistic patient goals and expectations must be agreed upon by the patient and all team members. There are few absolute contraindications, but intrathecal baclofen should be used cautiously in those (1) who need the spasticity to sustain upright posture and balance in locomotion, (2) with impaired renal function, (3) who are pregnant or breastfeeding, (4) who have a history of uncontrolled seizures, (5) with major psychologic or psychotic disorders.

Baclofen injection is delivered to the cerebrospinal fluid (CSF) and is believed to act at $GABA_B$ receptor sites in the spinal cord, similar to the oral form, but, at approximately one-hundredth the oral dose.[42] Intrathecal baclofen is eliminated by bulk CSF turnover with a half-life 4 to 5 hours. Given the effects of gravity, the concentration of intrathecal baclofen will be significantly higher in the lumbar region with less benefit in cervical innervated muscles. An intrathecal trial is always performed to assess the response. A 50-μg dose is injected through a lumbar puncture procedure, and the patient is assessed at 2 to 4 hours for effect. A comprehensive neurologic examination is performed before and after injections, and physical and occupation therapy is used to assess the patient for potential functional benefit. Those with incomplete injures who are ambulatory may find that standing and ambulation are more difficult with reduced tone. Videotaping is performed in these patients while ambulating on even surfaces and on stairs to review later with the team and the patient. If there is not an adequate response of reduced spasticity, a repeat dose of 100 μg can be given at a later date. Implantation involves placement of the baclofen pump subcutaneously in the abdomen, and the catheter is tunneled subcutaneously to enter in the intrathecal space. The catheter enters into a lumbar interspace and is advanced to approximately T6 to T8 in most cases. More cephalad placement can be attempted to get enhanced upper extremity spasticity control, but one must be cautious of potential respiratory compromise. Dosing is highly variable and adjustable but generally starts with a simple continuous infusion of 100 μg and is gradually titrated by 10% to 20% until effective spasticity control is obtained. Average dosing is generally between 200 to 400 μg per day but has been as high as 1500 μg per day.

The use of an intrathecal delivery system is an excellent choice for many patients, but it does have occasional adverse effects and requires absolute compliance with follow-up because abrupt discontinuation from either failure or from the drug running out can lead to acute life-threatening events. Intrathecal baclofen withdrawal is generally considered a medical emergency and will present most commonly with increased pruritus, increased tone, and irritability. Additional features of withdrawal are noted in **Box 3**. If not reversed this may lead to severe rhabdomyolysis, multiple organ failure, and death. The syndrome of withdrawal may closely resemble malignant hyperthermia or neuroleptic malignant syndrome. Treatment in reestablishing intrathecal delivery that most commonly involves disruption of catheter flow can be identified with dye-based radiologic study of the pump system. In the acute period of withdrawal, oral baclofen in doses up to 40 mg given 4 times daily and intermittent intravenous benzodiazepines may be necessary to control the severe spasticity.[43] Less-severe adverse events of intrathecal baclofen use include hypotonia, sedation, nausea, vomiting, headaches, paresthesia, and dizziness. Intrathecal baclofen overdose is rare and generally iatrogenic related to incorrect concentration or inadvertent excessive dosing. Treatment of overdose is supportive.

Several randomized controlled studies have supported the use of test-dose[44–46] intrathecal baclofen to decrease spasticity as measured by Ashworth scale and spasm frequency scales. Studies have also shown improvement in functional activities such as activities of daily living, the functional impairment measure, transfers, and bladder function.[46–48]

Intrathecal clonidine has been used with some success. However, it can have problematic hemodynamic side effects.

Box 3
Intrathecal baclofen withdrawal

Early symptoms and findings

- Pruritus without rash
- Increasing spasticity
- Irritability
- Diaphoresis

Additional symptoms may include

- Paresthesia
- Tachycardia
- Hypotension
- Elevated temperature
- Dysphoria, malaise, decreased consciousness
- Seizures
- Rhabdomyolysis
- Multiple organ failure

SURGICAL PROCEDURES

Surgical options can be considered for those who do not respond to typical physical, pharmacologic, and intrathecal options but are quite uncommon in the adult population with spasticity of spinal origin. Laminectomy, cordectomy, and adhesiolysis can be considered, particularly the last one when there is development of impaired cerebrospinal flow from a spinal cord tethering of syringomyelia leading to an increase in spasticity. Selective rhizotomies are commonly performed in the pediatric cerebral palsy population but are rarely performed in adults with spinal cord injury.[49] Similarly, orthopedic procedures such as Achilles tendon lengthening or hamstring lengthening are rarely performed in the adult population but tendon transfers for functional actions can be considered.

SUMMARY

Spasticity is a common component of those with spinal cord dysfunction. Spasticity can lead not only to pain and potential secondary complications such as contracture and pressure sores but also to significant functional impairment. The clinician must identify specific goals of spasticity treatment and assess the potential benefit of spasticity, particularly as it pertains to transfers and ambulation. Conservative treatment measures that include avoidance and identification of potential noxious stimuli and a daily stretching program that can be performed by the patient or caregivers are initiated in all patients. Additional treatment of more-diffuse spasticity will initially include oral pharmacologic agents, beginning with those having the least side effect potential. In the author's experience, this drug is usually Lioresal or tizanidine. Additional oral agents can then be added, with many patients requiring a multiple drug regimen. For more focal areas of increased spasticity, local chemodenervation with either botulinum toxin or phenol may also be a component of the multifaceted treatment. In those with severe spasticity that is refractory to conservative and pharmacologic treatments, or those with unacceptable side effects from oral medication, intrathecal delivery of baclofen can have a marked therapeutic effect. Each patient's care with regard to spasticity management is individual, and the clinician needs to understand the mechanisms and implementation strategies of these multiple treatment options.

REFERENCES

1. Lance J. Pathophysiology of spasticity and clinical experience with baclofen. In: Lance J, Feldman R, Young R, editors. Spasticity: disordered motor control. Chicago: Yearbook; 1980. p. 185–204.
2. Pandyan AD, Gregoric M, Barnes MP, et al. Spasticity: Clinical perceptions, neurological realities and meaningful measurement. Disabil Rehabil 2005; 27(1/2):2–6.
3. Kumru H, Murillo N, Samso JV, et al. Reduction of spasticity with repetitive transcranial magnetic stimulation in patients with spinal cord injury. Neurorehabil Neural Repair 2010;24(5):435–41.
4. Levi R, Hultling C, Seiger A. The Stockholm Spinal Cord Injury Study: 2. Association between clinical patient characteristics and post-acute medical problems. Paraplegia 1995;33:585–94.
5. Elia EA, Filippini G, Calandrella D, et al. Botulinum neurotoxins for post-stroke spasticity in adults: a systemic review. Mov Disord 2009;24(6):801–12.
6. Maynard FM, Karunas RS, Waring WP III. Epidemiology of spasticity following traumatic spinal cord injury. Arch Phys Med Rehabil 1990;71(8):566–9.

7. Rizzo MA, Hadjimichael OC, Preiningerova J, et al. Prevalence and treatment of spasticity reported by multiple sclerosis patients. Mult Scler 2004;10(5):589–95.
8. Elbasiouny SM, Moroz D, Bakr MM, et al. Management of spasticity after spinal cord injury: current techniques and future directions. Neurorehabil Neural Repair 2010;24(1):23–33.
9. Rushworth G. Spasticity and rigidity: an experimental study and review. J Neurol Neurosurg Psychiatry 1960;23:99–118.
10. Bohannon R, Smith M. Interrater reliability of a modified Ashworth scale of muscle spasticity. Phys Ther 1987;67(2):206.
11. Ashworth B. Preliminary trial of carisoprodal in multiple sclerosis. Practitioner 1964;192:540–2.
12. Beiring-Sorensen F, Neilsen JB, Klinge K. Spasticity-assessment; a review. Spinal Cord 2006;44:708–22.
13. Linsenmeyer TA. Acute management of Autonomic Dysreflexia: Individual with spinal cord injury presenting to health-care facilities. Clinical practice guidelines. 2nd edition. Consortium for Spinal Cord Medicine. Paralyzed Veterans Association; 2001.
14. Merritt JL. Management of spasticity in spinal cord injury. Mayo Clin Proc 1981; 56(10):614–22.
15. Schmit BD, Dewald JPA, Rymer WZ. Stretch reflex adaptation in elbow flexors during repeated passive movements in unilateral brain-injured patients. Arch Phys Med Rehabil 2000;81:269–78.
16. Bohannon RW. Tilt table standing for reducing spasticity after spinal cord injury. Arch Phys Med Rehabil 1993;74(10):1121–2.
17. Kunkel CF, Scremin AM, Eisenberg B, et al. Effect of "standing" on spasticity, contracture, and osteoporosis in paralyzed males. Arch Phys Med Rehabil 1993;74:73–8.
18. Shields RK, Dudley-Javoroski S. Monitoring standing wheelchair use after spinal cord injury: a case report. Disabil Rehabil 2005;27:142–6.
19. Abramson AS. Exercise in paraplegia. In: Basmajian JV, editor. Therapeuptic exercise. 3d edition. Baltimore (MD): WiHas s end Wilkins; 1985.
20. Elovic EP, Eisenberg ME, Jasey NN. Spasticity and muscle overactivity as components of the upper motor neuron syndrome. In: Frontera W, editor. Delisa's physical medicine and rehabilitation. Principles and practice. 5th edition. Philidelphia: Lippincott Williams and Wilkins; 2010. p. 1319–44.
21. Brouwer B, Davidson LK, Olney S. Serial casting in idiopathic toe-walkers and children with spastic cerebral palsy. J Pediatr Orthop 2000;20(2):221–5.
22. Krause P, Szecsi J, Straube A. Changes in spastic muscle tone increase in patient with spinal cord injury using functional electrical stimulation and passive leg movements. Clin Rehabil 2008;22(7):627–34.
23. Murillo N, Kumru H, Vidal-Samso J, et al. Decrease of spasticity with muscle vibration in patients with spinal cord injury. Clin Neurophysiol 2011;122:1183–9.
24. Van der Salm A, Veltink PH, Ijzerman MJ, et al. Comparison of electric stimulation methods for reduction of triceps surae spasticity in spinal cord injury. Arch Phys Med Rehabil 2006;87(2):222–8.
25. Granat MH, Ferguson AC, Andrews BJ, et al. The role of functional electrical stimulation in the rehabilitation of patients with incomplete spinal cord injury–observed benefits during gait studies. Paraplegia 1993;31(4):207–15.
26. Robinson CJ, Kett NA, Bolam JM. Spasticity in spinal cord injured patients: 1. Short-term effects of surface electrical stimulation. Arch Phys Med Rehabil 1988;69(8):598–604.

27. Gracies JM, Nance P, Elovic E, et al. Traditional pharmacological treatments for spasticity. Part II: General and regional treatments. Muscle Nerve Suppl 1997; 6:S92–120.
28. Gillis MC, editor. CPS Compendium of pharmaceuticals and specialties. 33rd edition. Ottawa (Ontario): Canadian Pharmacists Association; 1998. p. 883–4.
29. Aydin G, Tomruk S, Keles I, et al. Transcutaneous electrical stimulation versus baclofen in spasticity: clinical and electrophysiologic comparison. Am J Phys Med Rehabil 2005;84(8):584–92.
30. Tseng TC, Wang SC. Locus of action of centrally acting muscle relaxants, diazepam and tybamate. J Pharmacol Exp Ther 1971;178(2):350–60.
31. Bass B, Weinshenker B, Rice GP, et al. Tizanidine versus baclofen in the treatment of spasticity in patients with multiple sclerosis. Can J Neurol Sci 1988; 15(1):15–9.
32. Eyssette M, Rohmer F, Serratrice G, et al. Multi-center, double-blind trial of a novel antispastic agent, tizanidine, in spasticity associated with multiple sclerosis. Curr Med Res Opin 1988;10(10):699–708.
33. Nance PW, Bugaresti J, Shellenberger K, et al. Efficacy and safety of tizanidine in the treatment of spasticity in patients with spinal cord injury. North American Tizanidine Study Group. Neurology 1994;44:S44–51.
34. Nance PW, Shears AH, Nance DM. Clonidine in spinal cord injury. Can Med Assoc J 1985;133:41–2.
35. Yablon SA, Sipski ML. Effect of transdermal clonidine on spinal spasticy. Am J Phys Med Rehabil 1993;72:154–7.
36. Ward A, Chaffman MO, Sorkin EM. Dantrolene: a review of it's pharmacokinetic properties and therapeutic use in malignant hyperthermia, the neuroleptic malignant syndrome and an update of it's use in muscle spasticity. Drugs 1986;32:130–68.
37. Gruenthal M, Mueller M, Olson WL, et al. Gabapentin for the treatment of spasticity in patients with spinal cord injury. Spinal Cord 1997;35(10):686–9.
38. Collin C, Davies P, Mutiboko IK, et al. Randomized controlled trial of cannabis-bases medicine in spasticity caused by multiple sclerosis. Eur J Neurol 2007; 14(3):290–6.
39. Pooyania S, Ethans K, Szturm T, et al. A randomized, double-blinded, crossover pilot study assessing the effect of nabilone on spasticity in persons with spinal cord injury. Arch Phys Med Rehabil 2010;91(5):703–7.
40. Hayes KC. Fampridine-SR for multiple sclerosis and spinal cord injury. Expert Rev Neurother 2007;7(5):453–61.
41. Wenzel R, Jones D, Borrego JA. Comparing two botulinum toxin type A formulations using manufacturers' product summaries. J Clin Pharm Ther 2007;32(4):387–402.
42. Dralle D, Muller H, Zierski J, et al. Intrathecal baclofen for spasticity. Lancet 1985; 2(8462):1103.
43. Coffey RJ, Edgar TS, Francisco GE, et al. Abrupt withdrawal from intrathecal baclofen: recognition and management of a potentially life threatening syndrome. Arch Phys Med Rehabil 2002;83:735–41.
44. Penn RD, Savoy SM, Corcos D, et al. Intrathecal baclofen for severe spinal spasticity. N Engl J Med 1989;320:1517–21.
45. Coffey JR, Cahill D, Steers W, et al. Intrathecal baclofen for intractable spasticity of spinal origin: results of a long-term multicenter study. J Neurosurg 1993;78: 226–32.
46. Nance PW, Schreyvers O, Schmidt B, et al. Intrathecal baclofen therapy for adults with spinal spasticity: therapeutic efficacy and effect on hospital admissions. Can J Neurol Sci 1995;22:22–9.

47. Azouvi P, Mane M, Thiebaut JB, et al. Intrathecal baclofen administration for control of severe spinal spasticity: functional improvement and long-term follow-up. Arch Phys Med Rehabil 1996;77:35–9.
48. Broseta J, Garcia-March G, Sanchez-Ledesma MJ, et al. Chronic intrathecal administration in severe spasticity. Stereotact Funct Neurosurg 1990;54–55: 147–53.
49. Falci SP, Indeck C, Lammertse DP. Posttraumatic spinal cord tethering and syringomyelia; surgical treatment and long-term outcome. J Neurosurg Spine 2009; 11:445–60.

Cervical Spondylotic Myelopathy

Michel Toledano, MD, J.D. Bartleson, MD*

KEYWORDS

- Spondylosis • Myelopathy • Cervical spondylotic myelopathy
- Cervical spinal stenosis

KEY POINTS

- The presence of spondylotic changes is very common in the general population, but only a minority of patients are symptomatic.
- Clinically, cervical spondylosis can result in neck pain, cervical radiculopathy, and myelopathy.
- Cervical spondylotic myelopathy (CSM) is the most common form of myelopathy in patients older than 55 years of age.
- MRI is the most useful diagnostic tool. The use of MRI for predicting prognosis and surgical outcome is an evolving field.
- Conservative management with close observation can be considered in mild CSM. In patients with significant and/or progressive neurologic deficit, surgery should be considered.
- About 50% to 75% patients undergoing surgery for CSM improve. Benefit from surgery plateaus at 6 months.

INTRODUCTION

The differential diagnosis of cervical spondylotic myelopathy (CSM) is broad and includes multiple conditions that can cause and mimic myelopathy. In adults older than 55 years of age, CSM is the most common cause of myelopathy. The pathophysiology, clinical presentation, differential diagnosis, diagnostic evaluation, natural history, and treatment options are summarized in this article.

EPIDEMIOLOGY AND PATHOPHYSIOLOGY

Age-related, wear-and-tear changes affecting the vertebrae, intervertebral disks, the facets, and other true joints, as well as the associated ligaments, result in a degenerative cascade known as spondylosis. The presence of degenerative changes is very

Department of Neurology, Mayo Clinic College of Medicine, 200 First Street SW, Rochester, MN 55905, USA
* Corresponding author.
E-mail address: Bartleson.John@mayo.edu

Neurol Clin 31 (2013) 287–305
http://dx.doi.org/10.1016/j.ncl.2012.09.003
0733-8619/13/$ – see front matter © 2013 Elsevier Inc. All rights reserved.

common in the general population and becomes more prevalent with increasing age. Imaging studies of asymptomatic individuals older than the age of 60 show degenerative changes at one or more levels of the cervical spine in up to 95% of men and 89% of women.[1-3] These studies also showed that the most common level of involvement was C5-C6, then in decreasing order of frequency, C6-C7, C4-C5, C3-C4, and C2C-3.[2,3] Similarly, a consecutive autopsy series of 200 adults showed cervical spondylosis in 53.5% and evidence of myelopathy in 7.5%.[4] The mean age of the patients with spondylosis was significantly greater than the age of those without spondylosis (70.2 vs 57.3 years, respectively).[4] Cervical spondylosis usually affects multiple spinal levels.

Cervical spondylosis can be completely symptomless or cause neck and regional pain alone. If the cervical nerve roots are affected, a radiculopathy can ensue. Spinal cord involvement can result in neurologic dysfunction of the extremities, torso, and sphincters. CSM occurs when there is narrowing of the vertebral foramen at one or more levels with compression of the spinal cord. Although the primary mechanism of CSM may be compression of nervous tissue, there is some evidence that ischemia is a contributing factor.[5,6] Factors that can lead to spinal and intervertebral foramen narrowing include disk degeneration and bulging, osteophyte formation, ligamentous hypertrophy, congenital or acquired subluxation in which one vertebra is displaced forward or backward on its neighbor below, decreased disk height, uncovertebral joint thickening, and osteoarthritis (**Fig. 1**).

However, spondylotic changes alone do not account for the development of symptomatic CSM and the pathophysiology is thought to depend on both static factors causing stenosis and dynamic factors resulting in repetitive injury to the cord.

Static Factors

A significant predisposing factor to CSM is a congenitally narrow cervical spinal canal with the thought being that vertebral foramen narrowing is more likely to cause compression if there is already less room for the spinal cord.[7-11] However, dynamic MRI studies of 295 patients with symptomatic CSM by Morishita and colleagues[12] showed increased segmental mobility in the cervical spine of patients with a congenitally narrow canal (<13 mm anteroposteriorly), suggesting that segmental instability may also contribute to accelerated spondylosis in these patients.

Congenital anomalies of the cervical spine such as Klippel-Feil syndrome, which is characterized by fusion of any two cervical vertebrae, can lead to accelerated spondylosis.[13] Similarly, patients who have undergone surgical fusion of cervical vertebrae can have exaggerated spondylosis in adjacent segments.[14,15] Both congenital and iatrogenic fusions likely result in excessive motion of adjacent unfused spinal levels, which leads to increased spondylosis.

Dynamic Factors

Cervical nerve root and spinal cord irritation and compression are exacerbated by neck motion. The spinal cord stretches with flexion of the neck and it can be compressed against osteophytic spurs and intervertebral disks protruding into the spinal canal. Hyperextension can pinch the spinal cord between the posterior margin of the vertebral body anteriorly and the laminae or ligamentum flavum posteriorly.[16,17] Repetitive neck movements and trauma can also accelerate spondylosis. An animal study in which rabbits were exposed to repeated forcible neck extension and flexion movements showed early development of osteophytes.[18] Similarly, rugby players[19,20] and patients with dystonic cerebral palsy that included their cervical muscles[21] developed accelerated spondylosis.

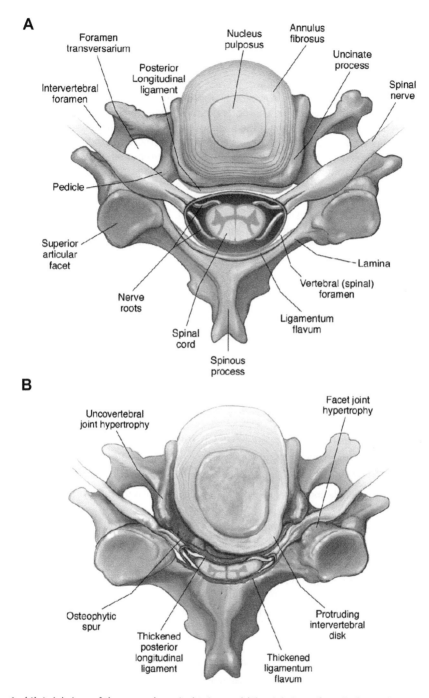

Fig. 1. (*A*) Axial view of the normal cervical spine and (*B*) axial view of cervical spinal stenosis with spinal cord impingement due to the combination of a congenitally narrow cervical spinal canal and superimposed cervical spondylosis. Encroachment on the cervical spinal canal is caused by bulging disks often with osteophytic spurring, thickening of the posterior longitudinal ligament and ligamenta flava, subluxation of one vertebra forward or backward on its neighbor, thickening of the posterior aspect of the uncovertebral joints, and osteoarthritis of the facet joints. (*From* Tracy JA, Bartleson JD. Cervical spondylotic myelopathy. Neurologist 2010;16(3):177. Copyrighted and used with permission of Wolters Kluwer Health, all rights reserved.)

CLINICAL PRESENTATION

The presenting signs and symptoms of CSM are variable and depend on the predominance of motor versus sensory symptoms, upper versus lower limb symptoms, changes in muscle tone, upper versus lower motor neuron phenomena in the upper extremities, and sphincter complaints (**Box 1**). The onset of symptoms is usually after the age of 40, often between 50 and 70 years, but can begin in the elderly. Men predominate at a rate of 3 to 2.[22,23] Typically, the onset is insidious, although symptoms can develop acutely or subacutely, often after minor head and neck trauma (such as from a fall or whiplash injury in a motor vehicle accident). Symptoms in CSM are characteristically persistent and not transient (eg, carpal tunnel syndrome) or fluctuating (eg, multiple sclerosis [MS]).

There are numerous scales for assessing CSM. The Nurick scale,[10] Harsh scale,[24] Cooper scale,[25] modifications of the Japanese Orthopedic Association Scale (mJOA),[26,27] and the Prolo scale.[28] Most often, however, these scales and scores are used in research settings instead of in everyday clinical practice.

Box 1
Symptoms and signs of myelopathy

Symptoms associated with myelopathy
- Neck pain
- Unilateral or bilateral upper limb pain
- Upper limb weakness, numbness, or loss of dexterity
- Lower limb stiffness, weakness, or sensory loss
- Urgency of bladder more often than bowel, urgency incontinence, frequency of urination
- Lhermitte sign (electric shock-like sensations extending down the spine and into the limbs with neck flexion)

Findings associated with myelopathy
- Increased lower and/or upper deep tendon reflexes
- Loss of superficial reflexes below the neck
- Positive Hoffmann signs (thumb adduction and thumb and finger flexion after forced flexion and sudden release of the tip of the long finger)
- Positive finger flexor reflex (brisk flexion of the patient's fingers when the examiner taps on the back of their own fingers while holding the patient's flexed fingertips)
- Babinski and/or Chaddock signs
- Upper limb weakness beyond the bounds of a single nerve root on one or both sides
- Weakness in the lower limbs in an upper motor neuron distribution
- Sensory loss in lower and/or upper limbs and/or torso
- Spasticity in the limbs, especially the lower extremities
- Gait disturbance, especially if suggestive of spasticity

From Bartleson JD, Deen HG. *Spine disorders: medical and surgical management.* Chapter 2. New York: Cambridge University Press; 2009:36. Copyrighted and used with permission of Mayo Foundation for Medical Education and Research, all rights reserved.

DIFFERENTIAL DIAGNOSIS

When evaluating a patient with CSM, it is important to determine whether they truly have a myelopathy. Parasagittal cerebral lesions, multiple strokes, and brainstem strokes can mimic CSM, although onset tends to be acute. Carpal tunnel syndrome, brachial plexopathy, ulnar neuropathy, Guillain-Barré syndrome, or other peripheral processes can also simulate CSM and use of electromyography (EMG) and nerve conduction studies (NCS) are helpful in ruling these conditions out. Motor neuron disease, chiefly amyotrophic lateral sclerosis (ALS) with its combination of upper and lower motor neuron findings, can be easily mistaken for CSM, and vice versa. Sensory symptoms and pain are not usually part of ALS, although they can also be absent in CSM. The presence of sphincter dysfunction argues in favor of CSM, whereas bulbar signs and symptoms are characteristic of ALS.

Once the presence of a myelopathy is established, it is important to ensure that entities other than CSM are ruled out by clinical judgment or ancillary testing (**Fig. 2**). This is especially important given the frequency of asymptomatic degenerative changes and cervical spinal stenosis in the general population.

Vascular causes of myelopathy include spinal cord infarction, spinal epidural hematoma, and vascular malformations of the cord, all of which can be ruled out by MRI. Dural arteriovenous fistulas primarily affect the thoracic cord but can cause symptoms that may be confused with CSM and may be missed unless MRI of the thoracic cord with and without gadolinium is performed.[29]

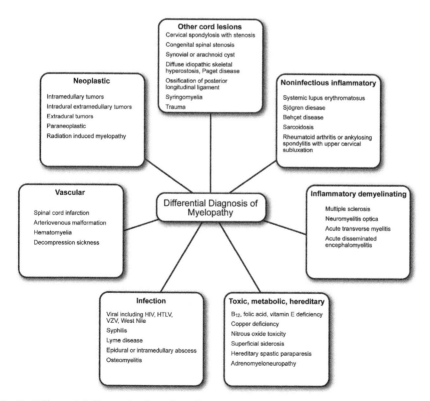

Fig. 2. Differential diagnosis of myelopathy.

Infectious causes of myelopathy are more commonly seen in immunosuppressed patients but can occur in immunocompetent hosts. Possibilities include abscess, human immunodeficiency-related vacuolar myelopathy,[30] human T-cell lymphotropic virus type 1, West-Nile virus infection,[31] cytomegalovirus, varicella zoster virus, syphilis, Lyme disease, and several enteroviruses.[32] Commonly, these patients will have a history of fevers, chills, and malaise, and may have an elevated white blood cell count.

Demyelinating causes of myelopathy include MS, acute disseminated encephalomyelitis (ADEM), transverse myelitis, and neuromyelitis optica (NMO). MRI of the spine usually shows T2 hyperintense lesions in the cervical cord suggestive of an inflammatory process. Patients with MS usually have evidence of multiple neurologic insults on examination and MRI of the brain. The presence of oligoclonal bands on CSF analysis is also helpful. ADEM also has multifocal neurologic manifestation, usually with an abrupt or subacute onset. Clues to NMO include longitudinally extensive spinal cord lesions on MRI, the presence of humoral NMO IgG antibodies, and a history of optic neuritis.

Rheumatologic disease can also be associated with inflammatory spinal cord lesions. These include systemic lupus erythematosus,[33] Sjögren syndrome,[34] and rheumatoid arthritis.[35] These can usually be differentiated from CSM by radiologic findings and by the presence of systemic manifestations and serologic markers. Patients with rheumatoid arthritis and ankylosing spondylitis can develop craniocervical and C1-C2 subluxation with myelopathy that should be evident on imaging. Other inflammatory disorders, such as sarcoidosis, can also present with a myelopathy.[36]

In cases when imaging of the spinal cord is negative or when nutritional deficiency is suspected (eg, inflammatory bowel disease, gastric bypass surgery), blood tests for vitamin and mineral levels should be considered. Vitamin B12 deficiency can produce subacute combined degeneration primarily affecting the dorsal and lateral spinal tracts. Copper deficiency can produce both myelopathy and peripheral neuropathy. Both of these deficiencies can show increased signal intensity involving the dorsal columns on T2-weighted MRI. Vitamin E deficiency and folic acid deficiency can rarely result in myelopathy.

Tumors intrinsic or extrinsic to the spinal cord can produce myelopathy. Tumors involving the vertebral bodies, such as metastatic cancer, can cause severe pain, bony destruction, and spinal cord compression. Meningeal carcinomatosis typically produces a painful polyradicular pattern of signs and symptoms. The above can usually be detected by MRI. Paraneoplastic disorders can present with myelopathy and have been reported with collapsin response-mediator protein-5,[37] glutamic acid decarboxylase-65,[38] amphiphysin,[39] antineuronal nuclear antibody (ANNA)-1,[40] ANNA-2,[41] and ANNA-3[42] antibodies. Postradiation myelopathy is also a known entity that can present months to years after radiation with mild to severe sensorimotor deficits. When it occurs early, transient sensory symptoms predominate.[43]

DIAGNOSTIC TESTING

Imaging of patients with CSM may include radiographs, computed tomography (CT), CT myelography, and MRI, which remains the most useful diagnostic test. MRI can confirm the diagnosis, document the extent and severity of degenerative changes, and rule out common mimics. MRI can also play a role in selection of patients for therapeutic intervention, although this remains an evolving field. Historically, lateral plain radiographs of the cervical spine were used to assess spinal canal narrowing by measuring from the most posterior aspect of one vertebral body to the closest spinolaminar line. A sagittal diameter of less than 13 mm was associated with an increased risk for myelopathy; absolute stenosis was defined as less than 10 mm.[11]

With the advent of cross-sectional imaging, the diameters and cross-sectional areas of the cervical spinal canal and the cervical cord can be measured directly. A recent study showed that both MRI and CT myelography provided reproducible measurements of cervical intracanalar dimensions.[44] MRI provides additional information because of its superior ability to image soft tissues such as disks and ligaments, and fluids such as water (**Fig. 3**). CT myelography however, is the test of choice when MRI is contraindicated.[45] In addition, CT myelography can be a helpful adjunct to MRI in delineating bony abnormalities and spinal cord deformation.

NCS and EMG can help identify spondylotic injury to the neural elements. Compression of the anterior spinal cord can result in damage to the anterior horn cells. On EMG this will manifest as long duration, high amplitude, and polyphasic motor units with

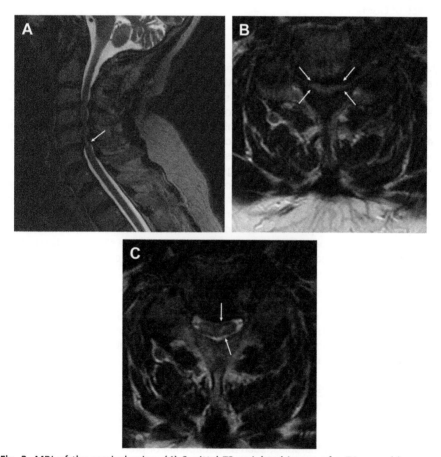

Fig. 3. MRI of the cervical spine. (*A*) Sagittal T2-weighted image of a 74-year-old woman with multilevel cervical spinal stenosis worse at C5-6, more than C4-5, more than C3-4. There is very little spinal fluid in front of or in back of the spinal cord at these levels. There is increased T2 signal intensity within the spinal cord just below the C5-6 interspace level (*arrow*). (*B*) Axial T2-weighted image at the level of maximal stenosis and spinal cord deformity (C5-6 interspace). The spinal cord is deformed and thinned (banana-shaped) by a bulging disk and osteophytic spurring anteriorly and the laminae and ligamenta flava posteriorly (*arrows*). (*C*) Axial T2-weighted image at a level between the interspaces below the area of maximal stenosis showing T2 signal hyperintensity (*arrows*).

reduced recruitment. Abnormal spontaneous activity such as fibrillations and positive sharp waves can occur if the denervation is subacute or not fully compensated. Spondylotic compression of the cervical nerve roots can cause similar EMG changes. The main role of NCS and EMG is to rule out other diagnoses such as peripheral neuropathy, peripheral nerve entrapment, and brachial plexopathy.

Somatosensory evoked potentials (SEP) and motor-evoked potentials can be useful in assessing the degree of central conduction impairment in CSM, and one study reported sensitivity and specificity equal to MRI.[46] One study suggested that motor-evoked potentials (MEP) may be more sensitive than SEP in early myelopathy.[47] Although evoked potentials are not routinely used in the diagnosis of CSM, they are very commonly used for electrophysiologic monitoring during surgery.

As discussed above blood and CSF tests can help diagnose or eliminate common mimics of CSM.

NATURAL HISTORY

The natural history of CSM has not been clearly defined, and many of the existing studies are limited. In a study of 120 cases of CSM by Clarke and Robinson,[48] 75% of patients without or before treatment worsened in a stepwise fashion, 20% slowly worsened, and 5% experienced a rapid onset of symptoms followed by a stable course. Lees and Turner[49] reported on 44 subjects with clinical and radiographic evidence of CSM who were followed for 3–40 years. Most subjects experienced long periods of stability with sporadic exacerbations whereas progressive deterioration was rare.[49] Conversely, Symon and Lavender[50] reported in a surgical series that 67% of their patients experienced a steadily progressive course before surgery. In a series of 37 cases treated conservatively, Nurick[51] reported that, for most subjects, there was an initial phase of deterioration followed by stabilization. A recent systematic review of the literature by Matz and colleagues[52] suggests a mixed course with a sizable number of patients having stable disease for long periods of time with others experiencing a slow stepwise decline. The clinical course of individual patients, however, is hard to predict.[53]

CONSERVATIVE TREATMENT

Nonsurgical treatment is a viable option in patients with radiographic evidence of cervical stenosis without clinical signs or symptoms of myelopathy (**Fig. 4**). Conservative management is aimed at controlling pain if needed, maintaining function, and protecting the spinal cord from additional injury.

Strategies for Managing Pain

- Analgesic medications, such as nonsteroidal antiinflammatory agents (NSAIDs) can be to control neck and radicular pain. NSAIDs are probably not disease modifying.
- Neuromodulating therapies, such as gabapentin or pregabalin, tricyclic agents, such as amitriptyline or nortriptyline, and duloxetine can be tried for persistent pain.
- Transforaminal epidural steroid injections can also be used, but these are not without side effects.[54]

Strategies for Neck Stabilization and Protecting the Cervical Spine from Injury

- Use of a soft cervical collar or rigid brace holding the neck in a slightly flexed position can be considered in patients with radiographic evidence of severe

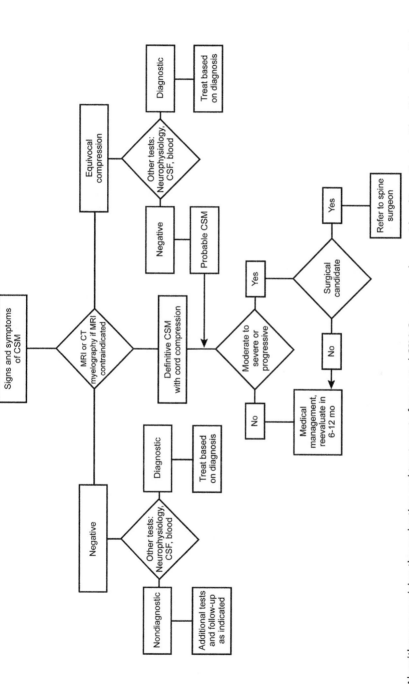

Fig. 4. Algorithm summarizing the evaluation and treatment of suspected CSM. Surgery can be considered in patients with mild myelopathy to prevent progression.

stenosis and mild symptoms; however, there is a paucity of evidence supporting their use.

- Cervical pillows are also available; however, there is no good evidence supporting their effectiveness.
- Patients should be advised to avoid injury to the spine by making appropriate safety modifications to their home, wearing supportive footwear, avoiding risky behaviors, such as high-impact sports or excessive alcohol consumption, and eliminating medications (eg, benzodiazepines and hypnotic drugs) that could increase the risk of falling.
- Physical therapy, including balance and gait training and strengthening exercises, as well as gait aids can be recommended for patients with neurologic impairment.

Studies comparing conservative versus surgical treatment in mild CSM are contradictory. Some studies show no difference between the two groups[55,56] and others show worsening in patients treated conservatively.[52] A recent prospective study of 60 patients with mild CSM showed that conservative treatment was successful at preventing progression in 70% of patients at 1-year follow-up.[57] A Cochrane review of randomized controlled trials for the role of surgery in mild CSM could find only one small controlled trial.[58] This trial found no significant differences between surgical and conservative management in 68 patients after 3 years of follow-up.[56,58] Given the paucity of data regarding the natural history of CSM, physicians should have a frank discussion with patients regarding their symptoms, degree of disability, and risk of progression of CSM before recommending conservative versus surgical treatment. If conservative treatment is recommended, the patient should be reevaluated every 6 to 12 months or sooner if the patient experiences progressive symptoms. Once the diagnosis of CSM is established, repeat imaging is not needed unless there has been significant clinical worsening or to aid in planning surgery.

SURGICAL MANAGEMENT

Surgery for CSM should be considered in patients with moderate to severe or progressive neurologic deficits. The decision to proceed with surgery must take into account the patient's age, baseline function, severity of symptoms, and the historical rate of progression, if any (see **Fig. 4**). Spinal cord decompression can be performed from either an anterior or a posterior approach. A combined approach can also be considered, especially in patients with spine deformity. The appropriate choice depends on the level and degree of spondylotic change; sagittal alignment and stability of the spine; individual characteristics, including previous surgery; and surgical expertise and preference.[59] Regardless of the procedure chosen, the goals of operative treatment are decompression of the spinal cord and its circulation, preservation of alignment and stability of the spine, and prevention of further neural injury. Anterior decompression procedures include single or multilevel discectomy and/or corpectomy and fusion with autologous or bone bank bone usually with plate and screw fixation. Anterior discectomy is usually recommended for 1 to 3 disk level disease and in patients with fixed cervical kyphosis. Posterior decompression procedures include laminectomy, in which laminae are removed completely at one or more levels, and laminoplasty, in which the lateral edges of several laminae are cut completely on one side and partially cut on the other so that several connected laminae can be swung open to decompress the spinal cord. Laminectomy or laminoplasty is often performed on patients requiring decompression of three or more levels, those with a congenitally narrowed canal, and those whose anterior vertebral column is already fused.[59]

Cervical disk arthroplasty is a new surgical treatment option. Currently, two artificial cervical disks have been approved by the US Food and Drug Administration.[60] Several studies have shown equivalence of disk arthroplasty to anterior cervical discectomy and interbody fusion for single-level CSM,[61,62] with reduced risk of subsequent symptomatic adjacent level spondylosis.[63] A recent multicenter randomized controlled trial comparing cervical disk arthroplasty with anterior cervical decompression showed similar improvement in neurologic status at 2-year follow-up.[64]

Predictors of Surgical Outcome

There is considerable interest in determining factors which can identify good surgical candidates by predicting who will progress without surgery and who will and will not benefit from surgery (**Box 2**). A sizable body of literature examines the role of imaging in predicting clinical response to therapeutic intervention. There is general consensus that patients with a smaller cross-sectional area of the cord at the site of compression have more severe symptoms and tend to do less well postoperatively.[65,66] Another area of consensus is that patients with no intramedullary signal change on MRI tend to do better postoperatively than patients who exhibit T2 hyperintensity.[66–71] However, there is contradictory evidence regarding the predictive power of T2 hyperintensity. Some studies suggest that focal T2 hyperintensity does not greatly affect prognosis.[72–74] The studies of Yukawa and colleagues,[75] Shin and colleagues,[76] Zhang and colleagues,[77] and Mastronardi and colleagues[69] suggest that patients with increased signal intensity within the spinal cord on T2-weighted MRI are older, have longer duration of disease, and/or have less neurologic recovery after surgery. Conversely, Okada and colleagues[65] found that increased T2 signal hyperintensity was associated with an improved recovery rate. Mummaneni and colleagues[78] noted that multilevel intramedullary T2 hyperintensity is associated with worse prognosis than a single focus. T2 hyperintensity regression after surgery, however, has more consistently been associated with postoperative neurologic improvement compared with patients in whom T2 hyperintensity remains stable.[65,69,71,73,79]

It is not necessary for patients with increased signal intensity on T2-weighted MRI of the cervical spinal cord to undergo surgery. Bednarik and colleagues[80] found that in patients with "presymptomatic spondylotic cervical cord compression" with MRI evidence of cord compression but no signs or symptoms of myelopathy, T2-weighted signal abnormality did not predict development of myelopathy.[80]

Diminished signal intensity on T1-weighted MRI is uncommon but is associated with a poor prognosis following surgical decompression. This is likely due to the occurrence of irrevocable spinal cord damage. Ohshio and colleagues[81] compared

---

Box 2
Predictors of adverse surgical outcome

Imaging characteristics

- Smaller cross-sectional area on MRI or CT myelography
- Presence of T2 hyperintensity, particularly at multiple levels or if persistent after surgery
- Intramedullary T1 hypointensity
- Intramedullary gadolinium enhancement

Patient-related factors

- Older age
- Longer duration of symptoms before surgery

postmortem spinal cord MRI to histopathologic spinal cord findings in normal controls. Areas of combined T1 hypointensity and T2 hyperintensity correlated with areas of gray matter necrosis, myelomalacia, and spongiform change.[81] Patients with signal intensity on T2-weighted images alone had milder pathologic changes or edema only.[81]

Intramedullary gadolinium enhancement may also have predictive value. Ozawa and colleagues[82] and Cho and colleagues[68] compared patients with CSM who exhibited gadolinium enhancement with a nonenhancing group and found that patients with preoperative enhancement had a poorer postoperative prognosis. Floeth and colleagues[83] studied 20 patients with CSM using 18F-fluorodeoxyglucose positron emission tomography. Patients with increased metabolic activity at the site of compression did better postoperatively than those with no increased activity. Finally, some recent studies suggest that diffusion tensor imaging may provide a better means of identifying symptomatic cord injury than T2 hyperintensity and/or T1 hypointensity. The parameters used are fractional anisotropy, mean diffusivity, and apparent diffusion coefficient.[84] Although promising, these new imaging techniques remain experimental.

Unfortunately, to date imaging studies can diagnose CSM but they cannot predict who will and will not benefit from surgery. Other factors thought to possibly affect prognosis include patient age and duration of symptoms. Matsuda and colleagues[85] studied 17 CSM patients older than 70 years (average age 77.2 years) and reported a recovery rate of 48.4% compared with 69.4% in 24 control patients younger than 65 (average age 50.2 years). Conversely, Hasegawa and colleagues[86] compared surgical outcomes in 40 patients older than 70 years and 50 patients younger than 60, and found no difference between the groups. However, the neurologic complication rate (defined in the study by any decrease in muscle strength by more than one grade or new sensory deficit) was higher in the older group of patients (15% vs 8%).[86] Holly and colleagues[87] reported similar findings when comparing surgical outcomes in 36 patients older than 75 years and 34 patients younger than 65. Naderi and colleagues[88] reported that patients younger than 60 improved more after surgery than older patients do. Furlan and colleagues,[89] in a recent prospective study of 81 patients who underwent surgical treatment of CSM, reported that older patients had less favorable outcomes after surgery.

Okada and colleagues,[65] Suri and colleagues,[73] Phillips,[90] Ebersold and colleagues,[91] Lee and colleagues,[92] and Morio and colleagues[79] all reported that longer duration of symptoms before surgery had an adverse effect on outcome. However, Lunsford and colleagues[93] and Arnasson and colleagues[94] did not find this to be the case. In general, it seems that older patients with CSM can benefit from surgery, but less so than younger patients, and they have a higher complication rate. Longer duration of symptoms before decompression seems to be a negative predictor of postoperative improvement.

Surgical Outcomes

Although it remains unclear whether patients with mild CSM benefit from surgery when compared with conservative management, patients with moderate and severe CSM benefit from surgical intervention. Several retrospective studies[91,93,95] have shown that between 50% to 75% of patients undergoing surgery for CSM improve, with some patients later declining with or without evidence of recurrent cervical spinal stenosis. In one study by Cheung and colleagues[96] 71% of 55 patients undergoing surgery for CSM improved, although improvement leveled off at 6 months postoperatively. Similarly, a recent prospective study of 81 patients who underwent cervical decompression reported by Furlan and colleagues[89] showed that there was significant functional recovery (measured by the Nurick and mJOA scales) 6 months after surgery.

However, no significant additional recovery was noted at 1 year.[89] The duration of symptoms, surgical approach (anterior vs posterior), and the number of spine levels treated did not affect functional outcome.[89] Older patients with a greater number of preexisting medical comorbidities, however, had less favorable outcomes.[89] In general, most of the benefit from surgery can be expected in the first 6 months postoperatively. Some patients who do not improve may experience stabilization of a previous downhill course.

Surgical intervention is associated with risks (**Box 3**). Two large reports have assessed this question by making use of the Nationwide Inpatient Sample, a nationally representative sample of hospital discharges in the Unites States. Wang and colleagues[97] reviewed 932,009 hospital discharges from 1992 to 2001 associated with cervical spine surgery for degenerative disease. Fifty-six percent were for herniated disk, 19% for cervical for cervical spondylosis with myelopathy, 18% for cervical spondylosis without myelopathy, and 6% for spinal stenosis. Those undergoing surgery for cervical spondylosis with myelopathy had the highest complication rate (6.5%) and the highest in-hospital mortality rate (0.39%).[97] Using the same database, Boakye and colleagues[98] reviewed 58,115 patients with CSM undergoing surgery between 1993 and 2002 and reported a complication rate of 13.4% (16.4% for posterior fusion and 11.9% for anterior fusion) with an in-hospital mortality rate of 0.6%. More recently, a large prospective study by Fehlings and colleagues[99] looked at perioperative (within 30 days of surgery) and delayed (31 days–2 years following surgery) complications in 302 patients who underwent surgical treatment of symptomatic CSM. The overall perioperative complication rate was 15.6% and the overall delayed complication rate was 4.4%.[99] Perioperative worsening of myelopathy occurred in 1.3% and the mortality rate was 0.33%.[99] Most of the reported complications were treatable and without long-term impact.[99] There was no significant difference in outcome between anterior versus posterior approaches but a combined approach correlated with a less favorable outcome.[99] The only patient factor that was associated with the occurrence of complications was patient age.[99]

Box 3
Surgical complications

Perioperative complications

- Infection

- Bleeding

- Dural leak or fistula

- Worsened myelopathy

- Nerve root injury

- Esophageal injury, hoarseness, transient dysphagia (with anterior approach)

- Death

Delayed complications

- Pseudoarthrosis

- Hardware breakage and/or migration

- Graft dislodgement

- Postlaminectomy kyphosis or restenosis

SUMMARY

The presence of spondylotic changes in the cervical spine is very common in the general population, but only a minority develops symptoms. Clinically, spondylosis can result in neck pain, cervical radiculopathy, and myelopathy. CSM is the most common cause of myelopathy in patients older than 55 years of age. Careful clinical evaluation with ancillary testing, including neuroimaging and, possibly, electrophysiologic studies, is warranted in patients presenting with cervical myeloradiculopathy. MRI is the most useful diagnostic test. The effectiveness of conservative treatment remains unproven, although it is an option, especially in patients with mild CSM. In patients with significant and/or progressive neurologic deficits, operative management should be strongly considered. Predictive factors for a good surgical outcome include younger age and shorter duration symptoms and signs. Imaging characteristics that predict good surgical outcomes are still being investigated. Surgery can result in clinical improvement in 50% to 75% of patients. Although not without risk, most perioperative and delayed postoperative complications from surgery are treatable and do not have long-term impact.

Case report

A 68-year-old woman presented with an 8-month history of worsening unsteadiness when walking. She also noted a sensation of numbness in her feet and ankles that had spread to her thighs. Recently she has had some clumsiness with use of her upper limbs and some frequency and mild urgency of urination. She reports no pain and has no constitutional symptoms or cognitive difficulties. Examination shows a mildly spastic-ataxic gait, weakness in both hands and in both lower limbs in an upper motor neuron distribution, decreased joint position and vibration sense in the lower extremities, generalized hyperreflexia, and bilateral Hoffmann and Babinski signs. MRI of the cervical spine showed advanced degenerative changes resulting in multilevel spinal canal stenosis (C3 through C7) and abnormal cord T2 signal at C3-C4 and C4-C5.

This patient clearly had evidence of myelopathy localized to the cervical spine. She had progressive symptoms as well as multilevel T2 hyperintensity on MRI. She underwent a C3 through superior C6 laminectomy with significant improvement in her gait and sensory symptoms.

REFERENCES

1. Gore DR, Sepic SB, Gardner GM. Roentgenographic findings of the cervical spine in asymptomatic people. Spine 1986;11(6):521–4.
2. Boden SD, McCowin PR, Davis DO, et al. Abnormal magnetic-resonance scans of the cervical spine in asymptomatic subjects. A prospective investigation. J Bone Joint Surg Am 1990;72(8):1178–84.
3. Matsumoto M, Okada E, Ichihara D, et al. Modic changes in the cervical spine: prospective 10-year follow-up study in asymptomatic subjects. J Bone Joint Surg Br 2012;94(5):678–83.
4. Hughes JT, Brownell B. Necropsy observations on the spinal cord in cervical spondylosis. Riv Patol Nerv Ment 1965;86(2):196–204.
5. Brain R. Cervical spondylosis. Ann Intern Med 1954;41(3):439–46.
6. Doppman JL. The mechanism of ischemia in anteroposterior compression of the spinal cord 1975. Invest Radiol 1990;25(4):444–52.
7. Bernhardt M, Hynes RA, Blume HW, et al. Cervical spondylotic myelopathy. J Bone Joint Surg Am 1993;75(1):119–28.

8. Ferguson RJ, Caplan LR. Cervical spondylitic myelopathy. Neurol Clin 1985;3(2): 373–82.
9. Ogino H, Tada K, Okada K, et al. Canal diameter, anteroposterior compression ratio, and spondylotic myelopathy of the cervical spine. Spine 1983;8(1):1–15.
10. Nurick S. The pathogenesis of the spinal cord disorder associated with cervical spondylosis. Brain 1983;95(1):87–100.
11. Edwards WC, LaRocca H. The developmental segmental sagittal diameter of the cervical spinal canal in patients with cervical spondylosis. Spine 1983; 8(1):20–7.
12. Morishita Y, Naito M, Hymanson H, et al. The relationship between the cervical spinal canal diameter and the pathological changes in the cervical spine. Eur Spine J 2009;18(6):877–83.
13. Guille JT, Miller A, Bowen JR, et al. The natural history of Klippel-Feil syndrome: clinical, roentgenographic, and magnetic resonance imaging findings at adulthood. J Pediatr Orthop 1995;15(5):617–26.
14. Bartolomei JC, Theodore N, Sonntag VK. Adjacent level degeneration after anterior cervical fusion: a clinical review. Neurosurg Clin N Am 2005;16(4): 575–87.
15. Hilibrand AS, Carlson GD, Palumbo MA, et al. Radiculopathy and myelopathy at segments adjacent to the site of a previous anterior cervical arthrodesis. J Bone Joint Surg Am 1999;81(4):519–28.
16. Penning L, van der Zwaag P. Biomechanical aspects of spondylotic myelopathy. Acta Radiol Diagn 1966;5:1090–103.
17. Bohlman HH, Emery SE. The pathophysiology of cervical spondylosis and myelopathy. Spine 1988;13(7):843–6.
18. Wada E, Ebara S, Saito S, et al. Experimental spondylosis in the rabbit spine. Overuse could accelerate the spondylosis. Spine 1992;17(Suppl 3):S1–6.
19. Quarrie KL, Cantu RC, Chalmers DJ. Rugby union injuries to the cervical spine and spinal cord. Sports Med 2002;32(10):633–53.
20. Berge J, Marque B, Vital JM, et al. Age-related changes in the cervical spines of front-line rugby players. Am J Sports Med 1999;27(4):422–9.
21. el-Mallakh RS, Rao K, Barwick M. Cervical myelopathy secondary to movement disorders: case report. Neurosurgery 1989;24(6):902–5.
22. Bartleson JD, Deen HG. Spine disorders: medical and surgical management. New York: Cambridge University Press; 2009.
23. Northover JR, Wild JB, Braybrooke J, et al. The epidemiology of cervical spondylotic myelopathy. Skeletal Radiol 2012;17:17.
24. Harsh GR IV, Sypert GW, Weinstein PR, et al. Cervical spine stenosis secondary to ossification of the posterior longitudinal ligament. J Neurosurg 1987;67(3): 349–57.
25. Cooper PR, Epstein F. Radical resection of intramedullary spinal cord tumors in adults. Recent experience in 29 patients. J Neurosurg 1985;63(4):492–9.
26. Hukuda S, Mochizuki T, Ogata M, et al. Operations for cervical spondylotic myelopathy. A comparison of the results of anterior and posterior procedures. J Bone Joint Surg Br 1985;67(4):609–15.
27. Benzel EC, Lancon J, Kesterson L, et al. Cervical laminectomy and dentate ligament section for cervical spondylotic myelopathy. J Spinal Disord 1991; 4(3):286–95.
28. Prolo DJ, Oklund SA, Butcher M. Toward uniformity in evaluating results of lumbar spine operations. A paradigm applied to posterior lumbar interbody fusions. Spine 1986;11(6):601–6.

29. Atkinson JL, Miller GM, Krauss WE, et al. Clinical and radiographic features of dural arteriovenous fistula, a treatable cause of myelopathy. Mayo Clin Proc 2001;76(11):1120–30.
30. McArthur JC, Brew BJ, Nath A. Neurological complications of HIV infection. Lancet Neurol 2005;4(9):543–55.
31. Sejvar JJ, Leis AA, Stokic DS, et al. Acute flaccid paralysis and West Nile virus infection. Emerg Infect Dis 2003;9(7):788–93.
32. Berger JR, Sabet A. Infectious myelopathies. Semin Neurol 2002;22(2):133–42.
33. Provenzale J, Bouldin TW. Lupus-related myelopathy: report of three cases and review of the literature. J Neurol Neurosurg Psychiatry 1992;55(9):830–5.
34. Delalande S, de Seze J, Fauchais AL, et al. Neurologic manifestations in primary Sjögren syndrome: a study of 82 patients. Medicine 2004;83(5):280–91.
35. Shen FH, Samartzis D, Jenis LG, et al. Rheumatoid arthritis: evaluation and surgical management of the cervical spine. Spine J 2004;4(6):689–700.
36. Saleh S, Saw C, Marzouk K, et al. Sarcoidosis of the spinal cord: literature review and report of eight cases. J Natl Med Assoc 2006;98(6):965–76.
37. Keegan BM, Pittock SJ, Lennon VA. Autoimmune myelopathy associated with collapsin response-mediator protein-5 immunoglobulin G. Ann Neurol 2008;63(4):531–4.
38. Pittock SJ, Yoshikawa H, Ahlskog JE, et al. Glutamic acid decarboxylase autoimmunity with brainstem, extrapyramidal, and spinal cord dysfunction. Mayo Clin Proc 2006;81(9):1207–14.
39. Pittock SJ, Lucchinetti CF, Parisi JE, et al. Amphiphysin autoimmunity: paraneoplastic accompaniments. Ann Neurol 2005;58(1):96–107.
40. Lucchinetti CF, Kimmel DW, Lennon VA. Paraneoplastic and oncologic profiles of patients seropositive for type 1 antineuronal nuclear autoantibodies. Neurology 1998;50(3):652–7.
41. Pittock SJ, Lucchinetti CF, Lennon VA. Anti-neuronal nuclear autoantibody type 2: paraneoplastic accompaniments. Ann Neurol 2003;53(5):580–7.
42. Chan KH, Vernino S, Lennon VA. ANNA-3 anti-neuronal nuclear antibody: marker of lung cancer-related autoimmunity. Ann Neurol 2001;50(3):301–11.
43. Rampling R, Symonds P. Radiation myelopathy. Curr Opin Neurol 1998;11(6):627–32.
44. Naganawa T, Miyamoto K, Ogura H, et al. Comparison of magnetic resonance imaging and computed tomogram-myelography for evaluation of cross sections of cervical spinal morphology. Spine 2011;36(1):50–6.
45. Houser OW, Onofrio BM, Miller GM, et al. Cervical spondylotic stenosis and myelopathy: evaluation with computed tomographic myelography. Mayo Clin Proc 1994;69(6):557–63.
46. Nakai S, Sonoo M, Shimizu T. Somatosensory evoked potentials (SEPs) for the evaluation of cervical spondylotic myelopathy: utility of the onset-latency parameters. Clin Neurophysiol 2008;119(10):2396–404.
47. Simo M, Szirmai I, Aranyi Z. Superior sensitivity of motor over somatosensory evoked potentials in the diagnosis of cervical spondylotic myelopathy. Eur J Neurol 2004;11(9):621–6.
48. Clarke E, Robinson PK. Cervical myelopathy: a complication of cervical spondylosis. Brain 1956;79(3):483–510.
49. Lees F, Turner JW. Natural history and prognosis of cervical spondylosis. Br Med J 1963;2(5373):1607–10.
50. Symon L, Lavender P. The surgical treatment of cervical spondylotic myelopathy. Neurology 1967;17(2):117–27.

51. Nurick S. The natural history and the results of surgical treatment of the spinal cord disorder associated with cervical spondylosis. Brain 1972;95(1):101–8.
52. Matz PG, Anderson PA, Holly LT, et al. The natural history of cervical spondylotic myelopathy. J Neurosurg Spine 2009;11(2):104–11.
53. LaRocca H. Cervical spondylotic myelopathy: natural history. Spine 1988;13(7):854–5.
54. Huston CW, Slipman CW, Garvin C. Complications and side effects of cervical and lumbosacral selective nerve root injections. Arch Phys Med Rehabil 2005;86(2):277–83.
55. Bednarik J, Kadanka Z, Vohanka S, et al. The value of somatosensory and motor evoked evoked potentials in pre-clinical spondylotic cervical cord compression. Eur Spine J 1998;7(6):493–500.
56. Kadanka Z, Bednarik J, Vohanka S, et al. Conservative treatment versus surgery in spondylotic cervical myelopathy: a prospective randomised study. Eur Spine J 2000;9(6):538–44.
57. Sumi M, Miyamoto H, Suzuki T, et al. Prospective cohort study of mild cervical spondylotic myelopathy without surgical treatment. J Neurosurg Spine 2012;16(1):8–14.
58. Nikolaidis I, Fouyas IP, Sandercock PA, et al. Surgery for cervical radiculopathy or myelopathy. Cochrane Database Syst Rev 2010;20(1):CD001466.
59. Rao RD, Gourab K, David KS. Operative treatment of cervical spondylotic myelopathy. J Bone Joint Surg Am 2006;88(7):1619–40.
60. Tracy JA, Bartleson JD. Cervical spondylotic myelopathy. Neurologist 2010;16(3):176–87.
61. Heller JG, Sasso RC, Papadopoulos SM, et al. Comparison of BRYAN cervical disc arthroplasty with anterior cervical decompression and fusion: clinical and radiographic results of a randomized, controlled, clinical trial. Spine 2009;34(2):101–7.
62. Riew KD, Buchowski JM, Sasso R, et al. Cervical disc arthroplasty compared with arthrodesis for the treatment of myelopathy. J Bone Joint Surg Am 2008;90(11):2354–64.
63. Robertson JT, Papadopoulos SM, Traynelis VC. Assessment of adjacent-segment disease in patients treated with cervical fusion or arthroplasty: a prospective 2-year study. J Neurosurg Spine 2005;3(6):417–23.
64. Sasso RC, Anderson PA, Riew KD, et al. Results of cervical arthroplasty compared with anterior discectomy and fusion: four-year clinical outcomes in a prospective, randomized controlled trial. J Bone Joint Surg Am 2011;93(18):1684–92.
65. Okada Y, Ikata T, Yamada H, et al. Magnetic resonance imaging study on the results of surgery for cervical compression myelopathy. Spine 1993;18(14):2024–9.
66. Takahashi M, Yamashita Y, Sakamoto Y, et al. Chronic cervical cord compression: clinical significance of increased signal intensity on MR images. Radiology 1989;173(1):219–24.
67. Ramanauskas WL, Wilner HI, Metes JJ, et al. MR imaging of compressive myelomalacia. J Comput Assist Tomogr 1989;13(3):399–404.
68. Cho YE, Shin JJ, Kim KS, et al. The relevance of intramedullary high signal intensity and gadolinium (Gd-DTPA) enhancement to the clinical outcome in cervical compressive myelopathy. Eur Spine J 2011;20(12):2267–74.
69. Mastronardi L, Elsawaf A, Roperto R, et al. Prognostic relevance of the postoperative evolution of intramedullary spinal cord changes in signal intensity on

magnetic resonance imaging after anterior decompression for cervical spondy-lotic myelopathy. J Neurosurg Spine 2007;7(6):615–22.

70. Matsuda Y, Miyazaki K, Tada K, et al. Increased MR signal intensity due to cervical myelopathy. Analysis of 29 surgical cases. J Neurosurg 1991;74(6): 887–92.

71. Mehalic TF, Pezzuti RT, Applebaum BI. Magnetic resonance imaging and cervical spondylotic myelopathy. Neurosurgery 1990;26(2):217–26.

72. Wada E, Ohmura M, Yonenobu K. Intramedullary changes of the spinal cord in cervical spondylotic myelopathy. Spine 1995;20(20):2226–32.

73. Suri A, Chabbra RP, Mehta VS, et al. Effect of intramedullary signal changes on the surgical outcome of patients with cervical spondylotic myelopathy. Spine J 2003;3(1):33–45.

74. Fernandez de Rota JJ, Meschian S, Fernandez de Rota A, et al. Cervical spondylotic myelopathy due to chronic compression: the role of signal inten-sity changes in magnetic resonance images. J Neurosurg Spine 2007;6(1): 17–22.

75. Yukawa Y, Kato F, Yoshihara H, et al. MR T2 image classification in cervical compression myelopathy: predictor of surgical outcomes. Spine 2007;32(15): 1675–8.

76. Shin JJ, Jin BH, Kim KS, et al. Intramedullary high signal intensity and neurolog-ical status as prognostic factors in cervical spondylotic myelopathy. Acta Neuro-chir 2010;152(10):1687–94.

77. Zhang L, Zeitoun D, Rangel A, et al. Preoperative evaluation of the cervical spon-dylotic myelopathy with flexion-extension magnetic resonance imaging: about a prospective study of fifty patients. Spine 2011;36(17):E1134–9.

78. Mummaneni PV, Kaiser MG, Matz PG, et al. Preoperative patient selection with magnetic resonance imaging, computed tomography, and electroencephalog-raphy: does the test predict outcome after cervical surgery? J Neurosurg Spine 2009;11(2):119–29.

79. Morio Y, Teshima R, Nagashima H, et al. Correlation between operative outcomes of cervical compression myelopathy and mri of the spinal cord. Spine 2001; 26(11):1238–45.

80. Bednarik J, Kadanka Z, Dusek L, et al. Presymptomatic spondylotic cervical cord compression. Spine 1999;29(20):2260–9.

81. Ohshio I, Hatayama A, Kaneda K, et al. Correlation between histopathologic features and magnetic resonance images of spinal cord lesions. Spine 1993; 18(9):1140–9.

82. Ozawa H, Sato T, Hyodo H, et al. Clinical significance of intramedullary Gd-DTPA enhancement in cervical myelopathy. Spinal Cord 2010;48(5):415–22.

83. Floeth FW, Stoffels G, Herdmann J, et al. Prognostic Value of 18F-FDG PET in Monosegmental Stenosis and Myelopathy of the Cervical Spinal Cord. J Nucl Med 2011;52(9):1385–91.

84. Maus TP. Imaging of spinal stenosis: neurogenic intermittent claudication and cervical spondylotic myelopathy. Radiol Clin North Am 2012;50(4):651–79.

85. Matsuda Y, Shibata T, Oki S, et al. Outcomes of surgical treatment for cervical myelopathy in patients more than 75 years of age. Spine 1999;24(6):529–34.

86. Hasegawa K, Homma T, Chiba Y, et al. Effects of surgical treatment for cervical spondylotic myelopathy in patients > or = 70 years of age: a retrospective comparative study. J Spinal Disord Tech 2002;15(6):458–60.

87. Holly LT, Moftakhar P, Khoo LT, et al. Surgical outcomes of elderly patients with cervical spondylotic myelopathy. Surg Neurol 2008;69(3):233–40.

88. Naderi S, Ozgen S, Pamir MN, et al. Cervical spondylotic myelopathy: surgical results and factors affecting prognosis. Neurosurgery 1998;43(1):43–9.

89. Furlan JC, Kalsi-Ryan S, Kailaya-Vasan A, et al. Functional and clinical outcomes following surgical treatment in patients with cervical spondylotic myelopathy: a prospective study of 81 cases. J Neurosurg Spine 2011;14(3):348–55.

90. Phillips DG. Surgical treatment of myelopathy with cervical spondylosis. J Neurol Neurosurg Psychiatry 1973;36(5):879–84.

91. Ebersold MJ, Pare MC, Quast LM. Surgical treatment for cervical spondylitic myelopathy. J Neurosurg 1995;82(5):745–51.

92. Lee TT, Manzano GR, Green BA. Modified open-door cervical expansive laminoplasty for spondylotic myelopathy: operative technique, outcome, and predictors for gait improvement. J Neurosurg 1997;86(1):64–8.

93. Lunsford LD, Bissonette DJ, Zorub DS. Anterior surgery for cervical disc disease. Part 2: treatment of cervical spondylotic myelopathy in 32 cases. J Neurosurg 1980;53(1):12–9.

94. Arnasson O, Carlsson CA, Pellettieri L. Surgical and conservative treatment of cervical spondylotic radiculopathy and myelopathy. Acta Neurochir 1987; 84(1–2):48–53.

95. Emery SE, Bohlman HH, Bolesta MJ, et al. Anterior cervical decompression and arthrodesis for the treatment of cervical spondylotic myelopathy. Two to seventeen-year follow-up. J Bone Joint Surg Am 1998;80(7):941–51.

96. Cheung WY, Arvinte D, Wong YW, et al. Neurological recovery after surgical decompression in patients with cervical spondylotic myelopathy—a prospective study. Int Orthop 2008;32(2):273–8.

97. Wang MC, Chan L, Maiman DJ, et al. Complications and mortality associated with cervical spine surgery for degenerative disease in the United States. Spine 2007; 32(3):342–7.

98. Boakye M, Patil CG, Santarelli J, et al. Cervical spondylotic myelopathy: complications and outcomes after spinal fusion. Neurosurgery 2008;62(2):455–61.

99. Fehlings MG, Smith JS, Kopjar B, et al. Perioperative and delayed complications associated with the surgical treatment of cervical spondylotic myelopathy based on 302 patients from the AOSpine North America Cervical Spondylotic Myelopathy Study. J Neurosurg Spine 2012;16(5):425–32.

Paraneoplastic Myelopathy

Eoin P. Flanagan, MBBCh*, B. Mark Keegan, MD, FRCP(C)

KEYWORDS

- Paraneoplastic • Myelopathy • Autoimmune • Spinal cord

KEY POINTS

- Paraneoplastic myelopathies are an uncommon but important category of spinal cord disease to recognize because the neurologic presentation often precedes the detection of cancer.
- The hallmark MRI finding in paraneoplastic myelopathy is longitudinally extensive, symmetric, tract-specific signal changes within the spinal cord that often enhance after gadolinium administration.
- The two most common neural autoantibodies found are amphiphysin-IgG and colapsin-response-mediator-protein-5-IgG and the two most common oncological associations reported are breast and lung cancer.
- The initial treatment of paraneoplastic myelopathies involves detection and treatment of the underlying cancer, typically followed by consideration of a trial of immunotherapy.
- Despite treatment, only a minority of patients improves and, although treatment may confer some stability and delay time to wheelchair, most patients ultimately become wheelchair dependent.

INTRODUCTION

Paraneoplastic myelopathies are an uncommon but important category of spinal cord disease to recognize because the neurologic presentation often precedes the detection of cancer. Most patients present clinically with an insidiously progressive myelopathy with fewer patients presenting subacutely over a few weeks and even fewer with a relapsing remitting course. The recent discovery of novel neural specific autoantibodies, such as collapsin response-mediator protein-5 (CRMP-5) IgG,[1] has led to an increased recognition and improved understanding of the pathogenesis of paraneoplastic myelopathies. Autoimmune myelopathies may also occur in association with neural-specific antibodies, such as aquaporin-4 IgG,[2] without the presence of an underlying cancer and the myelopathic presentation is typically that of a transverse

Financial Disclosure Statements: Dr Flanagan has no disclosures; Dr Keegan has served as a consultant to Novartis, Bionest, and Bristol Meyers Squibb and has research funded by Caridian BCT.
Department of Neurology, Mayo Clinic, 200 First Street South West, Rochester, MN 55905, USA
* Corresponding author.
E-mail address: flanagan.eoin@mayo.edu

myelitis that is often recurrent. Neuromyelitis optica is discussed by Dr Sahraian in more detail elsewhere in this issue. Although myelopathies may occur in the context of a systemic autoimmune disease or with other inflammatory diseases of uncertain causes (eg, sarcoid), the focus of this article is paraneoplastic myelopathies.

CASE

A 54-year-old, previously healthy, right-handed woman developed lower extremity weakness. Three years before presentation, the patient had midthoracic pain followed by insidiously progressive gait impairment due to lower extremity weakness and spasticity with neurogenic bladder and bowel impairment. Her weakness progressed and she became wheelchair-dependent 18 months after symptom onset. She was initially diagnosed with primary progressive multiple sclerosis (MS) and treated with β-interferon. She reported some mild temporary improvement with corticosteroid treatments for presumed MS. She required a baclofen pump for severe spasticity. She was a lifelong nonsmoker without family history of autoimmunity. Her past medical history was notable only for remote pulmonary coccidiomycosis. Her neurologic examination revealed spastic-paraplegia with distal lower extremity pin and vibratory sensory loss. Spinal cord MRI spine revealed longitudinally extensive T2-signal hyperintensity with symmetric gadolinium enhancement in the lateral columns from T2 through T7, similar to that seen in **Fig. 1**. Brain MRI was normal. Cerebrospinal fluid (CSF) had revealed elevated white blood cells, but further results were not available.

Given the tract-specific findings on MRI (tractopathy), a paraneoplastic cause was suspected and a serum paraneoplastic autoantibody panel revealed elevated amphiphysin-IgG. CT of the chest, abdomen, and pelvis were normal. Mammogram results were equivocal but, considering the very high positive predictive value of amphiphysin-IgG positivity for cancer presence (~80%–90%), breast ultrasound and MRI were performed. These revealed a right breast lesion and subsequent breast biopsy confirmed an estrogen-receptor-positive adenocarcinoma. The patient underwent right mastectomy and sentinel lymph node biopsy revealed no metastatic disease. She received adjuvant hormonal therapy. The patient was placed on oral mycophenolate mofetil as maintenance immunotherapy without neurologic improvement.

The patient later developed cognitive impairment thought to be related to paraneoplastic syndrome, after other causes were excluded. The patient's neurologic condition remained stable; however, 4 years later she developed breast carcinoma in the left breast that was treated with surgery. Additional chemotherapy and radiation treatment were recommended; no further follow-up was available.

Discussion

Most commonly, paraneoplastic myelopathy presents with a progressive myelopathy manifesting before detection of underlying cancer. Additional multifocal neurologic symptoms, such as encephalopathy (as in this case), cranial neuropathies, and cerebellar ataxia are often present. Tract-specific spinal cord MRI signal abnormalities should raise suspicion for a paraneoplastic cause. The presence of neural specific autoantibodies confirms the autoimmune neurologic disease and guides the search for cancer. Some neural autoantibodies, such as amphiphysin-IgG, have a high positive predictive value for cancer and an aggressive search for malignancy is required. If initial cancer screening is negative, cancer surveillance screening every 6 to 12 months may be warranted because cancer may be detected long after the myelopathy occurred. Despite oncological and immunosuppressant treatments, morbidity is high and most patients remain wheelchair dependent.

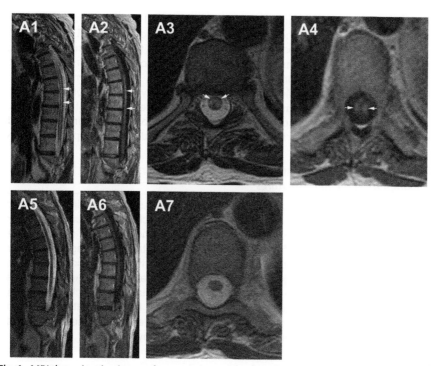

Fig. 1. MRI thoracic spine images from a patient with a tonsillar carcinoma shows longitudinally extensive T2-signal abnormality (*A1, white arrows*) extending over seven spinal segments with associated gadolinium enhancement (*A2, white arrows*) on sagittal section. Symmetric tract-specific T2-signal abnormality (lateral columns) on axial section (*A3, white arrows*) enhances after gadolinium administration (*A4, white arrows*) on T1-weighted axial images. Repeat MRI after cancer and immunosuppressant treatment demonstrates almost complete resolution (*A5–A7*) of MRI abnormalities; this was associated with clinical improvement from dependence on a walker to a cane. (*Adapted from* Flanagan EP, McKeon A, Lennon VA, et al. Paraneoplastic isolated myelopathy: clinical course and neuroimaging clues. Neurology 2011;76(24):2089–95; with permission.)

PATHOGENESIS OF PARANEOPLASTIC DISORDERS

Paraneoplastic neurologic disorders are thought to result from the expression of antigens in tumors that are not expressed by normal cells and, therefore, recognized as foreign by the immune system. These antigens are also present in mature cells in the nervous system, including neurons and glia; therefore, they are known as onconeural antigens. In the nervous system these onconeural antigens may be intracellular (nuclear, nucleolar, or cytoplasmic) or may be located on the cell surface (in the plasma membrane).[3] Intracellular antigens are generally hidden from the immune system but peptides from these intracellular antigens may be expressed on the cell surface by upregulated MHC class-1 molecules in the proinflammatory state of cytokine release and proteasomal degradation. These proteins mark these cells (neurons or glia) for cytotoxic T-cell destruction in the setting of the autoantibodies produced to onconeural antigens.

Antibodies targeting intracellular nuclear or cytoplasmic antigens (eg, anti-amphiphysin antibodies) are thought to be merely a marker of a related CD8+ cytotoxic T-cell response and thus, in themselves, are not considered directly pathogenic.[3] Patients with this type of immune response tend to not respond well to B-cell antibody depleting therapies and, whereas immunotherapy choices tend to focus more on T-cell depleting agents, overall patients respond poorly to oncological treatment and/or immunotherapy. Conversely, in patients with antibodies targeting cell surface onconeural antigens (eg, aquaporin-4 IgG or voltage gated potassium channel complex IgG) the antibodies are thought to be directly pathogenic. They may result in agonist or antagonistic affects on the cell, activation of complement, and internalization of the antigens.[3] As such, these patients are more likely to respond favorably to B-cell and/or antibody depleting immunotherapy and, if the cancer is identified, to direct antineoplastic therapy.

PATIENT EVALUATION OVERVIEW
Demographics and Clinical Features

Paraneoplastic myelopathies may occur with exclusive spinal cord involvement or with accompanying multifocal neurologic impairment, such as optic neuritis, encephalopathy, movement disorders, cerebellar symptoms, and peripheral nerve involvement.[4] Approximately 60% of patients are women and the median age is 62 years (range 37–79).[5] Because the usual clinical presentation is that of an insidious progressive myelopathy, patients may be misdiagnosed as primary progressive MS.[5] Occasionally they may have acute or even relapsing presentations mimicking relapsing remitting MS.[4] In approximately two-thirds of patients, the myelopathy symptoms begin before the detection of cancer. One study reported a median time of 12 months (range 2–44 months) to cancer detection from myelopathy onset.[5]

Laboratory Features

CSF examination typically reveals a moderate lymphocytic pleocytosis (0–100 white cells/μL) and a mild to moderately elevated protein. Unique CSF oligoclonal bands are present in approximately 30%. CSF cytology and flow cytometry is particularly indicated if a known malignancy exists.

MRI Features

The hallmark MRI finding in paraneoplastic myelopathy is longitudinally extensive, symmetric, tract-specific signal changes within the spinal cord that often enhance after gadolinium administration (see **Fig. 1**).[5] This is seen in up to a third to half of patients and is suggestive of the diagnosis in the correct context. This pattern most commonly involves the lateral columns (see **Fig. 1**) but dorsal columns or central gray matter patterns have also been reported.[5] It is important to ask for axial images with gadolinium because this is often helpful in revealing this pattern and may not be performed routinely in spinal cord MRI. However, it should also be noted that the MRI may be normal in up to half of cases. MRI imaging of the brain is usually unrevealing and patterns suggestive of MS are not seen.

Tract-specific changes on MRI may be seen in some nutritional deficiencies and other metabolic myelopathies. It is important to test vitamin B12 and copper in these patients.[6,7] Dorsal column signal abnormalities have been reported in patients with leukoencephalopathy with brain stem and spinal cord involvement and lactate elevation associated with the autosomal recessive DARS2 gene on chromosome 1, which results in mitochondrial aspartyl-tRNA synthetase deficiency.[8] Tract-specific changes in an owl-eye pattern may also be seen in ischemic myelopathies; however, the presentation would be much more acute than with paraneoplastic myelopathies.[9]

In patients with a known diagnosis of cancer, it is important to exclude intramedullary spinal cord metastases because it may present similarly. MRI may also be helpful to suggest alternative causes of chronic progressive myelopathy with flow voids and central T2 signal hyperintensity suggestive of a dural arteriovenous fistula[10] and pial enhancement suggesting neurosarcoidosis.[11]

Neural Autoantibodies

Numerous neural autoantibodies are associated with paraneoplastic myelopathies and, therefore, a comprehensive autoantibody panel is indicated rather than selecting individual serum autoantibodies (**Table 1**). Autoantibodies predict cancer presence rather than particular neurologic presentation in most cases.[12] The two most common neural autoantibodies found are amphiphysin-IgG and CRMP-5-IgG, and the two most common oncological associations reported are breast and lung cancer.[4,5,13] Neuromyelitis optica spectrum disorders with aquaporin-4 IgG rarely occur in a paraneoplastic context.[14] CSF paraneoplastic autoantibody evaluation may complement serologic testing and enhance detection of paraneoplastic autoantibodies.[15] Negative autoantibody evaluation does not exclude paraneoplastic myelopathy because undiscovered antibodies exist and known antibody levels may be reduced by immunosuppressive therapy.

Cancer detection

Evaluation of a suspected paraneoplastic myelopathy requires a detailed clinical history regarding cancer risk factors such as cigarette smoking and family history of cancer. Constitutional symptoms, such as unexplained weight loss, enlarged lymph glands, hemoptysis, bloody stools, change in color or size of a nevus or a recent history of venous thromboembolism, should be sought. The authors recommend initial imaging with a CT of the chest, abdomen, and pelvis. Gender-specific tests, including mammography and ovarian or testicular ultrasound, are appropriate. Whole body [18]flourodeoxyglucose positron emission tomography (FDG-PET) may improve the sensitivity for detecting a cancer for which routine evaluations are unrevealing.[16]

TREATMENT AND PROGNOSIS
Oncological Treatment

The initial treatment of paraneoplastic myelopathies involves detection and treatment of the underlying cancer, typically followed by consideration of a trial of immunotherapy. A multidisciplinary approach to paraneoplastic myelopathy is appropriate and the assistance of an oncologist and surgeon may be necessary to help with oncologic treatment. The oncological treatment is tailored toward the type of malignancy. Certain chemotherapy agents also function as potent immunosuppressants (eg, cyclophosphamide) and, if a reasonable choice for the underlying cancer, may be a good choice to work as a dual immunotherapy and chemotherapy agent. Treatment of the underlying cancer alone or in combination with immunotherapy may result in improvement in the neurologic syndrome.[5,17]

Pharmacologic Treatment Options

There are no randomized controlled trials evaluating immunotherapy in paraneoplastic myelopathies and evidence for treatment is based on case series,[5] case reports,[18,19] and expert opinion.[20] There have been reports of stability or improvements with the following treatments alone or in combination: corticosteroids,[4,5,18,19] plasma exchange,[5] cyclophosphamide,[4,5] mycophenolate,[4,5] and azathioprine.[4,5]

Because the most neural-specific autoantibodies in paraneoplastic myelopathies reflect a cytotoxic CD8+ T-cell response, the authors tend to avoid treatments that only deplete B cells (eg, rituximab) and focus on agents that deplete T cells alone or

Table 1
Neural-autoantibodies, clinical features and cancer associations in paraneoplastic myelopathy

Neural Autoantibody	Association with Cancer[a]	Other Neurological Features	Most Frequent Cancer Associations
Amphiphysin-IgG[13]	Strong	Neuropathy, encephalopathy, stiff-person syndrome and ataxia	Breast, small-cell lung
ANNA-1 (anti-Hu)[21]	Strong	Sensory neuropathy, autonomic neuropathy, limbic and brainstem encephalitis, ataxia.	Small-cell lung
ANNA-2 (anti-Ri)[22]	Strong	Opsoclonus-myoclonus, brainstem encephalitis, laryngospasm, jaw opening dystonia, neuropathy	Breast, lung
ANNA-3[23]	Strong	Limbic encephalitis, ataxia, neuropathy	Lung
AQP4 (NMO)-IgG[14]	Weak	Optic neuritis, intractable nausea and vomiting	Breast, lung, thymoma
Calcium channel (N and P/Q-types)[3]	Weak	Lambert-Eaton syndrome, ataxia	Breast, lung
CRMP-5-IgG[1]	Strong	Neuropathy, chorea, optic neuropathy, dementia, ataxia, neuromuscular junction disorder	Small-cell lung, thymoma
Glutamic acid decarboxylase 65 (GAD-65)[27]	Weak	Stiff-person syndrome, ataxia, PERM, limbic encephalitis	Thymoma, renal cell, breast, colon
Glycine receptor antibodies[3]	Weak	Progressive encephalomyelitis rigidity and myoclonus (PERM)	Thymoma
Ma1 (anti-Ma)[26]	Strong	Limbic encephalitis, brainstem encephalitis	Lung, GI tract, breast, germ cell, non-Hodgkin lymphoma
Ma2 (anti-Ta)[26]	Strong	Limbic encephalitis, brainstem encephalitis	Germ cell of testis
PCA-1 (anti-Yo)[24]	Strong	Ataxia, brainstem encephalitis, neuropathy	Ovary, breast, fallopian tube
PCA-2[25]	Strong	Ataxia, encephalitis, Lambert-Eaton syndrome, neuropathy	Lung
Voltage-gated potassium channel complex[28]	Weak	Limbic encephalitis, neuromyotonia, motor neuron disease	Lung, breast

Abbreviations: AQP4(NMO)-IgG, Aquaporin-4(neuromyelitis optica)-IgG; ANNA-1, anti-neuronal nuclear autoantibody type 1; ANNA-2, anti-neuronal nuclear autoantibody type 2; ANNA-3, anti-neuronal nuclear autoantibody type 3; CRMP-5 IgG, collapsin response-mediator protein-5 IgG; GI, gastrointestinal; PCA-1, Purkinje-cell cytoplasmic autoantibody type 1 (anti-Yo); PCA-2, Purkinje-cell cytoplasmic autoantibody type 2; PERM, progressive encephalomyelitis rigidity and myoclonus.
[a] Strong = >70% associated with cancer; weak = <30% associated with cancer.
Data from Flanagan EP, Lennon VA, Pittock SJ. Autoimmune myelopathies. Continuum (Minneap Minn) 2011;17:776–99.

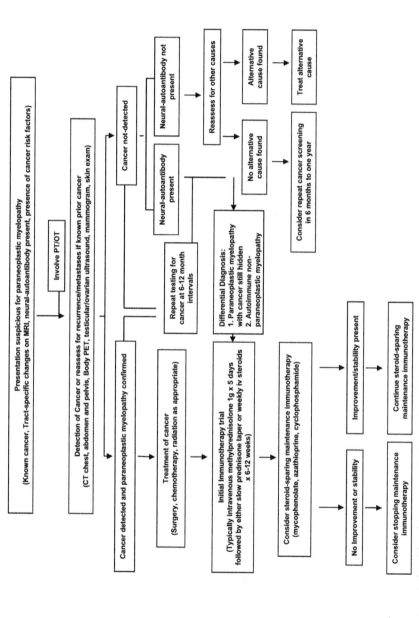

Fig. 2. Treatment algorithm for paraneoplastic myelopathies. OT, occupational therapy; PT, physical therapy.

Table 2
Paraneoplastic immunotherapy regimens, monitoring necessary and associated side effects

Medication, Dose, and Regimen Used	Mechanism of Action	Precautions or Monitoring or Prophylaxis	Common and Important Side Effects
IV methylprednisolone or oral prednisone Initial Rx • Typically 1000 mg IV × 3–5 d • Consider slow oral steroid taper vs once weekly IV 1 g infusions of methylprednisolone Maintenance Rx Oral prednisone 60 mg daily with slow taper as tolerated	Complex: • Stabilize neutrophil lysosomes preventing degranulation • Alter gene transcription by inhibiting cytokines, upregulation of antiinflammatory proteins • Decreased T-cell, mast cell and eosinophil activation	Precautions/Monitoring: • Assess for hyperglycemia if diabetic or at risk • Consider baseline bone density scan in at risk Prophylaxis: • Calcium 1200 mg/d and vitamin D 1200 IU/d • Trimethoprim-sulfamethoxazole 1 double-strength tablet (800 mg–160 mg) daily • Proton pump inhibitor or histamine-2 receptor blocker if at risk for gastric ulceration	Infection, osteoporosis, avascular necrosis of the hip, cushingoid appearance, skin thinning and easy bruising, insomnia, psychosis, depression, cataracts, hypertension, weight gain and edema Caution when discontinuing due to risk of addisonian crisis when discontinued abruptly
IVIG Initial Rx: 0.4 g/kg × 3–5 d Maintenance Rx: 0.4 g/kg once weekly for 6–12 weeks followed by slow weaning by increasing the interval between doses as tolerated	• Block Fc receptors on macrophages preventing phagocytosis • May neutralize pathogenic autoantibodies	Precautions: • Measure IgA as IgA deficient at risk of anaphylaxis (or use non-IgA formulation)	Headache, aseptic meningitis, renal failure, increased risk myocardial infarct (avoid in at risk patients), and deep venous thrombosis
Mycophenolate mofetil Maintenance Rx Oral dose: 250 mg bid by mouth to 1000 mg bid by mouth	B- and T-cell proliferation prevented by its inhibiting of inosine monophosphate dehydrogenase, which inhibits production of purines and, therefore, DNA formation	Monitoring: • Blood counts, renal function and liver function as a baseline, then weekly for 1 mo, every other week for 2 mo and monthly thereafter	Infection, increased risk of malignancy (lymphoma, skin cancers, etc), diarrhea, hypertension, hepatitis, myelosuppression, and renal failure

Drug/Dosing	Mechanism	Precautions/Monitoring	Adverse Effects
Azathioprine Maintenance Rx 1–2 mg/kg/d in divided doses by mouth	B- and T-cell proliferation prevented by inhibiting purine synthesis through metabolite 6-mercaptopurine	Precautions/Monitoring: • Measure thiopurine S-methyltransferase enzyme activity before starting • Low activity increases risk for drug toxicity and may require increased monitoring or use of alternative agent • Blood counts, renal function, and liver function as a baseline then weekly for 1 mo, every other week for 2 mo and monthly thereafter • Consider monitoring MCV because increases of >5 points may correlate with improved efficacy	Infection, malignancy (lymphoma, skin cancers and others), nausea, macrocytic anemia, skin rash, hypersensitivity reaction, pancreatitis, and elevated liver function tests
Cyclophosphamide Maintenance Rx Oral: 1–2 mg/kg/d (once daily dosing) IV: 1000 mg/square meter monthly	Alkylating agent that predominantly depletes T cells	Monitoring • Blood count initially every wk for 1 mo, every 2 wk for 2 mo and monthly thereafter • Regular urinalyses, encourage liberal hydration, and consider mesna use to monitor for and prevent hemorrhagic cystitis	Infection, malignancy (lymphoma, skin cancers and others), hemorrhagic cystitis, infertility, alopecia and nausea and vomiting

Abbreviations: MCV, mean corpuscular volume; Rx, treatment.

in combination (eg, corticosteroids, mycophenolate, azathioprine, and cyclophospha-mide). In rare cases of paraneoplastic myelopathies with antibodies to cell-surface antigens (eg, paraneoplastic neuromyelitis optica spectrum disorders) it may be reasonable to consider agents that only deplete B-cells, such as rituximab.

The use of immunotherapy involves a twofold approach. The initial treatment aims to obtain the maximal reversibility. This usually involves high-dose intravenous (IV) meth-ylprednisolone 1000 mg for 3 to 5 days. In patients who are intolerant to corticoste-roids, IV immunoglobulin (IVIG) is a reasonable alternative. In patients with rapid deterioration despite corticosteroids, plasma exchange could also be considered. After the acute treatment, maintenance oral corticosteroids may be considered orally for 6 to 12 weeks or, alternatively, some physicians advocate once weekly IV methyl-prednisolone for this time period. The patients can then be reassessed and decisions on tapering the medications could be made at follow-up visits. Once the maximal reversibility has been obtained consideration for the use of a steroid-sparing agent could be given. In the authors' practice, we tend to use mycophenolate, azathioprine, or cyclophosphamide. A suggested, non–evidence-based, treatment algorithm has been provided (**Fig. 2**). The dosage of medications has been provided in **Table 2**.

Nonpharmacologic Treatment Options

The treatment of paraneoplastic myelopathies is multidisciplinary and involvement of a physical medicine and rehabilitation specialist to coordinate physical and occupa-tional therapy is important. This is well illustrated in the case provided, in which a baclofen pump was necessary to treat the spasticity. Treatment of spasticity is dis-cussed in more detail by Dr Strommen elsewhere in this issue. Other complications of myelopathy, including bowel and bladder difficulties, need to be evaluated and treated (further discussion of this is beyond the scope of this article).

Treatment Complications, Prophylaxis, and Monitoring

Immunosuppressant treatments often require initial blood tests to assess the safety of starting the medication, regular blood monitoring, and prophylactic treatments while on the medications. **Table 2** outlines the initial testing necessary before starting certain immunosuppressants, monitoring needed while on immunotherapy, prophy-lactic treatments recommended, and the side effects of the immunotherapies used in paraneoplastic myelopathies.

Evaluation of Outcome and Long-term Recommendations

In patients with a neural autoantibody strongly associated with cancer, repeated surveillance imaging at 6-month to yearly intervals should be considered to look for the emergence of cancer. Follow-up to assess for improvement in ambulation and the neurologic syndrome is important. Despite treatment, only a minority of patients improves, and, although treatment may confer some stability and delay time to wheel-chair, ultimately most patients become wheelchair dependent.[5] In one study, 50% of patients were wheelchair-dependent by 16 months, despite treatment.[5] Younger patients are more likely to respond to treatment. Death may result from the underlying cancer, progression of the neurologic disorder (especially if multifocal), treatment side effects, or complications associated with immobility.

SUMMARY

In summary, paraneoplastic myelopathies cause a slowly progressive myelopathy often manifesting before the detection of cancer. Longitudinally extensive, symmetric, tract-specific T2-signal hyperintensities that enhance gadolinium when evident on MRI are suggestive of the diagnosis. Detection of neural-specific autoantibodies may help confirm the diagnosis and guide the cancer search. Initial management involves detection and treatment of the underlying cancer. Combinations of T-cell depleting immunotherapies are recommended; however, only a minority of patients improves and most become wheelchair dependent.

REFERENCES

1. Yu Z, Kryzer TJ, Griesmann GE, et al. CRMP-5 neuronal autoantibody: marker of lung cancer and thymoma-related autoimmunity. Ann Neurol 2001;49:146–54.
2. Lennon VA, Wingerchuk DM, Kryzer TJ, et al. A serum autoantibody marker of neuromyelitis optica: distinction from multiple sclerosis. Lancet 2004;364:2106–12.
3. McKeon A, Pittock SJ. Paraneoplastic encephalomyelopathies: pathology and mechanisms. Acta Neuropathol 2011;122:381–400.
4. Keegan BM, Pittock SJ, Lennon VA. Autoimmune myelopathy associated with collapsin response-mediator protein-5 immunoglobulin G. Ann Neurol 2008;63: 531–4.
5. Flanagan EP, McKeon A, Lennon VA, et al. Paraneoplastic isolated myelopathy: clinical course and neuroimaging clues. Neurology 2011;76:2089–95.
6. Hemmer B, Glocker FX, Schumacher M, et al. Subacute combined degeneration: clinical, electrophysiological, and magnetic resonance imaging findings. J Neurol Neurosurg Psychiatry 1998;65:822–7.
7. Kumar N, Ahlskog JE, Klein CJ, et al. Imaging features of copper deficiency myelopathy: a study of 25 cases. Neuroradiology 2006;48:78–83.
8. Scheper GC, van der Klok T, van Andel RJ, et al. Mitochondrial aspartyl-tRNA synthetase deficiency causes leukoencephalopathy with brain stem and spinal cord involvement and lactate elevation. Nat Genet 2007;39:534–9.
9. Masson C, Pruvo JP, Meder JF, et al. Spinal cord infarction: clinical and magnetic resonance imaging findings and short term outcome. J Neurol Neurosurg Psychiatry 2004;75:1431–5.
10. McKeon A, Lindell EP, Atkinson JL, et al. Pearls & oy-sters: clues for spinal dural arteriovenous fistulae. Neurology 2011;76:e10–2.
11. Junger SS, Stern BJ, Levine SR, et al. Intramedullary spinal sarcoidosis: clinical and magnetic resonance imaging characteristics. Neurology 1993;43:333–7.
12. Pittock SJ, Kryzer TJ, Lennon VA. Paraneoplastic antibodies coexist and predict cancer, not neurological syndrome. Ann Neurol 2004;56:715–9.
13. Pittock SJ, Lucchinetti CF, Parisi JE, et al. Amphiphysin autoimmunity: paraneoplastic accompaniments. Ann Neurol 2005;58:96–107.
14. Pittock SJ, Lennon VA. Aquaporin-4 autoantibodies in a paraneoplastic context. Arch Neurol 2008;65:629–32.
15. McKeon A, Pittock SJ, Lennon VA. CSF complements serum for evaluating paraneoplastic antibodies and NMO-IgG. Neurology 2011;76:1108–10.
16. McKeon A, Apiwattanakul M, Lachance DH, et al. Positron emission tomography-computed tomography in paraneoplastic neurologic disorders: systematic analysis and review. Arch Neurol 2010;67:322–9.
17. Anderson DW, Borsaru A. Case report: lymphoma-related resolving paraneoplastic myelopathy with MRI correlation. Br J Radiol 2008;81:e103–5.
18. Leypoldt F, Eichhorn P, Saager C, et al. Successful immunosuppressive treatment and long-term follow-up of anti-Ri-associated paraneoplastic myelitis. J Neurol Neurosurg Psychiatry 2006;77:1199–200.

19. Rajabally YA, Qaddoura B, Abbott RJ. Steroid-responsive paraneoplastic demyelinating neuropathy and myelopathy associated with breast carcinoma. J Clin Neuromuscul Dis 2008;10:65–9.
20. Graber JJ, Nolan CP. Myelopathies in patients with cancer. Arch Neurol 2010;67: 298–304.
21. Sillevis Smitt P, Grefkens J, de Leeuw B, et al. Survival and outcome in 73 anti-Hu positive patients with paraneoplastic encephalomyelitis/sensory neuronopathy. J Neurol 2002;249:745–53.
22. Pittock SJ, Lucchinetti CF, Lennon VA. Anti-neuronal nuclear autoantibody type 2: paraneoplastic accompaniments. Ann Neurol 2003;53:580–7.
23. Chan KH, Vernino S, Lennon VA. ANNA-3 anti-neuronal nuclear antibody: marker of lung cancer-related autoimmunity. Ann Neurol 2001;50:301–11.
24. McKeon A, Tracy JA, Pittock SJ, et al. Purkinje cell autoantibody type 1 accompaniments: the cerebellum and beyond. Arch Neurol 2011;68:1282–9.
25. Vernino S, Lennon VA. New Purkinje cell antibody (PCA-2): marker of lung cancer-related neurological autoimmunity. Ann Neurol 2000;47:297–305.
26. Hoffmann LA, Jarius S, Pellkofer HL, et al. Anti-Ma and anti-Ta associated paraneoplastic neurological syndromes: 22 newly diagnosed patients and review of previous cases. J Neurol Neurosurg Psychiatry 2008;79:767–73.
27. Pittock SJ, Yoshikawa H, Ahlskog JE, et al. Glutamic acid decarboxylase autoimmunity with brainstem, extrapyramidal, and spinal cord dysfunction. Mayo Clin Proc 2006;81:1207–14.
28. Tan KM, Lennon VA, Klein CJ, et al. Clinical spectrum of voltage-gated potassium channel autoimmunity. Neurology 2008;70:1883–90.

Stiff Person Syndrome

Giuseppe Ciccotto, MD, MPH, Maike Blaya, MD,
Roger E. Kelley, MD*

KEYWORDS

- Stiff person syndrome • Axial spasm • Anti-GAD antibodies
- Autoimmune neuromuscular disorder

KEY POINTS

- Stiff person syndrome (SPS) is a rare autoimmune neurologic disorder presenting with muscular rigidity and trigger-induced painful muscle spasms predominantly affecting the proximal limb and axial muscles.
- SPS is associated with autoantibodies to glutamic acid decarboxylase (anti-GAD).
- Because SPS is frequently underdiagnosed or misdiagnosed, there is limited accurate epidemiologic data.
- Persons suffering from SPS typically do not have pyramidal and extrapyramidal signs.
- There have numerous reports of response of the stiffness and spasms to agents in the benzodiazepine class, such as diazepam or clonazepam.

INTRODUCTION

Stiff person syndrome (SPS) is a rare autoimmune neurologic disorder presenting with muscular rigidity and trigger-induced painful muscle spasms predominantly affecting the proximal limb and axial muscles, with emphasis on the paraspinal muscles, leading to gait difficulties and progressive disability. Sudden death due to autonomic dysfunction may also occur in these patients.[1] The condition was first described by Moersch and Woltman[2] in 1924 based on 14 cases. The term stiff-man syndrome was coined by Moersch and Woltman after their patients used descriptions such as "falls as a wooden man," "falls like a wax dummy," "stiff," or "board like."[2] The term "stiff" was also maintained because of the lack of extrapyramidal features, pyramidal tract dysfunction, or any other known neurologic disorder that could explain the characteristic muscular contractions seen in the patients with the disease.[3]

In 1958, Asher[4] reported the first woman with similar complaints to those reported by Moersch and Woltman.[2] Shortly after this report, Bowler[5] reported the first child with stiff-man syndrome. As the nature of the disease became better understood, it was recommended that the word "person" be used in recognition that the disease can affect both genders.[6]

Department of Neurology, Tulane University School of Medicine, 1430 Tulane Avenue 8065, New Orleans, LA 70112, USA
* Corresponding author.
E-mail address: rkelley2@tulane.edu

Neurol Clin 31 (2013) 319–328
http://dx.doi.org/10.1016/j.ncl.2012.09.005   neurologic.theclinics.com

PATHOPHYSIOLOGY

SPS is associated with autoantibodies to glutamic acid decarboxylase (anti-GAD).[6–8] GAD is the key enzyme that converts glutamate to gamma-aminobutyric acid (GABA) and exists in two isoforms: GAD65 and GAD67. Both GAD65 and GAD67 function synchronously to produce and regulate physiologic levels of GABA.[9,10] GAD67 produces the basal level of GABA, whereas GAD65 seems to play a role when extra GABA neurotransmitter is required (eg, in times of stress).[9] The production of autoantibodies seen in SPS is primarily against GAD65 and not GAD67. GAD65 is reported to be the target antigen in about 60% of the patients with SPS.[11,12] The structural differences between GAD65 and GAD67 may explain this contrasting antigenicity. GAD65 structure inherent flexibility not present in GAD67 may be the cause of its increase B-cell antigenicity. Also, GAD65 structure displays a strong negative electrostatic field in the C-terminal domain, not seen in the structure of GAD67.[13,14]

Autoantibodies (autoAb) to GAD65 that are found in patients with SPS can inhibit the enzymatic activity of GAD65 and impair the syntheses of GABA, resulting in low levels of this neurotransmitter. GABA is the major inhibitory neurotransmitter of the brain and its impairment seen in SPS may explain the symptoms of stiffness and excessive muscle spasms.[8] GAD65 autoantibodies are detectable in the cerebrospinal fluid and sera of patients with SPS; however, their titers do not seem to correlate with the severity of the disease.[8,14] GAD is also found in nonneuronal tissues, such as beta cells of pancreatic islets, testes, and oviducts. Interestingly, SPS is occasionally associated with endocrine disorders. Thirty percent of patients with SPS have insulin-dependent diabetes and both diseases share autoantibodies to the same isoform GAD65.[8]

GAD65-specific autoantibodies are also seen in some patients with other neurologic diseases, such as myoclonus, cerebellar ataxia, epilepsy, and Batten disease; however, studies suggest that these GAD65 autoAb are organ and disease-specific.[15] IgG from GAD65 Ab-positive patients with SPS administered to the cerebellum of rats induced SPS-like effects in the animals; however, an epitope-specific GAD65-Ab is not yet identified in SPS patients.[8] Despite increasing reports of SPS throughout the world, little is known about the pathophysiological mechanism of the disease. Other known autoantigens described in SPS include amphiphysin, gephyrin, and GABA(A) receptor–associated protein (GABARAP).[16,17] What induces the development of autoimmunity is still not well understood. The autoimmune response to an antigenic stimulus is possibly triggered by a combination of appropriate interactive genetic and environmental factors that culminate in the disease.

EPIDEMIOLOGY

Because SPS is frequently underdiagnosed or misdiagnosed, there are limited accurate epidemiologic data. The literature reveals it has a tendency to occur predominately in the mid-fifth decade of life and, more often, insidiously following an especially stressful event in life. The incidence is estimated to be equal to or less than one person per million with a 2:1 female/male ratio. There has not been evidence of predominance between races or ethnicities; however, there seems to be a link between diabetes mellitus and SPS.[18,19] Antibodies to amphiphysin have been implicated in paraneoplastic variants of SPS. Antibodies to gephyrin was described in one patient.[17] GABARAP is a protein involved in the trafficking and assembly of GABA(A) receptor, and it is another target antigen in 70% of the subjects with SPS studied.[20] The lack of uniform anti-GAD antibody presence, the lack of what was once viewed as the classic manifestation of axial stiffness and spasms, as well as other variations on a theme, such as restriction to the lower limbs,[21] confounds accurate compilation of the true incidence and distribution of this disorder. Furthermore, the case report of SPS in a patient after West Nile virus infection suggests possible cross-reactivity and molecular mimicry.[22] SPS manifestations in association with antiamphiphysin antibodies were also found in some patients who had breast cancer or lung cancer, predominately small cell lung cancer.[16,23]

CLINICAL FEATURES

SPS is a disease characterized by muscle rigidity and episodic spasms, often insidious in onset. Stiffness is predominately in the thoracolumbar paraspinal muscles or abdominal muscles with progressive spread to proximal limb muscles over time.[21] Sporadic stiffening and, often painful, muscle spasms can lead to functional impairment with inability to walk and care for oneself. The anxiety of unpredictable exacerbations results in fear of leaving the house and becoming stranded should an attack occur. There is resultant phobia about leaving the home[24,25] and, not unexpected, situational depression. Triggers reflect heightened response to external stimuli, including emotional stressors, sudden unexpected external stimuli (eg, sound or touch), or fast movement in affected muscle groups.[26,27] Though the spasms and rigidity may be localized and sporadic at onset, with improvement during sleep, as the disease progresses the symptoms become static, ultimately leading to loss of independence in daily activities, assistance in walking, and inability to bend at the waist resulting in major functional impairment and disability.[28] A summary of potential features of SPS is provided in **Box 1**.

VARIATIONS ON A THEME

Some patients manifest clinical characteristics localized to a specific region of the body with designations of stiff limb syndrome and stiff trunk syndrome. Barker and colleagues[21] have reported on the association of rigidity with a subacute encephalomyelitis seen at autopsy. In addition, one can see a paraneoplastic syndrome consisting of progressive encephalomyelitis in combination with rigidity and myoclonus (PERM).[29]

Stiff infant syndrome (SIS), or infantile hyperexplexia,[30] manifests at birth or early in infancy and is associated with at least five different genes in a both autosomal-dominant and autosomal-recessive form. These infants will present with hypotonia and diminished rigidity during sleep contrasted with generalized muscle stiffness

---

Box 1
Potential features of SPS

1. Rigidity which can be generalized or localized

2. Painful muscle spasms

3. The finding of anti-GAD antibodies in up to 60% of patients

4. Lack of an alternative explanation for the rigidity and muscle spasm

5. Potential overlap with other autoimmune disorders

6. Potential relationship with a progressive subacute encephalomyelitis

7. Potential component of a paraneoplastic syndrome

8. Hyperexcitability of spinal motor neurons on neurophysiological studies

and increased rigidity on awakening, including episodes of apnea and exaggerated startle response. As in SPS, these infants will have brisk deep tendon reflexes, though infants with SIS will have a generalized spread of the response. Most patients with SIS will have resolved their stiffness before the end of infancy, with most children being normal by age 3. Recurring episodes of stiffness throughout adolescence and adulthood are not, however, uncommon. Such episodes can be triggered by cold exposure, pregnancy, or startle.

Patients with SPS continue to be prone to exaggerated startle response to visual, tactile, or auditory stimuli, more so than the average individual is, throughout their lives. This can lead to inability to protect themselves from falls during an unexpected generalized stiffness response. Later in life, they may also exhibit hypnagogic myoclonus as well as periodic limb movements during sleep.[31] One reported form of hypokinetic rigid syndrome in a neonate was attributed to mitochondrial DNA depletion in association with secondary defect in neurotransmission and was progressive and fatal.[32]

ELECTROPHYSIOLOGICAL CORRELATES

Persons suffering from SPS typically do not have pyramidal and extrapyramidal signs. The stiffness occurs from involuntary firing of muscle motor units that will reveal itself as voluntary contraction on electromyography (EMG).[3,33] This is manifested by normal motor unit potential (MUP) configurations and firing rates with lack of denervation.[34] EMG typically reveals continuous MUP firing that can be reduced by administration of benzodiazepines.[34] Muscle spasms can occur spontaneously or by triggering events. Such spasms involve co-contraction of antagonist muscles.[21,26] Subnoxious stimulation of cutaneous or mixed nerves will cause disproportionate spread of reflexes and spasms to distant muscles from the stimulation site that, if confirmed by EMG, can support the diagnosis of SPS.[34] As in hereditary hyperekplexia, which involves loss of glycinergic transmission resulting in disinhibition at brainstem and spinal cord levels, SPS patients have an exaggerated startle response. This can lead to prolonged spasms after loud, or sudden, noises.[34,35] However, unlike hereditary hyperekplexia patients, SPS patients have exaggerated acoustic responses manifested as prolonged spasm of distant muscles, often major motor groups, such as the lumbar paraspinal muscles, neck, and proximal extremities.

The characteristic EMG finding of continuous firing of motor unit activity in SPS is not a result of motor unit disease nor of aberrations in the monosynaptic reflex arc because firing rates and recruitment of MUPs are maintained, as well as conduction velocities, F-waves, H-reflex, and the silent period induced by muscle stretch and mixed nerve stimulation.[34,36] Also, there tends to be a normal interference pattern seen during the spasms. Clinically, patients often have hyperactive deep tendon reflexes and some have clonus, although the Babinski reflex tends to be flexor.[34] The rigidity and the continuous motor unit activity disappear during sleep, as well as during peripheral nerve block and during anesthesia, which seems to indicate a central origin.[2,37]

DIFFERENTIAL DIAGNOSIS

The more typical manifestations of SPS versus variants are being increasingly recognized, as highlighted in a recent review by McKeon and colleagues.[33] As mentioned previously, SPS can reflect an isolated subacute progressive encephalomyelitis with rigidity[21] as well as a paraneoplastic syndrome in combination with PERM.[29] PERM is a rare condition seen in patients with cancer, especially small cell carcinoma of the lung. Unlike SPS, these patients often will have brainstem dysfunction, myoclonus, and spinal rigidity. The clinical features are a result of widespread central nervous system dysfunction, with the cervical spinal cord most commonly affected. Isaacs syndrome, or acquired neuromyotonia, is an autoimmune channelopathy[38] that manifests as a result of antibodies to voltage-gated potassium channel (VGKC) found along the peripheral motor never axons. This syndrome can be paraneoplastic in origin. VGKC play an important role in nerve cell repolarization after action potential firing. Autoantibodies to the VGKC result in a decrease in higher than normal membrane potential by disrupting potassium efflux leading to inappropriate action potential firing and overrelease of acetylcholine responsible for the muscle cramps, slow postcontraction muscle relaxation, and myoclonus. Other clinical features of Isaacs syndrome include hyperhidrosis, lacrimation, and salivation, which are thought to be a result of antibodies to VGKC in autonomic fibers. An important distinction between SPS and Isaacs syndrome is demonstrated on EMG. Unlike SPS, the EMG in Isaacs syndrome has spontaneous muscle activity as a result of abnormal peripheral nerve firing.[39] In a possible overlap syndrome, Brown and colleagues[40] reported on subjects with lower limb rigidity and spasms without associated anti-GAD antibodies. It was speculated that this variant might be more reflective of a chronic spinal interneuronitis.

Painful rigidity can also be seen with tetanus. Painful muscle spasms are also part of the clinical spectrum of both neuroleptic malignant syndrome and the malignant hyperpyrexia that can been seen with certain anesthetic agents such as suxamethonium and halothane. The serotonin syndrome is characterized by the clinical triad of mental status changes, autonomic hyperactivity, and neuromuscular manifestations that can include rigidity.[41] A compilation of potential challenges in the differential diagnosis of SPS is provided in **Box 2**.

TREATMENT

There have numerous reports of response of the stiffness and spasms to agents in the benzodiazepine class, such as diazepam or clonazepam. In addition, antispasmodic agents, such as baclofen or dantrolene, can also provide some measure of relief. In view of the autoimmune nature of SPS, efforts have been made at immunosuppression with agents such as steroids and rituximab, as well as plasma exchange and intravenous gammaglobulin.[42] No positive controlled clinical trial to establish optimal therapy on evidence-based criteria has been achieved. This is certainly understandable given the rare nature of this disorder as well as the variations on a theme in terms of

---

Box 2
Differential diagnosis of stiff-person syndrome

1. Hyperekplexia in pediatric population
2. Neuroleptic malignant syndrome
3. Malignant hyperpyrexia related to certain anesthetic agents in genetically susceptible Individuals
4. Tetanus
5. Isaacs syndrome
6. Serotonin syndrome
7. Overlap with paraneoplastic process
8. Component of a subacute progressive encephalomyelitis
9. Chronic spinal interneuronitis

Box 3
Potential treatment options in SPS

1. Benzodiazepines including diazepam and clonazepam
2. Alternative muscle relaxants including baclofen (including intrathecal), dantrolene, and tizanidine
3. Corticosteroid therapy
4. Plasma exchange
5. Intravenous gamma globulin
6. Other immunosuppressive agents, such as mycophenolate, cyclophosphamide, azathioprine, methotrexate, and rituximab
7. Vigabatrin
8. Gabapentin
9. Sodium valproate
10. Levetiracetam
11. Botulinum toxin injections

---

pathogenesis. Sevy and colleagues[43] reported on successful treatment using rituximab with an intractable patient with SPS who had failed alternative immunosuppressive therapy. Of interest, despite clinical improvement in terms of reduced stiffness and spasm frequency, the blood and cerebrospinal fluid levels of anti-GAD antibodies increased during the course of treatment. A 12-year-old patient was also recently reported to have a significant response to rituximab.[44] However, in a recently reported controlled clinical trial, rituximab was not found to be superior to alternative therapy.[45]

An example how the overlap of manifestations can affect therapeutic response was provided by Cabo-López and colleagues.[46] They described a 28-year-old woman with psychogenic mutism. While hospitalized, this patient developed axial and proximal limb stiffness with hyperreflexia and prominent muscle spasms. She was found to have anti-GAD antibodies, as well as antibodies to parietal cells, microsomal thyroid peroxidase, and thyroglobulin. A partial response was observed with a combination of benzodiazepines, muscle relaxants, and corticosteroids.

Other immunosuppressive agents that have been tried include cyclophosphamide and mycophenolate. Additional agents reported in the literature include tizanidine, piracetam, and phenobarbital, as well as sodium valproate,[47] levetiracetam,[48] gabapentin,[49] vigabatrin,[50] and propofol.[51] Also, there have been reports of some response to botulinum toxin injections.[52] Potential treatment approaches are provided in **Box 3**.

SUMMARY

The recognition of an intriguing, but disabling, neuromuscular disorder, SPS, is vitally important in the clinical realm. SPS is an uncommon, if not rare, disorder characterized by a sense of body stiffness associated with painful muscle spasms. Like many illnesses, the manifestations can vary in terms of location and severity. The syndrome has been subdivided into stiff trunk versus stiff limb presentation as well as a progressive encephalomyelitis associated with rigidity. Stiff person-type syndrome can also reflect a paraneoplastic picture. Most patients demonstrate exaggerated lumbar lordosis. Roughly 60% of patients have anti-GAD antibodies in the blood and the cerebrospinal fluid. The differential diagnosis includes tetanus, serotonin syndrome, encephalomyelitis, neuroleptic malignant syndrome, and malignant hyperpyrexia. There have been reports of response to muscle relaxants, including benzodiazepines, immunosuppressants, intravenous gamma globulin, plasma exchange, several anticonvulsants, and botulinum toxin.

Case study

A 54 year old right-handed African-American woman is referred to you because of increasing sense of "stiffness" and painful spasms. She has a several year history of type II diabetes mellitus and hypertension. She has been in otherwise good health, but reports a several month history of diminished appetite with a 20 lb. weight loss. She is being treated with an oral hypoglycemic agent for her diabetes and an angiotensin converting enzyme inhibitor for her hypertension. She has never smoked, drank alcohol or used illicit drugs. She has had a total abdominal hysterectomy with retention of her ovaries and this was related to uterine fibroids.

Family history is pertinent for hypertension and diabetes with both of her parents dying in their 60's from recurrent stroke. She has a brother, age 47, who is on hemodialysis for end-stage renal disease attributed to hypertensive nephropathy. Review of systems is pertinent for a generalized sense of weakness, a sense of "stiffness" of her axial musculature, and increasing painful muscle spasms of her extremities, especially her legs, along with the diminished appetite and weight loss.

On exam, her vital signs are stable except for a blood pressure of 154/94 mm Hg. She has no rash. Funduscopic exam reveals arteriolar narrowing. You noted some cervical lymphadenopathy. She also has some abdominal distension. Her mental status and speech are intact. Cranial nerve exam is normal. She has fairly good tone and strength throughout but muscle spasms of her lower torso and proximal lower extremities are noted during the exam. There is no evidence of cerebellar dysfunction. Her sensory exam reveals somewhat diminished vibratory sensation in a stocking-type distribution which you attribute to her diabetes. No sensory level is noted. The deep tendon reflexes are prominent in the 3/4 range with the Babinski response flexor on both sides. Her gait is somewhat antalgic related to her muscle spasms, but no actual truncal ataxia is noted.

Your differential diagnosis includes possible demyelinating disease, possible Lyme disease with spinal cord involvement, diabetic amyotrophy, or a paraneoplastic syndrome. The creatine kinase is normal at 154 with normal thyroid profile, normal B12 and folate level but a surprisingly elevated sedimentation rate of 87. A diligent medical student has been assigned this patient and does an extensive review of of possible explanations for the sense of body stiffness with painful muscle spasms. A diligent medical student has been assigned this patient and does an extensive review of possible explanations for the sense of body stiffness and painful muscle spasms. This leads to the sending off of a serum anti-glutamic acid decarboxylase antibody titer which comes back elevated at 1.2 nmol/L (normal = $\leq$ 0.02 Nmol/L). Unfortunately, the chest x-ray reveals multiple lesions felt to reflect metastatic disease and the CT scan of the abdomen reveals advanced ovarian carcinoma.

During presentation at Neurology Grand Rounds, at the medical center where the patient was admitted, it is felt by most attendees that his presentation represented stiff person syndrome as paraneoplastic manifestation of her metastatic ovarian carcinoma.

REFERENCES

1. Mitsumoto H, Schwartzman MJ, Estes ML, et al. Sudden death and paroxysmal autonomic dysfunction in stiff-man syndrome. J Neurol 1991;238:91–6.
2. Moersch FP, Woltman HW. Progressive fluctuating muscular rigidity and spasm (stiff-man syndrome); report of a case and some observations in 13 other cases. Proc Staff Meet Mayo Clinic 1956;31:421–7.

3. Toro C, Jacobowitz DM, Hallett M. Stiff-man syndrome. Semin Neurol 1994;14: 154–8.

4. Asher RA. Woman with stiff-man syndrome. Br Med J 1958;1:265–6.

5. Bowler D. The 'stiff-man syndrome' in a boy. Arch Dis Child 1960;35:289–92.

6. Fatima A, Merrill R, Bindu J, et al. Stiff-person syndrome (SPS) and anti-GAD-related CNS degenerations: protean additions to the autoimmune central neuropathies. J Autoimmun 2011;37:79–87.

7. Levy LM, Dalakas MC, Floeter MK. The stiff-person syndrome: an autoimmune disorder affecting neurotransmission of gamma-aminobutyric acid. Ann Intern Med 1999;131:522–30.

8. Raju R, Hampe CS. Immunology of stiff-person syndrome. Int Rev Immunol 2008; 27:79–92.

9. Fenalti G, Buckle AM. Structural biology of the GAD autoantigen. Autoimmun Rev 2010;9:148–52.

10. Battaglioli G, Liu H, Martin DL. Kinetic differences between the isoforms of glutamate decarboxylase: implications for the regulation of GABA synthesis. J Neurochem 2003;86:879–87.

11. Solimena M, Folli F, Denis-Donini S, et al. Autoantibodies to glutamic acid decarboxylase in a patient with stiff-man syndrome, epilepsy, and type I diabetes mellitus. N Engl J Med 1988;318:1012–20.

12. Solimena M, Folli F, Aparisi R, et al. Autoantibodies to GABA-ergic neurons and pancreatic beta cells in stiff-man syndrome. N Engl J Med 1990;322:1555–60.

13. Levy LM, Levy-Reis I, Fujii M, et al. Brain gamma-aminobutyric acid changes in stiff-person syndrome. Arch Neurol 2005;62:970–4.

14. Rakocevic G, Raju R, Dalakas MC. Anti-glutamic acid decarboxylase antibodies in the serum and cerebrospinal fluid of patients with stiff-person syndrome: correlation with clinical severity. Arch Neurol 2004;61:902–4.

15. Manto MU, Laute MA, Aguera M, et al. Effects of anti-glutamic acid decarboxylase antibodies associated with neurological diseases. Ann Neurol 2007;61:544–51.

16. Rosin L, De Camilli P, Butler M, et al. Stiff-man syndrome in a woman with breast cancer: an uncommon central nervous system paraneoplastic syndrome. Neurology 1998;50:94–8.

17. Butler M, Hayashi A, Ohkoshi N, et al. Autoimmunity to gephyrin in stiff-man syndrome. Neuron 2000;26:307–12.

18. Bilic E, Bilic E, Sepec BI, et al. Stiff-person syndrome, type 1 diabetes, dermatitis herpetiformis, celiac disease, microcytic anemia and copper deficiency. Just a coincidence or an additional shared pathophysiological mechanism? Clin Neurol Neurosurg 2009;111:644–5.

19. Egwuonwu S, Chedebeau F. Stiff-person syndrome: a case report and review of the literature. J Natl Med Assoc 2010;102:1261–3.

20. Raju R, Rakocevic G, Chen Z, et al. Autoimmunity to GABA-receptor associated protein in stiff-person syndrome. Brain 2006;129:3270–6.

21. Barker RA, Revesz T, Thom M, et al. Review of 23 patients affected by the stiff man syndrome: clinical subdivision into stiff trunk (man) syndrome, stiff limb syndrome, and progressive encephalomyelitis with rigidity. J Neurol Neurosurg Psychiatry 1998;65:633–40.

22. Hassin-Baer S, Kirson ED, Shulman L, et al. Stiff-person syndrome following West Nile fever. Arch Neurol 2004;61:938–41.

23. Dalmau J, Rosenfeld M. Paraneoplastic neurologic syndromes. In: Daroff RB, Fenichel GM, Jankovic J, et al, editors. Bradley's neurology in clinical practice. 6th edition. Philadelphia: Elsevier; 2012. p. 767–75.

24. Ameli R, Snow J, Rakocevic G, et al. A neuropsychological assessment of phobias in patients with stiff person syndrome. Neurology 2005;64:1961–3.
25. Henningsen P, Meinck HM. Specific phobias is a frequent non-motor feature in stiff person syndrome. J Neurol Neurosurg Psychiatry 2003;74:462–5.
26. Meinck HM, Thompson PD. Stiff man syndrome and related conditions. Mov Disord 2002;17(5):853–66.
27. Matsumoto JY, Caviness JN, McEvoy KM. The acoustic startle reflex in stiff-man syndrome. Neurology 1994;44:1952–5.
28. Mamoli B, Heiss WD, Maida E, et al. Electrophysiological studies on the "stiff-man" syndrome. J Neurol 1977;217:111–21.
29. Hutchinson M, Waters P, McHugh J, et al. Progressive encephalomyelitis, rigidity, and myoclonus: a novel glycine receptor antibody. Neurology 2008;71:1291–2.
30. Tohier C, Roze JC, David A, et al. Hyperexplexia or stiff baby syndrome. Arch Dis Child 1991;66:46–51.
31. Fenichel GM. Paroxysmal disorders. In: Fenichel GM, editor. Clinical pediatric neurology. 6th edition. Philadelphia: Elsevier; 2009. p. 1–48.
32. Moran MM, Allen NM, Treacy EP, et al. "Stiff neonate" with mitochondrial DNA depletion and secondary neurotransmitter defects. Pediatr Neurol 2011;45:403–5.
33. McKeon A, Robinson MT, McEvoy KM, et al. Stiff-man syndrome and variants. Arch Neurol 2012;69:230–8.
34. Rakocevic G, Floeter MK. Autoimmune stiff person syndrome and related myelopathies: understanding of electrophysiological and immunological processes. Muscle Nerve 2012;45:623–34.
35. Berger C, Meinck HM. Head retraction reflex in stiff-man syndrome and related disorders. Mov Disord 2003;18:906–11.
36. Correale J, Garcia Erro M, Kosac S, et al. An electrophysiological investigation of the "stiff-man" syndrome. Electromyogr Clin Neurophysiol 1988;28:215–21.
37. Gershanik OS. Stiff-person syndrome. Parkinsonism Relat Disord 2009;15:S130–4.
38. Rana SS, Ramanathan RS, Small G, et al. Paraneoplastic Isaacs' syndrome: a case series and review of the literature. J Clin Neuromuscul Dis 2012;13:228–33.
39. Kerchner GA, Ptacek LJ. Channelopathies: episodic and electrical disorders of the nervous system. In: Daroff RB, Fenichel GM, Jankovic J, et al, editors. Bradley's neurology in clinical practice. 6th edition. Philadelphia: Elsevier; 2012. p. 1488–507.
40. Brown P, Rothwell JC, Marsden CD. The stiff-leg syndrome. J Neurol Neurosurg Psychiatry 1997;62:31–7.
41. Boyer EW, Shannon M. The serotonin syndrome. N Engl J Med 2005;352:1112–20.
42. Holmoy T, Geis C. The immunological basis for treatment of stiff person syndrome. J Neuroimmunol 2011;231:55–60.
43. Sevy A, Fraques J, Chiche L, et al. Successful treatment with rituximab in a refractory stiff-person syndrome. Rev Neurol (Paris) 2012;168:375–8 [in French].
44. Fekete R, Jankovic J. Childhood stiff-person syndrome improved with rituximab. Case Rep Neurol 2012;4:92–6.
45. Dalakas M, Rakocevic G, Dambrosia J, et al. Double-blind, placebo-controlled study of rituximab in patients with stiff-person syndrome (SPS). Ann Neurol 2009;66:S21.
46. Cabo-López I, Negueruela-López M, Garcia-Bermejo P, et al. Stiff-person syndrome a case-report. Rev Neurol 2008;15:249–52.

47. Spehlmann R, Norcross K, Rasmus SC, et al. Improvement in stiff-man syndrome with sodium valproate. Neurology 1981;31:1162–3.
48. Sechi G, Barrocu M, Piluzza MG, et al. Levetiracetam in stiff-person syndrome. J Neurol 2008;255:1721–5.
49. Holmoy T. Long-term effect of gabapentin in stiff limb syndrome: a case report. Eur Neurol 2007;58:251–2.
50. Vermeij FH, van Doorn PA, Busch HF. Improvement of stiff-man syndrome with vigabatrin. Lancet 1996;348:612.
51. Hattan E, Angle MR, Chalk C. Unexpected benefit of propofol in stiff-person syndrome. Neurology 2008;70:1641–2.
52. Liquori R, Cordivari C, Lugaresi E, et al. Botulinum toxin A improves muscle spasms and rigidity in stiff-person syndrome. Mov Disord 1997;12:1060–3.

Index

Note: Page numbers of article titles are in **boldface** type.

Neurol Clin 31 (2013) 329–341
http://dx.doi.org/10.1016/S0733-8619(12)00109-0
0733-8619/13/$ – see front matter © 2013 Elsevier Inc. All rights reserved.

neurologic.theclinics.com

Moving?

Make sure your subscription moves with you!

To notify us of your new address, find your **Clinics Account Number** (located on your mailing label above your name), and contact customer service at:

Email: journalscustomerservice-usa@elsevier.com

800-654-2452 (subscribers in the U.S. & Canada)
314-447-8871 (subscribers outside of the U.S. & Canada)

Fax number: 314-447-8029

Elsevier Health Sciences Division
Subscription Customer Service
3251 Riverport Lane
Maryland Heights, MO 63043

ELSEVIER

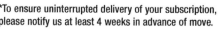

Printed and bound by CPI Group (UK) Ltd, Croydon, CR0 4YY

03/10/2024

01040440-0014